Peptides and Non Peptides of Oncologic and Neuroendocrine Relevance

From Basic to Clinical Research

Springer-Verlag Italia Srl.

E.E. Müller (Ed)

Peptides and Non Peptides of Oncologic and Neuroendocrine Relevance

From Basic to Clinical Research

Springer

Eugenio E. Müller
Department of Pharmacology
University of Milan
Milan, Italy

Originally published by Springer-Verlag Italia, Milano in 2003
Softcover reprint of the hardcover 1st edition 2003

ISBN 978-88-470-2170-9

Library of Congress Cataloging-in-Publication Data:
Peptides and non peptides in neuroendocrinology and oncology: from basic to clinical research/editor, E.E. Muller.
p. cm.
Includes bibliographical references and index.
ISBN 978-88-470-2170-9 ISBN 978-88-470-2085-6 (eBook)
DOI 10.1007/978-88-470-2085-6
1. Neuroendocrine tumors-Chemotherapy. 2. Hormone antagonists-Therapeutic use. 3. Peptide hormones. I. Müller, E.E.

RC280. E55P47 2003
616.99'28-dc22

2003057317

Typesetting: Color Point Srl (Milan)

Cover design: Simona Colombo

SPIN: 10937754

Preface

Antineoplastic chemotherapy has been, and still is, the most efficient form of tumor treatment. It has, however, the major drawback that a great many cytotoxic drugs non selectively alter the function of healthy cells as well as that of diseased cells. Greater specificity of the action of substances endowed with antineoplastic mechanisms and activity, targeted exclusively at tumor cells, the old Paul Ehrlich concept of the "magic bullet", provides an antineoplastic approach free of the constraints of the traditional chemotherapy. The development of monoclonal antibodies directed exclusively against a tumoral cell clone, sparing healthy cells, brings a new therapeutic strategy to counter a metastatic breast cancer, as does the use of an anti-tumoral DNA vaccine.

The "old" endocrine-based therapy of tumors, too, is putting out promising signals for a targeted antineoplastic therapy. It is well known that tumors arising from hormone-sensitive tissues maintain a state of hormone dependency that can be exploited to inhibition of growth. However, major progress in antineoplastic hormone therapy has been achieved by substituting hormones produced by peripheral endocrine glands with peptides synthesized in the brain. These molecules (hypothalamic regulatory hormones, RHs), in most cases originally identified in the hypothalamus, have been subsequently found in many organs and tissues of the body, especially in the gastrointestinal tract. RHs provide a physiologic stimulus to the pituitary when they are secreted in a physiologic pulsatile fashion, desensitizing and down-regulating their pituitary receptors when are secreted or, more commonly, administered either continuously, or in the form of superactive agonists. As an example, LHRH, the physiologic stimulus for the function of the ovary and the testis when is secreted intermittently, induces a state of "medical castration" when it is secreted or administered in a way that allows permanent occupancy of its pituitary receptors. This mechanism explains the successful use of LHRH or its superactive analogues in hormone-sensitive-tumors (breast, ovary, uterus, prostate). Medical castration functionally inactivates a tumor that has estrogen or testosterone receptors, blocks cellular proliferation, and, in the most sensitive forms, induces regression of metastases. In addition to this indirect mechanism, exerted via the pituitary, there also is the possibility of a direct action of the RH, acting directly on receptor sites embedded in the tumor, a feature typical, for instance, of another RH, somatostatin (SS).

For SS, the ubiquitous location of its receptors lent credence to the idea that, besides inhibiting GH secretion in acromegalic subjects and inducing shrinkage of some GH secreting tumors, it may be helpful to counter the growth of tissues and organs harboring SS receptors, as shown by an antitumoral action exerted on neuroendocrine tumors, and, more recently, by promising results on cell lines from solid tumors (breast, prostate, ovary, kidney, brain). Development of synthetic analogues of SS more stable in plasma than the native peptide led to the discovery that the sensitivity of a particular intact or tumoral tissue is based not only on the presence, but also on the number and the subtype of SS receptors expressed. Hence, the need to develop "universal" SS analogues that, like the native peptide, can act on the full panoply of SS tissue receptors.

In the case of SS, the multiplicity of RH mechanisms of action is best testified to by the additional ability of this peptide to exert an indirect, inhibitory action, i.e. to restrain GH secretion, with ensuing reduction of circulating and tissue titers of IGF-1, a potent mitogenic factor. Finally, another antineoplastic action of SS is its antiangiogenic action, mediated by peritumoral vascular receptors, which, when activated, curtail the vascular supply to the tumor. A similar multiplicity of mechanisms of action is shared by another class of RH-derived peptides, the GHRH antagonists.

The "magic bullet" approach of Ehrlich has been strengthened with the development of targeted hybrids in which a chemotherapeutic compound is coupled to an analogue of an RH.

The present volume, structured in 17 chapters, discussess the many aspects and problems of this new antineoplastic approach. Excellent preclinical and clinical researchers of the field, first among them Andrew V. Schally, one of the discoverers of RHs, extensively and critically review and update our knowledge of the diagnostic and therapeutic use of endocrine-derived compounds not only hypothalamic or pituitary (LHRH agonists and antagonists, GHRH antagonists, suppressors of GH secretion, such as somatostatin, corticostatin, or GH receptors antagonists), but also selective estrogen receptor modulators, antiandrogens, and enzyme inhibitors aimed at exerting antineoplastic activity or potentiating the activity of traditional chemotherapy on neuroendocrine and/or solid tumors. In addition, four chapters of the book are devoted to the physiologic functions of a new class of potent GH releasers, ghrelin and ghrelin mimetics, their receptors, and to the important endocrine and non endocrine actions of these compounds.

Given the importance and novelty of the matter and the excellence of the authors, it is hoped that this book may be of appealing interest not only to basic and clinical oncologists, endocrinologists, gynecologists, and urologists, but also to students of cell biology worldwide.

Grateful thanks are due to Ardana Biosciences, Astra Zeneca, Consiglio Nazionale delle Ricerche, Keryos, Novartis Farma, Pharmacia-Upjohn, Sanofi-Synthelabo, Zentaris for the generous financial support, which made possible the publication of this book.

Milan, July 2003 *E.E. Müller*

Table of Contents

List of Contributors

E. Arvat
Division of Endocrinology and Metabolism, Department of Internal Medicine, University of Turin, Turin, Italy

R. Avallone
Department of Experimental and Environmental Medicine and Biotechnology, University of Milano-Bicocca, Monza, Italy

A. Benso
Division of Endocrinology and Metabolism, Department of Internal Medicine, University of Turin, Turin, Italy

F. Boccardo
Academic Department of Medical Oncology (Medical Oncology B), University and National Cancer Research Institute, Genoa, Italy

E. Bresciani
Department of Experimental and Environmental Medicine and Biotechnology, University of Milano-Bicocca, Monza, Italy

F. Broglio
Division of Endocrinology and Metabolism, Department of Internal Medicine, University of Turin, Turin, Italy

I. Bulgarelli
Department of Experimental and Environmental Medicine and Biotechnology, University of Milano- Bicocca, Monza, Italy

L. Buscail
INSERM Unit 531 and Department of Gastroenterology, CHU Rangueil, Toulouse, France

P. Cassoni
Department of Biomedical Sciences and Oncology, Department of Internal Medicine, University of Turin, Turin, Italy

F. Catapano
Department of Anatomy, Pharmacology, and Forensic Medicine, University of Turin, Turin, Italy

A.-M. Comaru-Schally
Endocrine, Polypeptide and Cancer Institute, VA Medical Center, and Section of Experimental Medicine, Tulane University School of Medicine, New Orleans, LA, USA

R. Deghenghi
Division of Endocrinology and Metabolism, Department of Internal Medicine, University of Turin, Turin, Italy

A. Demers
Faculty of Pharmacy,
University of Montreal,
Montreal, Quebec, Canada

W.W. de Herder
Department of Internal Medicine,
Section of Endocrinology,
Erasmus MC, Rotterdam,
The Netherlands

S. Destefanis
Division of Endocrinology and
Metabolism, Department of Internal
Medicine, University of Turin,
Turin, Italy

S.L. Dickson
Department of Physiology,
University of Cambridge,
Cambridge, UK

K. Diedrich
Department of Gynecology and
Obstetrics, University Clinic,
Lübeck, Germany

J.B. Engel
Department of Gynecology and
Obstetrics, University Clinic,
Lübeck, Germany

J. Epelbaum
U. 549 INSERM,
IFR 77 Broca-Sainte Anne,
Paris, France

L. Filtri
Division of Endocrinology and
Metabolism, Department of Internal
Medicine, University of Turin,
Turin, Italy

E. Ghigo
Division of Endocrinology and
Metabolism, Department of Internal
Medicine,University of Turin,
Turin, Italy

C. Gottero
Division of Endocrinology and
Metabolism, Department of Internal
Medicine,University of Turin,
Turin, Italy

P. Guglielmini
Academic Department of Medical
Oncology (Medical Oncology B),
University and National Cancer
Research Institute,
Genoa, Italy

A.K. Hewson
Department of Physiology,
University of Cambridge,
Cambridge, UK

S.W.J. Lamberts
Department of Internal Medicine,
Section of Endocrinology, Erasmus MC,
Rotterdam, The Netherlands

D. Lamontagne
Faculty of Pharmacy,
University of Montreal,
Montreal, Quebec, Canada

P. Limonta
Institute of Endocrinology,
Center for Endocrinological Oncology,
University of Milan,
Milan, Italy

V. Locatelli
Department of Experimental and
Environmental Medicine and
Biotechnology, University of Milano-
Bicocca, Monza, Italy

P. Magni
Institute of Endocrinology,
University of Milan,
Milan, Italy

S. Marleau
Faculty of Pharmacy,
University of Montreal,
Montreal, Quebec, Canada

M. Montagnani Marelli
Institute of Endocrinology,
Center for Endocrinological
Oncology, University of Milan,
Milan, Italy

R.M. Moretti
Institute of Endocrinology,
Center for Endocrinological
Oncology, University of Milan,
Milan, Italy

M. Motta
Institute of Endocrinology,
University of Milan,
Milan, Italy

G. Muccioli
Department of Anatomy, Pharmacology,
and Forensic Medicine,
University of Turin,
Turin, Italy

E.E. Müller
Department of Pharmacology,
University of Milan,
Milan, Italy

C. Netti
Department of Pharmacology,
University of Milan,
Milan, Italy

H. Ong
Faculty of Pharmacy,
University of Montreal,
Montreal, Quebec, Canada

M. Papotti
Department of Biomedical
Sciences and Oncology,
University of Turin,
Turin, Italy

F. Prodam
Division of Endocrinology and
Metabolism, Department of Internal
Medicine, University of Turin,
Turin, Italy

P. Pronzato
Department of Oncology,
S. Andrea Hospital,
La Spezia, Italy

G. Rindi
Department of Pathology and
Laboratory Medicine,
University of Parma,
Parma, Italy

A.V. Schally
Endocrine, Polypeptide and Cancer
Institute, VA Medical Center, and
Section of Experimental Medicine,
Tulane University School of Medicine,
New Orleans, LA, USA

V. Sibilia
Department of Pharmacology,
University of Milan,
Milan, Italy

E. Tanabra
Department of Anatomy,
Pharmacology, and Forensic Medicine,
University of Turin,
Turin, Italy

A. Tognoni
Department of Oncology,
S. Andrea Hospital,
La Spezia, Italy

A. Torsello
Department of Experimental and
Environmental Medicine and
Biotechnology, University of Milano-
Bicocca, Monza, Italy

L.Y.C. Tung
Department of Physiology,
University of Cambridge,
Cambridge, UK

A.J. van der Lely
Department of Medicine,
Erasmus MC, Rotterdam,
The Netherlands

E. Verri
Academic Department of Medical Oncology (Medical Oncology B), University and National Cancer Research Institute, Genoa, Italy

M. Volante
Department of Biomedical Sciences and Oncology, University of Turin, Turin, Italy

LHRH/SOMATOSTATIN

Twenty-five Years of Endocrine Oncology with Analogs of Hypothalamic Peptides: an Overview

A.V. Schally

In this chapter I will try to report to you what I have been doing for the past 25 years and what advancements in oncology have emanated so far from the work on the hypothalamus. The discovery of hypothalamic hormones, especially luteinizing hormone-releasing hormone (LHRH) and somatostatin, has led to practical clinical use of their analogs in the field of cancer treatment. LHRH, somatostatin, growth hormone-releasing hormone (GHRH), their mRNAs and their receptors are found in diverse tumors (Schally et al., 2001a, 2001b). Mammalian bombesin-like peptides, such as gastrin-releasing peptide (GRP) and neuromedin B, are likewise present in various tumors, and appear to produce mitogenic effects (Cuttitta, 1985; Sunday et al., 1988; Schally et al., 2001a). Antagonists of bombesin/GRP can be also used for the development of new methods for treatment of various tumors. In addition we have synthesized and evaluated cytotoxic analogs of LHRH, somatostatin and bombesin that can be targeted to various tumors. Moreover, we have made antagonists of GHRH, not discussed here. This chapter reviews some selected experimental and clinical findings on the use of analogs of LHRH, somatostatin and bombesin for treatment of various cancers.

LHRH Analogs

In 1971, our laboratory achieved the isolation, elucidation of structure and synthesis of hypothalamic luteinizing hormone-releasing hormone, or LHRH, winning the race against other groups (Schally et al., 1971a, 1971b, 1971c). We showed that both natural and synthetic LHRH possessed major FSH-releasing as well as LH-releasing activity. We also suggested that the name LHRH be changed to GnRH, for gonadotropin-releasing hormone (Schally et al., 1971b), but this led to confusion with GHRH, so we now prefer to use LHRH (Schally, 1999).

In the past 30 years, more than 3000 analogs of LHRH have been synthesized (Karten and Rivier, 1986). Agonistic analogs, such as Decapeptyl (triptorelin), Lupron (leuprolide), Zoladex (goserelin) and Suprefact (buserelin), much more active than the LHRH itself and available in depot preparations, have important clinical applications in gynecology and oncology (Schally et al., 2001a, 2001b). Potent antagonists of LHRH, such as cetrorelix, have also been synthesized (Bajusz et al., 1988; Molineaux et al., 1998; Schally 1999). In addition, cytotoxic analogs of LHRH, consisting of doxorubicin linked to

LHRH agonist [D-Lys^6]LHRH to form analog AN-152, or 2-pyrrolinodoxorubicin also linked to [D-Lys^6]LHRH to produce analog AN-207, that can be targeted to LHRH receptors on tumors, have been also developed in our laboratory (Nagy et al., 1996; Schally and Nagy, 1999).

The actions of LHRH and its analogs are mediated by high-affinity receptors for LHRH found on the membranes of the pituitary gonadotrophs (Schally et al., 2001b). Acute administration of agonists of LHRH induces a marked release of LH and FSH, but a continous stimulation of the pituitary by chronic administration of LHRH agonists produces an inhibition of the hypophyseal-gonadal axis through the process of down regulation of pituitary receptors for LHRH, desensitization of the pituitary gonadotrophs, and a suppression of circulating levels of LH and sex steroids (Emons and Schally, 1994; Schally, 1999). This downregulation of LHRH receptors, produced by sustained administration of LHRH agonists, provides the basis for clinical applications in gynecology and oncology. LHRH antagonists produce a competitive blockade of LHRH receptors and cause an immediate inhibition of the release of gonadotropins and sex steroids (Schally et al., 2001a, 2001b). Recently, we demonstrated that administration of the LHRH antagonist cetrorelix to rats also produces downregulation of pituitary LHRH receptors and a decrease in the levels of mRNA for LHRH receptors (Pinski et al., 1996; Kovacs et al., 2001).

Specific LHRH receptors are also found on various cancers (Dondi et al., 1994; Schally et al., 2001a, 2001b; Limonta et al., 1992). These LHRH receptors on tumor cells can mediate the direct effects of LHRH analogs. Thus, high-affinity binding sites for LHRH have been detected in 86% of human prostate cancer samples (Halmos et al., 2000a), more than 50% of human breast cancers, 78% of human ovarian epithelial cancer specimens and nearly 80% of human endometrial carcinomas (Emons and Schally, 1994; Schally et al., 2001b). The expression of LHRH receptor gene in human prostatic, breast, endometrial and ovarian tumors has also been demonstrated by RT-PCR (Dondi et al., 1994). The expression of mRNA for LHRH has also been demonstrated in human prostatic, mammary, endometrial and ovarian cancer lines (Dondi et al., 1994; Halmos et al., 2000a; Schally et al., 2001b). This suggests that local LHRH may be involved in the growth of these tumors. We will now summarize the findings on the effects of LHRH analogs on various tumors.

Prostate Cancer

The greatest therapeutic impact of LHRH analogs has been in the field of prostate cancer, which is the most common non-cutaneous malignant tumor in men (Schally et al., 2000). Pioneering work in the 1940s by Huggins established that carcinoma of the prostate is frequently testosterone-dependent (Huggins and Hodges, 1941). This discovery laid the foundations to all the present modalities for the treatment of advanced prostate cancer, which are based upon androgen deprivation. Endocrine therapy for adenocarcinoma of the prostate has included bilateral orchiectomy, administration of estrogens and anti-androgens, and even hypophysectomy. However, surgical castration is associated with a psychological and social impact, estrogens have serious cardiovascular, hepatic and mammotropic side effects, and anti-androgens are also toxic to the liver. In the early 1980s, we introduced a different hormonal therapy for prostate cancer based on the use of highly potent agonistic analogs of LHRH. First, we showed that chronic administration of agonist [D-Trp^6]LHRH suppressed tumor growth in rats with prostate cancer (Redding and Schally, 1981). We then demonstrated the efficacy of therapy with agonistic analogs of LHRH in men with advanced prostate cancer in a collaborative clinical trial at the Royal Victoria Hospital in Montreal (Tolis et al., 1982). Therapy with agonists of LHRH is currently the preferred treatment for men with advanced prostate cancer and in about 70% of cases LHRH agonists are selected for primary treatment (Schally et al., 2000). Administration of anti-androgens prior to and during early therapy with agonists can prevent flare-up of the disease.

Our clinical trials in patients with advanced prostate cancer show that the antagonist of LHRH, cetrorelix, can induce a clinical remission (Gonzales-Barcena et al., 1994, 1995). Cetrorelix and other LHRH antagonists could be beneficial as a monotherapy for patients with prostate cancer and metastases in the brain, spine, liver and bone marrow, in whom the LHRH agonists cannot be used as single drugs because of the possibility of flare-up. LHRH antagonists greatly reduce the time of onset of therapeutic effects. In addition, we showed that treatment with cetrorelix can produce long-term improvement in patients with symptomatic benign prostatic hyperplasia (BPH) (Comaru-Schally et al., 1998). Cetrorelix offers a therapeutic alternative to patients with BPH who are considered poor surgical risks.

Clinical evidence indicates that in patients with advanced prostate cancer, medical castration produced by chronic administration of LHRH analogs accounts for most benefits derived from the treatment (Schally et al., 2000). However, all hormonal therapies aimed at androgen deprivation, including LHRH analogs, can only provide a remission of limited duration and most patients eventually relapse and die of androgen-independent prostatic cancer. This androgen-independent growth of prostate cancer cells is apparently mediated or caused by various growth factors such as IGF-1 and IGF-2, EGF and others (Schally et al., 2000). Interestingly, LHRH analogs and other peptides can also exert direct effects on tumor cells. These direct effects of peptides on receptors for LHRH, somatostatin, GHRH and bombesin on prostate cancers may be used for the development of methods for treatment of hormone-refractory prostate cancer. Interference with endogenous growth factors and their receptors on tumors by bombesin/GRP antagonists, and GHRH antagonists or the use of targeted cytotoxic peptide analogs could inhibit the growth of androgen-independent prostate cancers and improve the tumor treatment outcome (Schally et al., 2000, 2001a).

Recent investigation of a large number of specimens of human prostate adenocarcinomas showed that 86% of cancers exhibited high-affinity binding sites for LHRH and expressed mRNA for LHRH receptors (Halmos et al., 2000a). Prostate cancers also contain a high percentage (63-65%) of binding sites for somatostatin and bombesin and express mRNA for somatostatin and bombesin receptor subtypes (Halmos et al., 2000b). This provides a rationale for the development of methods for therapy of this malignancy, based on targeted cytotoxic analogs. Investigations with cytotoxic analogs of LHRH were carried out in various models of prostate cancer. In rats bearing hormone-dependent Dunning R-3327-H prostate carcinomas, the tumors regressed to about one-half of their initial volume after three injections of AN-207. In a study on PC-82 human prostate cancers xenografted into nude mice, there was a major reduction in tumor volume and a fall in serum prostate-specific antigen (PSA) levels after administration of cytotoxic analog AN-207 (Koppan et al., 1999).

We also showed that cytotoxic LHRH analog AN-207 inhibits growth of MDA-PCa-2B prostate cancers xenografted subcutanecusly (s.c.) into nude mice. AN-207 inhibited final tumor volume by 63%, as compared with controls, and PSA levels in mice treated with AN-207 were lowered by 65%. Our work supports the concept that targeted chemotherapy based on hormone peptide analogs should be more efficacious and less toxic than the current systemic chemotherapeutic regimens. The use of targeted chemotherapy should permit an escalation of doses.

The side effects of targeted cytotoxic LHRH analogs are expected to be minor, because the receptors for LHRH are not widely distributed in normal tissues.

Breast Cancer

Breast cancer is the most common malignancy in women. About 30% of women with breast cancers have estrogen-dependent tumors and can be treated by hormonal manipulations, such as tamoxifen, raloxifene or oophorectomy. Experimental and clinical studies show that agonists of LHRH can be used for treatment of estrogen-dependent breast cancer. Clinical trials demonstrated regression of tumor mass and disappearance of metastases in premenopausal and some postmenopausal women with breast cancer treated with [D-Trp^6]LHRH, buserelin, goserelin, or leuprolide (Santen, 1990; Kaufmann et al., 1989; Schally, 1999). These studies showed that LHRH agonists are efficacious for the treatment of premenopausal women with estrogen-dependent, estrogen receptor-positive breast cancer. A recent clinical trial by Klijn et al. (2000) in 161 premenopausal women with advanced breast cancer revealed that combined treatment with LHRH agonists and tamoxifen was more effective and resulted in longer overall survival than treatment with either drug alone. The main effect of LHRH agonists on mammary carcinomas is based on estrogen deprivation, but some direct antitumor effects of LHRH analogs are also likely. Several groups found LHRH receptors on human breast cancer specimens and in breast cancer lines. About 52% of breast cancer biopsy samples are positive for LHRH receptors (Schally et al., 2001b). LHRH antagonists have so far been tested only in experimental models of breast cancer. Cetrorelix inhibited tumor growth of murine mammary carcinomas and human breast cancers transplanted into nude mice (Schally et al., 2001a, 2001b).

Targeted cytotoxic analogs of LHRH bind with high-affinity to LHRH receptors on human breast cancers. One injection of AN-207 caused a complete regression of MX-1 hormone-independent doxorubicin-resistant human breast cancers in nude mice, which remained tumor-free for at least 60 days after treatment (Kahan et al., 1999a).

Epithelial Ovarian Cancer

Epithelial ovarian cancer is the fourth most frequent cause of cancer-related deaths in women. The treatment based on surgery or chemotherapy is not very effective and new approaches are needed. Studies in vivo indicate that cetrorelix inhibits growth of human OV-1063 and ES-2 epithelial ovarian cancers xenografted into nude mice better than agonist [D-Trp^6]LHRH (Schally et al., 2001a), but in a multicenter trial no beneficial effects of therapy with [D-Trp6]LHRH could be found (Emons et al., 1996). Clinical trials with cetrorelix are in progress.

Specific membrane receptors for LHRH have been found in 78% of surgically removed human ovarian carcinomas and in various human ovarian cancer cell lines (Emons and Schally, 1994). These receptors mediate direct effects of LHRH analogs on the growth of ovarian cancer cell lines in vitro. The agonist [D-Trp^6]LHRH and antagonist cetrorelix reduce the proliferation of ovarian cancer cell lines in culture (Emons et al., 1993). However, the best approach may be based on targeted cytotoxic LHRH analogs. In the first study (Miyazaki et al., 1997), we showed that a single injection of cytotoxic analog AN-152 inhibited the growth of LHRH receptor-positive OV-1063 ovarian tumors in nude mice for at least 4 weeks. AN-152 did not inhibit the growth of LHRH receptor-negative UCI-107 human ovarian carcinomas, showing that the presence of receptors is essential. In other studies, we demonstrated that the growth of OV-1063 and ES-2 ovarian cancers could be suppressed by administration of cytotoxic LHRH analog AN-207 in doses 100 times smaller than those of AN-152 (Miyazaki et al., 1999). Targeted chemotherapy based on analogs such as AN-152 and AN-207 may improve the management of ovarian cancer. Clinical trials will start in the spring in Germany.

Endometrial Cancer

Endometrial cancer is a common gynecologic malignancy in the Western world. Surgery or radiotherapy is successful in 75% of cases, but new methods are needed for advanced or relapsed cancers (Emons and Schally, 1994). In view of the presence of LHRH receptors on nearly 80% of endometrial cancers, targeted cytotoxic analogs are being investigated (Schally et al., 1999, Schally et al., 2001a, 2001b).

Renal Cell Carcinoma (RCC)

The etiology of RCC is poorly understood and the present methods of treatment of RCC must be improved (Schally et al., 2001a). Sex steroids and growth factors may play a role in proliferation of kidney neoplasms. When we tested LHRH antagonist cetrorelix on CAKI-I RCC line in nude mice, the tumor volume was significantly decreased (Jungwirth et al., 1998). Clinical trials with cetrorelix in patients with RCC are in progress.

Somatostatin Analogs

Somatostatin (SST) was isolated from ovine (Brazeau et al., 1973) and later from porcine hypothalami and characterized as an inhibitor of growth hormone secretion from the pituitary gland. SST exists as a 14 amino acid peptide and an extended version consisting of 28 amino acids and other forms (Schally et al., 2001a). Because of the short plasma half-life of SST-14, more stable SST analogs were developed, including octreotide (SMS 201-995; sandostatin; Bauer et al., 1982) and vapreotide (RC-160; Cai et al., 1986). These analogs are about 50 times more potent than SST-14. SST and its octapeptide analogs exert their effects through specific membrane receptors. So far, five distinct receptor subtypes (sst_{1-5}) have been cloned and characterized (Patel, 1997). Native SST shows similar high affinity to sst_{1-5}, but the synthetic octapeptides, such as RC-160 and octreotide, bind preferentially to sst_2 and sst_5. SST analogs are used for the treatment of acromegaly, endocrine tumors of the gastroenteropancreatic system, including carcinoid tumors, insulinomas, glucagonomas and gastrinomas (Lamberts et al., 1991). RC-160 was shown to be a powerful tumor growth suppressor in experimental models of various cancers (Schally, 1988). Attempts have been made to use SST analogs for the therapy of human cancers, such as prostatic, breast, pancreatic and lung, but relevant palliative benefits have been obtained only in hepatocellular carcinoma. Poor therapeutic results with octapeptide SST analogs are likely due to the fact that in various cancers there is a loss of gene expression for sst_2, which is the preferred subtype for these analogs (Buscail et al., 1996). However, the expression of sst_5 and sst_3 should make possible therapy with SST analogs labeled with various radioisotopes or cytotoxic SST analogs.

The presence of SST receptors permits the localization of some tumors and metastases using scanning techniques (Krenning et al., 1993). Radiolabeled analogs of SST, such as ^{111}In-octreotide (OctreoScan), are used clinically for the localization of tumors expressing receptors for SST. Neuroendocrine tumors that could be localized with OctreoScan include carcinoids and small cell lung carcinoma (SCLC). Non-neuroendocrine tumors that could be localized by scintigraphy include breast cancer, brain tumors, astrocytomas and non-SCLC squamous cell carcinoma. Work is also in progress on application of somatostatin analogs labeled with appropriate radionuclides, such as ^{90}Yttrium in cancer therapy. Our approach consists of targeting chemotherapeutic agents linked to somatostatin analogs to receptors for somatostatin in certain cancers.

Cytotoxic SST Analogs

We developed a series of novel targeted cytotoxic SST conjugates that consist of carriers RC-121 and RC-160 coupled to 2-pyrrolino-doxorubicin (Nagy et al., 1998). Of these hybrid cytotoxic conjugates, analog AN-238, containing AN-201, was demonstrated to be very effective in experimental cancer models (Schally and Nagy, 1999).

Carcinoma of the Prostate

The prognosis of patients with androgen-refractory prostate cancer is very poor, and no effective treatment exists at present. High-affinity binding of radiolabeled RC-160 was demonstrated in 65% of primary prostate cancer specimens and we found the expression of sst_2 on 14% and sst_5 on 64% of 22 samples tested (Halmos et al., 2000b). SST analog AN-238 was first evaluated on the very aggressive androgen-independent Dunning R-3327-AT-1 prostate carcinoma in Copenhagen rats and produced a >80% decrease in tumor weight 4 weeks after therapy (Schally et al., 2001a).

A strong inhibition of growth of androgen-independent PC-3 human prostate cancers xenografted into nude mice was obtained after treatment with a single dose or two consecutive injections of AN-238 (Plonowski et al., 1999). In these experiments, AN-238 reduced final tumor volumes, tumor weights and tumor burden by more than 60%. In a metastatic model of PC-3, the treatment with AN-238 inhibited the weight of orthotopically grown tumors, producing a 77% reduction. In addition, no retroperitoneal or distant metastases could be observed 4 weeks after the initiation of the therapy with AN-238. Four injections of AN-238 also virtually arrested the proliferation of DU-145 prostate cancer.

Breast Cancer

The presence of SST receptor subtypes on human breast cancer specimens has been established by several research groups (Kahan et al., 1999b). Thus, patients with estrogen-independent metastatic breast cancer could benefit from treatment with cytotoxic somatostatin analogs such as AN-238.

To investigate the efficacy of SST receptor-targeting in human breast cancer, nude mice bearing xenografts of various breast cancer lines were treated with a single i.v. injection of AN-238. In the MCF-7-MIII model, several tumors showed constant regression and 60 days after the administration of AN-238 tumor volume was greatly decreased. In the MDA-MB-231 model and in the doxorubicin-resistant MX-1 model, many tumors also showed regression after treatment with AN-238 (Kahan et al., 1999b). In all three models, radical AN-201 was again more toxic and less effective than AN-238.

Epithelial Ovarian Cancer

Most surgical specimens of human epithelial ovarian cancer exhibit high-affinity binding sites for radiolabeled RC-160, and the expression of mRNA for sst_2, sst_3, and sst_5 has also been demonstrated (Schally et al., 2001a). Thus, ovarian cancers might be also targeted by cytotoxic SST analogs. In SST receptor-positive UCI-107 human ovarian cancers xenografted into nude mice, tumor weights were reduced by 67.3% after two intravenous (i.v.) injections of AN-238 (Schally et al., 2001a).

Renal Cell Carcinoma (RCC)

The prognosis for metastatic RCC is poor because of its resistance to both chemotherapy and radiotherapy. Since more than 70% of RCCs express high affinity binding sites for SST (Reubi and Kvols, 1992), we evaluated the effects of AN-238 on growth of xenografts of human RCC lines in nude mice (Plonowski et al., 2000b). High-affinity binding of AN-238 was found on membrane preparations of SW-839 and 786-0 and the growth of these tumors was inhibited significantly. A strong inhibition was also obtained with orthotopically grown 786-0 metastatic RCC. Three of seven mice treated with AN-238 were tumor-free at the end of the experiment and only one mouse developed lymphatic metastases. In contrast, metastases were observed in five of six animals in both the control and the AN-201-treated group. No significant antitumor effect of AN-238 was observed on SST receptor-negative CAKI-1 xenografts.

Brain Tumors

Glioblastomas represent the most common form of primary brain tumors and are considered incurable. Low-grade glioblastomas (astrocytomas) express sst_2 making this malignancy amenable for targeted chemotherapy with SST analogs (Kiaris et al., 2000). Because U-87 MG human glioblastomas express receptors for SST, we tested AN-238 in subcutaneous and orthotopic models in nude mice. A single injection of AN-238 induced an 82% inhibition of growth of subcutaneous tumors. In mice bearing orthotopically grown U-87 MG tumors, AN-238 produced a significant prolongation of survival time, indicating that the tumor blood-brain barrier is penetrable by cytotoxic SST analog AN-238.

Small Cell Lung Carcinoma (SCLC) and Non-SCLC

SCLC constitutes about 20% of all lung cancers and most cases are already metastatic at the time of diagnosis. Chemotherapy can be used for treatment but the long-term survival-rate is low (Schally et al., 2001a). A high percentage of primary SCLC tumors and metastatic lesions express SST receptors (Krenning et al., 1993).

When we treated nude mice bearing H-69 SCLC xenografts with AN-238, a single dose produced a >50% inhibition of tumor growth (Kiaris et al., 2001). Three doses of AN-238 inhibited tumor growth for more than 42 days. H-69 tumors expressed high levels of mRNA for sst_2. Treatment with AN-238 also produced a very strong 91% growth inhibition of H-157 non-SCLC because of the presence of SST receptors in the tumor vasculature (Kiaris et al., 2001).

Pancreatic Cancer

Some studies indicate a binding of a radionuclide SST octapeptide to pancreatic cancers in patients and the expression of mRNA for sst_5 and sst_3 was also reported (Buscail et al., 1996). Consequently, we tested AN-238 on human pancreatic cancer lines xenografted in nude mice (Szepeshazi et al., 2001). The growth of SW-1990 human pancreatic cancers containing SST_3 and SST_5 was significantly inhibited by AN-238.

Colorectal Cancers

The resistance of advanced colorectal cancers to therapy is often related to mutations in the *p53* tumor suppressor gene. Because at least the subtype 5 of somatostatin receptors (sst_5) is present in colorectal carcinomas, we tested the targeted cytotoxic SST analog AN-238 (Szepeshazi et al., 2002). AN-238 inhibited the growth of HCT-15 and HT-29 colorectal cancers that express mutant *p53*, whereas AN-201 and DOX showed no effect. Thus, cytotoxic SRIF analog AN-238 can inhibit the growth of experimental colon cancers that express ssts, regardless of their *p53* status.

All these studies demonstrate major differences in efficacy between a "straight" analog, such as RC-160, and a cytotoxic analog such as AN-238. Thus, it is possible that very potent cytotoxic SST analogs, such as AN-238, would be targeted even to tumors with a low concentration of SST-receptors, producing effective clinical responses.

Antagonists of Bombesin and Gastrin-releasing Peptide (GRP)

The family of bombesin-like peptides consists of a large number of peptides found in amphibians and mammals (Sunday et al., 1988). Bombesin is a tetradecapeptide isolated from frog skin. Gastrin-releasing peptide (GRP) was isolated from porcine stomach, has 27 amino acids and its carboxyl-terminal decapeptide is similar to that of bombesin (Sunday et al., 1988). Bombesin-like immunoreactivity and GRP are widely distributed in mammalian brain, including the hypothalamus, as well as in lung and the gastrointestinal tract (Sunday et al., 1998). From an oncologic point of view, the most important action of bombesin/GRP and neuromedin B is their ability to function as growth factors (Cuttita et al., 1985). In addition to SCLC, bombesin-like peptides are also produced in other cancers, such as breast, prostatic and pancreatic cancer (Schally et al., 2001a). Four receptor subtypes (BRS) associated with the bombesin-like peptide family have been identified and cloned so far (Nagy et al., 1997; Schally et al., 2001a; Kiaris et al., 1999; Sun et al., 2000).

The finding that bombesin or GRP can function as an autocrine growth factor for various tumors stimulated the development of bombesin/GRP antagonists. Various bombesin/GRP antagonists were synthesized in our laboratory including RC-3095 and RC-3940-II (Cai et al., 1994; Schally et al., 2001a). The main mechanism of tumor inhibitory action of bombesin/GRP antagonists appears to be the reduction in concentration of EGF receptors on tumors. The studies with bombesin/GRP antagonists in various cancers are described below.

Prostate Cancer

Neuroendocrine cells are widely distributed throughout the normal prostate. Neuropeptides such as bombesin and other growth factors produced by neuroendocrine cells may interact with non-neuroendocrine cells and activate mitogenic pathways. Interference with the autocrine/paracrine activity of bombesin may improve the management of androgen-refractory prostate cancer (Schally et al., 2001a). The expression of GRP receptors in prostate can be correlated with neoplastic transformation of the tissue (Markwalder and Reubi, 1999). High-affinity receptors for bombesin/GRP were detected on specimens of human prostate cancer and PC-3 and DU-145 human prostate cancer cell lines (Schally et al., 2000; Sun et al., 2000)

Our studies have demonstrated that bombesin antagonists RC-3940-II and RC-3950-II strongly inhibit growth of PC-3 and DU-145 androgen-independent prostate cancers in nude mice and cause down regulation of EGF receptors in the tumors (Schally et al., 2001a). Bombesin/GRP antagonists can also potentiate the inhibitory effects of GHRH antagonists on the growth of PC-3 prostate cancers (Schally et al., 2001a; Plonowski et al., 2000c). The combination of both classes of analogs interfere with both IGF and bombesin/EGF pathways and could be useful clinically for the management of androgen-independent prostate cancer.

Breast Cancer

Bombesin/GRP receptors were found by radioreceptor assay in about 33% of human breast cancer samples. Various studies in our laboratory have clearly demonstrated that bombesin/GRP antagonists can inhibit the growth of mammary cancers (Schally et al., 2001a). Thus, antagonists RC-3940-II and RC-3095 suppressed growth of estrogen-independent MDA-MB-231 human breast cancers in nude mice, RC-3940-II being the more powerful. The inhibition of tumor growth was associated with a decrease in EGF receptors in the tumors (Miyazaki et al., 1998). Therapy with RC-3940-II and RC-3095 also resulted in a regression of MDA-MB-468 estrogen-independent human breast cancers in nude mice (Kahan et al., 2000).

Growth of MDA-MB-435 breast cancers in nude mice was similarly inhibited by RC-3095 and RC-3940-II, with a reduction in the mRNA levels and protein for the ErbB receptor tyrosine kinase family (EGF-receptor and ErbB-2, 3 and 4; Bajo et al., 2002). Bombesin/GRP antagonists could provide a new treatment modality for breast tumors expressing bombesin receptors and ErbB-2/Her-2 oncogene and replace herceptin.

Ovarian Cancer

Human epithelial ovarian cancers express three subtypes of bombesin/GRP receptors (Schally et al., 2001a). Recent work shows that bombesin antagonists RC-3095 and RC-3940-II can inhibit the growth of OV-1063 and ES-2 tumors in nude mice. On the basis of these results, bombesin antagonists are being tested clinically in patients with ovarian cancer.

Lung Cancer (SCLC)

Lung cancer is the leading cause of cancer-related deaths in the Western world and new therapeutic modalities are needed for both SCLC and non-SCLC. SCLC secrete bombesin-like peptides (Cuttitta et al., 1985), including GRP and neuromedin B, which function as autocrine growth factors and stimulate tumor growth. Receptors for bombesin-like peptides are found in various SCLC lines (Kiaris et al., 1999). Bombesin/GRP receptor mechanisms may play a role in development of lung cancers in smokers. It was reported that the GRP receptor gene is activated in bronchial epithelial cells after long-term exposure to tobacco and makes the cells susceptible to the development of cancer (Shriver et al., 2000). New endocrine methods for treating SCLC, based on bombesin/GRP antagonists, are being developed. Antagonists RC-3095 and RC-3940-II inhibited growth of H-69 SCLC xenografted into nude mice (Koppan et al., 1998). Clinical trials with RC-3095 are in progress.

Pancreatic Cancer

The prognosis for patients with ductal carcinoma of the pancreas is very poor and it is essential to develop more effective therapies. Bombesin/GRP may function as autocrine growth factors in pancreatic cancer (Schally et al., 2001a) Bombesin/GRP antagonists RC-3095 and RC-3940-II inhibited the growth of various human pancreatic cancer cells xenografted in nude mice (Schally et al., 2001a).

Gastric Cancer

Carcinoma of the stomach ranks seventh in the USA among causes of cancer-related deaths. However, stomach cancer is an international health problem, being the leading cause of mortality from cancer in Japan, China and India and thus it ranks No. 2 overall in the world, second only to lung cancer. In patients with unresectable cancer of the stomach, the prognosis is dismal. New treatment modalities are needed for patients with locally advanced and metastatic gastric carcinoma. The receptors for bombesin and GRP are present in human gastric cancers and various gastric cell lines. The administration of bombesin/GRP antagonists inhibited the growth of MKN-45 and H_S746T human gastric cancers xenografted in nude mice (Schally et al., 2001a).

Colorectal Cancer

Advanced colon cancer is difficult to treat. Most colon cancers express GRP, GRP receptor and mRNA for GRP receptor. Thus, GRP could be an autocrine growth factor in colorectal cancer (Chave et al., 2000). Approaches based on the use of antagonists of bombesin/GRP are being tried in colorectal cancer. Bombesin antagonists can inhibit the growth of HT-29 human colon cancers in nude mice and downregulate EGF receptors (Schally et al., 2001a). Bombesin/GRP antagonists could be considered for therapy of pancreatic, gastric and colon cancer.

Renal Cell Carcinoma (RCC)

Bombesin/GRP receptors are expressed in human RCC and our work shows that bombesin/GRP antagonist RC-3940-II inhibits growth of CAKI-1 human renal cell cancers in nude mice (Jungwirth et al., 1998). This effect is accompanied by a decrease in EGF receptors on tumors. Based on these results, bombesin antagonists could be considered for the therapy of RCC.

Brain Tumors

About 13,000 deaths annually in the USA are attributed to brain tumors. Various brain tumors and human glioblastoma cell lines contain receptors for bombesin/GRP. Bombesin/GRP antagonists RC-3095 and RC-3940-II inhibit the proliferation of U-87MG and U-373MG human glioblastomas transplanted into nude mice or cultured in vitro (Schally et al., 2001a). This inhibition is associated with a downregulation of EGF receptors. Bombesin/GRP antagonists could be considered for the development of new approaches to the treatment of some brain tumors.

Cytotoxic Bombesin Analogs

Since bombesin/GRP receptors are expressed in various tumors, the application of radiolabeled bombesin analogs for tumor detection has been proposed (Markwalder and Reubi, 1999). ^{111}In-labeled analogs of bombesin allow a visualization of tumors.

We synthesized targeted cytotoxic bombesin conjugates using bombesin antagonists as carriers (Nagy et al., 1997). Thus, superactive cytotoxic bombesin conjugate AN-215 was prepared by linking radical AN-201 to the amino terminal of des-D-Tpi-RC-3095. We then demonstrated that the growth of SCLC H-69 tumors in nude mice was greatly inhibited by treatment with AN-215 (Kiaris et al., 1999). The effectiveness of cytotoxic bombesin analog AN-215 was also shown in nude mice bearing PC-3 androgen-independent human prostate cancers (Plonowski et al., 2000a). Treatment with AN-215 caused about 70% reduction in tumor volume and greatly extended tumor doubling time. Cytotoxic radical AN-201 was ineffective and more toxic. Because bombesin receptors are present on metastatic prostate cancers, targeted chemotherapy with AN-215 should benefit patients with advanced prostatic carcinoma who no longer respond to androgen deprivation.

Treatment of experimental U-87MG human glioblastoma in nude mice with AN-215 also effectively inhibited tumor growth (Szereday et al., 2002). Thus, patients with inoperable brain tumors, such as malignant gliomas may benefit from targeted chemotherapy based on cytotoxic bombesin analog AN-215.

Conclusions

We reviewed the use of peptide analogs for the therapy of various cancers. Some analogs of hypothalamic hormones already have major applications for the diagnosis and especially the treatment of diverse malignancies. These applications are certain to increase in the future. Many patients with various neoplastic diseases have already benefited from modern therapies based on hypothalamic hormones. It is gratifying to us that the discovery of hypothalamic hormones has led to practical clinical use of their analogs for cancer treatment. New generations of peptide analogs should improve the treatment of various tumors considered untreatable by current therapeutic modalities.

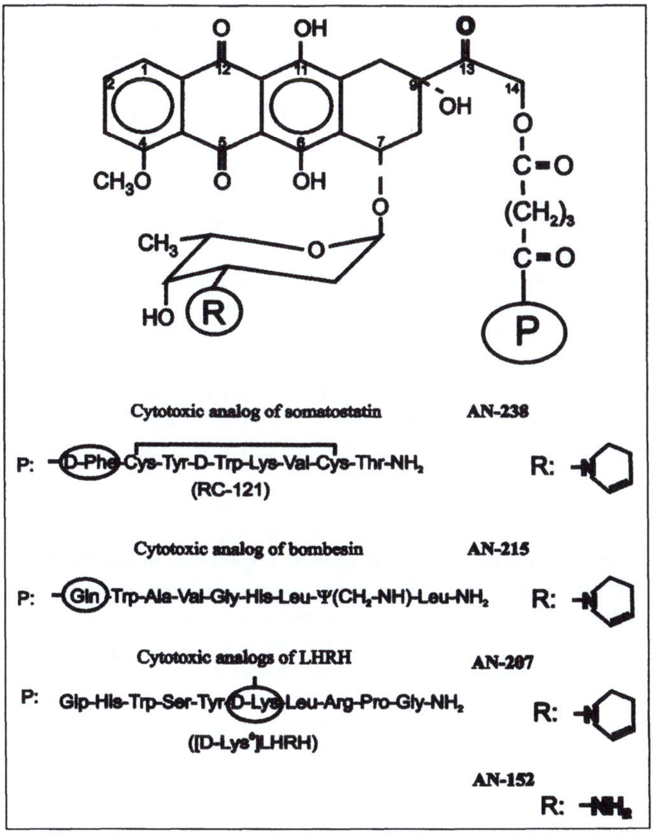

Fig. 1. Molecular structure of cytotoxic analogs of SST (AN-238) bombesin (AN-215), and LHRH (AN-152 and AN-207). The cytotoxic radicals doxorubicin (R=NH2) and 2-pyrrolinodoxorubicin (R=2-pyrrolino) are linked through a glutaric acid spacer to the free amino groups of amino acids (circled) in the peptide carriers (P). From Nagy A., Plonowsky A., Schally A.V., 2000. Copyright 2000 Natl. Acad. Sc. USA. Reprinted by permission from Nagy et al. 2000, National Academy of Science of the USA

References

Bajo A.M., Schally A.V., Krupa M., Hebert F., Groot K. and Szepeshazi K. (2002). Bombesin antagonists inhibit growth of MDA-MB-435 estrogen independent breast cancers and decrease the expression of ErbB-2/HER-2 oncoprotein and c-jun and c-fos oncogenes. Proc Nat Acad Sci NSA, 99, 3836-3841.

Bajusz S., Csernus V.J., Janaky T., Bokser L., Fekete M. and Schally A.V. (1988). New antagonists of LHRH: II. Inhibition and potentiation of LHRH by closely related analogues. Int J Peptide Prot Res, 32, 425-435.

Bauer W., Briner U., Doepfner W., Haller R., Huguenin R., Marbach P., Petcher T.J. and Pless J. (1982). SMS 201-995: a very potent and selective octapeptide analogue of somatostatin with prolonged action. Life Sci, 31, 1133-1140.

Brazeau P., Vale W., Burgus R., Ling N., Butcher M., Rivier J. and Guillemin R. (1973). Hypothalamic polypeptide that inhibits the secretion of immunoreactive pituitary growth hormone. Science, 179, 77-79.

Buscail L, Saint-Laurent N., Chastre E., Vaillant J.C., Gespach C., Capella G., Kalthoff H., Lluis F., Vaysse N. and Susini C. (1996). Loss of sst2 somatostatin receptor gene expression in human pancreatic and colorectal cancer. Cancer Res, 56, 1823-1827.

Cai R-Z, Reile H., Armatis P. and Schally A.V. (1994). Potent bombesin antagonists with C-terminal Leu ψ(CH2N)-Tac-NH_2 or its derivatives. Proc Natl Acad Sci USA, 91, 12664–12668.

Cai R-Z., Szoke B., Lu R., Fu D., Redding T.W. and Schally A.V. (1986). Synthesis and biological activity of highly potent octapeptide analogs of somatostatin. Proc Natl Acad Sci USA, 83, 1896-1900.

Chave H.S., Gough A.C., Palmer K., Preston S.R. and Primrose J.N. (2000). Bombesin family receptor and ligand gene expression in human colorectal cancer and normal mucosa. Br J Cancer, 82, 124-130.

Comaru-Schally A.M., Brannan W., Schally A.V., Colcolough M. and Monga M. (1998). Efficacy and safety of LHRH antagonist cetrorelix in the treatment of symptomatic benign prostatic hyperplasia. J Clin Endocrinol Metab, 83, 3826-3831.

Cuttitta F., Carney D.N., Mulshine J., Moody T.W., Fedorko J., Fischler A. and Minna J.D. (1985), Bombesin-like peptides can function as autocrine growth factors in human small-cell lung cancer. Nature, 316, 823-826

Dondi D., Limonta P., Moretti R.M., Marelli M.M., Garattini E. and Motta M. (1994). Antiproliferative effects of luteinizing hormone-releasing hormone (LHRH) agonists on human androgen-independent prostate cancer cell line DU 145: evidence for an autocrine-inhibitory LHRH loop. Cancer Res, 54, 4091-4095

Emons G., Ortmann O., Becker M., Irmer G., Springer B., Laun R., Holzel F., Schulz K-D. and Schally A.V. (1993). High affinity binding and direct antiproliferative effects of LHRH analogues in human ovarian cancer cell lines. Cancer Res, 53, 5439-5446.

Emons G., Ortmann O., Teichert H.M., Fassl H., Barreton G., Lohrs U., Kullander S., Kauppila A., Ayalon D., Schally A. V., Heinrich C., Schulz K.D. and Oberheuser F. (1996). Luteinizing hormone-releasing hormone agonist triptorelin in combination with cytotoxic chemotherapy in patients with advanced epithelial ovarian cancer - A prospective double blinded randomized trial. Cancer, 78, 1452-1460.

Emons G. and Schally A.V. (1994). The use of luteinizing hormone-releasing hormone agonists and antagonists in gynecological cancers. Hum Reprod, 9, 1364-1379.

Gonzalez-Barcena D., Vadillo-Buenfil M., Cortez-Morales A., Fuentes-Garcia M., Cardenas-Cornejo I., Comaru-Schally A.M. and Schally A.V. (1995). Luteinizing hormone-releasing hormone antagonist cetrorelix as primary single therapy in patients with advanced prostatic cancer and paraplegia due to metastatic invasion of spinal cord. Urology, 45, 275-281.

Gonzalez-Barcena D., Vadillo-Buenfil M., Gomez-Orta F., Fuentes Garcia M., Cardenas-Cornejo I., Graef-Sanchez A., Comaru-Schally A.M. and Schally A.V. (1994). Responses to the antagonistic analog of LHRH (SB-75, cetrorelix) in patients with benign prostatic hyperplasia and prostatic cancer. Prostate, 24, 84-92.
Halmos G., Arenciba J.M., Schally A.V., Davis R. and Bostwick D.G. (2000a). High incidence of receptors for luteinizing hormone-releasing hormone (LHRH) and LHRH receptor gene expression in human prostate cancers. J Urol, 163, 623-629.
Halmos G., Schally A.V., Sun B., Davis R., Bostwick D.G. and Plonowski A. (2000b). High expression of somatostatin receptors and ribonucleic acid for its receptor subtypes in organ-confined and locally advanced human prostate cancers. J Clin Endocrinol Metab, 85, 2564-2571.
Huggins C. and Hodges C.V. (1941). Studies of prostatic cancer. I. Effect of castration, estrogens and androgen injections on serum phosphatases in metastatic carcinoma of the prostate. Cancer Res, 1, 293-295
Jungwirth A., Schally A.V., Halmos G., Groot K., Szepeshazi K., Pinski J. and Armatis P. (1998). Inhibition of the growth of Caki-I human renal adenocarcinoma in vivo by LHRH antagonists cetrorelix, somatostatin analog RC-160 and bombesin antagonist RC-3940-II. Cancer, 82, 909-917.
Kahan Z., Nagy A., Schally A.V., Halmos G., Arencibia J.M. and Groot K. (1999a). Complete regression of MX- I human breast carcinoma xenografts after targeted chemotherapy with a cytotoxic analog of luteinizing hormone-releasing hormone, AN-207. Cancer, 85, 2608-2615.
Kahan Z., Nagy A., Schally A.V., Hebert F., Sun B., Groot K. and Halmos G. (1999b). Inhibition of growth of MX- I, MCF-7, MIII and MDA-MB-23I human breast cancer xenografts after administration of a targeted cytotoxic analog of somatostatin, AN-238. Int J Cancer, 82, 592-598.
Kahan Z., Sum Sun B., Schally A.V., Arencibia J.M., Cal R-Z., Groot K. and Halmos G. (2000). Inhibition of growth of MDA-MB-468 estrogen-independent human breast cancers by bombesin/gastrin-releasing peptide (GRP) antagonists RC-3095 and RC-3940-II. Cancer, 88, 1384-1392.
Karten M.J. and Rivier J.E. (1986) Gonadotropin-releasing hormone analog design. Structure-function studies toward the development of agonists and antagonists: rationale and perspective. Endocr Rev, 7, 44-66
Kaufmann M., Jonat W., Kleeberg U., Eiermann W., Janicke F., Hilfrich J., Kreienberg R., Albrecht M., Weitzel H.K., Schmid H., Strunz P., Schachner-Wunschmann E., Bastert G. and Maass H. (1989). Goserelin, a depot gonadotropin-releasing hormone agonist in the treatment of premenopausal patients with metastatic breast cancer. German Zoladex Trial Group. J Clin Oncol, 7, 1113-1119.
Kiaris H., Schally A.V., Nagy A., Sun B., Armatis P. and Szepeshazi K. (1999). Targeted cytotoxic analog of bombesin/gastrin-releasing peptide inhibits the growth of H-69 human small-cell lung carcinoma in nude mice. Br J Cancer, 81, 966-971.
Kiaris H., Schally A.V., Nagy A., Sun B., Szepeshazi K. and Halmos G. (2000). Regression of U-87MG human glioblastomas in nude mice after treatment with a cytotoxic somatostatin analog AN-238. Clin Cancer Res, 6, 709-717.
Kiaris H., Schally A.V., Nagy A., Szepeshazi K., Hebert F. and Halmos G. (2001) A targeted cytotoxic somatostatin (SST) analogue AN-238 inhibits the growth of H-69 small cell lung carcinoma (SCLC) and H-157 non-SCLC in nude mice. Eur J Cancer, 37, 620-628.
Klijn J.G., Beex L.V., Mauriac L., van Zijl J.A., Veyret C., Wildiers J., Jassem J., Piccart M., Burghouts J., Becquart D., Seynaeve C., Mignolet F. and Duchateau L. (2000). Combined treatment with buserelin and tamoxifen in premenopausal metastatic breast cancer: a randomized study. J Natl Cancer Inst, 92, 903-911.
Koppan M., Halmos G., Arencibia J.M., Lamharzi N. and Schally A.V. (1998). Bombesin gastrin-releasing peptide antagonists RC-3095 and RC-3940-11 inhibit tumor growth

and decrease the levels and mRNA expression of epidermal growth factor receptors in H-69 small cell lung carcinoma. Cancer, 83, 1335-1343.

Koppan M., Nagy A., Schally A.V., Plonowski A., Halmos G., Arencibia J.M. and Groot K. (1999). Targeted cytotoxic analog of luteinizing hormone-releasing hormone AN-207 inhibits the growth of PC-82 human prostate cancer in nude mice. Prostate, 38, 151-158.

Kovacs M., Schally A.V., Csernus B. and Rekasi Z. (2001). Luteinizing hormone-releasing hormone (LHRH) antagonist cetrorelix down regulates the mRNA expression of pituitary receptors for LHRH by counteracting the stimulatory effect of endogenous LHRH. Proc Natl Acad Sci USA, 98, 1829-1834.

Krenning E.P., Kwekkeboom D.J., Bakker W.H., Breeman W.A., Kooij P.P., Oei H.Y., van Hagen M., Postema P.T., de Jong M., Reubi J.C., Visser T.J., Reijs A.E.M., Hofland L.J, Koper J.W, Lamberts S.W.J. and Krenning E.P. (1993). Somatostatin receptor scintigraphy with [^{111}In-DTPA-D-Phe1]- and [^{123}I-Tyr3]-octreotide: the Rotterdam experience with more than 1000 patients. Eur J Nucl Med, 20, 716-731.

Lamberts S.W., Krenning E.P. and Reubi J.C. (1991). The role of somatostatin and its analogs in the diagnosis and treatment of tumors. Endocr Rev, 12, 450-82.

Limonta P., Dondi D., Moretti R.M., Maggi R. and Motta M. (1992). Antiproliferative effects of luteinizing hormone-releasing hormone agonists on the human prostatic cancer cell line LNCaP. J Clin Endocrinol Metab, 75, 207-212.

Markwalder R. and Reubi J.C. (1999). Gastrin-releasing peptide receptors in the human prostate: relation to neoplastic transformation. Cancer Res, 59, 1152-1159

Miyazaki M., Lamharzi N., Schally A.V, Halmos G., Szepeshazi K., Groot K. and Cai R-Z. (1998). Inhibition of growth of MDA-MB-231 human breast cancer xenografts in nude mice by bombesin/gastrin releasing peptide (GRP) antagonists RC-3940-II and RC-3095. Eur J Cancer, 34, 710-717.

Miyazaki M., Nagy A., Schally A.V., Lamharzi N., Halmos G., Szepeshazi K., Groot K. and Armatis P. (1997). Growth inhibition of human ovarian cancers by cytotoxic analogues of luteinizing hormone-releasing hormone. J Natl Cancer Inst, 89, 1803-1809

Miyazaki M., Schally A.V., Nagy A., Lamharzi N., Halmos G., Szepeshazi K. and Armatis P. (1999). Targeted cytotoxic analog of luteinizing hormone-releasing hormone AN-207 inhibits growth of OV-1063 human epithelial ovarian cancers in nude mice. Am J Obstet Gynecol, 180, 1095-1103,

Molineaux C.J., Sluss P.M., Bree M.P., Gefter M.L., Sullivan L.M. and Garnic M.B. (1998). Suppression of plasma gonadtrophs by abrelix: a potent new LHRH antagonist. Mol Urol, 2, 265-268.

Nagy A., Armatis P., Cai R-Z., Szepeshazi K., Halmos G. and Schally A.V. (1997). Design, synthesis and in vitro evaluation of cytotoxic analogs of bombesin-like peptides containing doxorubicin or its intensely potent derivative, 2-pyrrolinodoxorubicin. Proc Natl Acad Sci USA, 94, 652-656.

Nagy A., Plonowski A. and Schally A.V. (2000). Stability of cytotoxic hormone-releasing hormone conjugate (AN-152) containing doxorubicin-14-O-Hemiglutarate in mouse and human serum in vitro; implications for the design of preclinical studies. Proc Natl Acad Sci USA, 97, 829-834.

Nagy A., Schally A.V., Armatis P., Szepeshazi K., Halmos G., Kovacs M., Zarandi M., Groot K., Miyazaki M., Jungwirth A. and Horvath J. (1996). Cytotoxic analogs of luteinizing hormone-releasing hormone containing doxorubicin or 2-pyrrolinodoxorubicin, a derivative 500-1000 times more potent. Proc Natl Acad Sci USA, 93, 7269-7273.

Nagy A., Schally A.V., Halmos G., Armatis P., Cai R-Z., Csernus V., Kovacs M., Koppan M., Szepeshazi K. and Kahn Z. (1998). Synthesis and biological evaluation of cytotoxic analogs of somatostatin containing doxorubicin or its intensely potent derivative 2-pyrrolinodoxonubicin. Proc Natl Acad Sci USA, 95, 1794-1799.

Patel Y.C. (1997). Molecular pharmacology of somatostatin receptor subtypes. J Endocrinol Invest, 20, 348-367.

Pinski J., Lamharzi N., Halmos G., Groot K., Jungwirth A., Vadillo-Buenfil M., Kakar S.S. and Schally A.V. (1996). Chronic administration of luteinizing hormone-releasing hormone (LHRH) antagonist Cetrorelix decreases gonadotrope responsiveness and pituitary LHRH receptor messenger ribonucleic acid levels in rats. Endocrinology, 137, 3430-3436.

Plonowski A., Nagy A., Schally A.V., Sun B., Groot K. and Halmos G. (2000a). In vivo inhibition of PC-3 human androgen-independent prostate cancer by a targeted cytotoxic bombesin analogue AN-215. Int J Cancer, 88, 652-657.

Plonowski A., Schally A.V., Nagy A., Kiaris H., Hebert F. and Halmos G. (2000b). Inhibition of metastatic renal cell carcinomas expressing somatostatin receptors by a targeted cytotoxic analog of somatostatin AN-238. Cancer Res, 60, 2996-3001.

Plonowski A., Schally A.V., Nagy A., Sun B. and Szepeshazi K. (1999). Inhibition of PC-3 human androgen-independent prostate cancer and its metastases by cytotoxic somatostatin analogue AN-238. Cancer Res, 59, 1947-1953.

Plonowski A., Schally A.V., Varga J.L., Rekasi Z., Hebert F., Halmos G. and Groot K. (2000c). Potentiation of the inhibitory effect of growth hormone-releasing hormone antagonists on PC-3 human prostate cancer by bombesin antagonists indicative of interference with both IGF and EGF pathways. Prostate, 44, 172-180.

Redding T.W. and Schally A.V. (1981). Inhibition of prostate tumor growth in two rat models by chronic administration of D-Trp^{6}-LHRH. Proc Nat Acad Sci USA, 78, 6509-6512

Reubi J.C. and Kvols L. (1992). Somatostatin receptors in human renal cell carcinomas. Cancer Res, 52, 6074-6078.

Santen R.J., Manni A., Harvey H. and Redmond C. (1990). Endocrine treatment of breast cancer in women. Endocr Rev, 11, 221-265.

Schally A.V. (1988). Oncological applications of somatostatin analogs. Cancer Res, 48, 6977-6985.

Schally A.V. (1999). Luteinizing hormone-releasing hormone analogs: their impact on the control of tumorigenesis. Peptides, 20, 1247-1262.

Schally A.V., Arimura A., Baba Y., Nair R.M.G., Matsuo H., Redding T.W., Debeljuk L. and White W.F. (1971a). Isolation and properties of the FSH- and LH-releasing hormone. Biochem Biophys Res Commun, 43, 393-399.

Schally A.V., Arimura A., Kastin A.J., Matsuo H., Baba Y., Redding T.W., Nair R.M.G., Debeljuk L. and White W.F. (1971b). Gonadotropin-releasing hormone: one polypeptide regulates secretion of luteinizing and follicle-stimulating hormones. Science, 173, 1036-1038.

Schally A.V., Comaru-Schally A.M., Nagy A., Kovacs M., Szepeshazi K., Plonowski A., Varga J.L. and Halmos G. (2001a). Hypothalamic hormones and cancer. Frontiers Neuroendocrinol, 22, 248-291.

Schally A.V., Comaru-Schally A.M., Plonowski A., Nagy A., Halmos G. and Rekasi Z. (2000). Peptide analogs in the Therapy of Prostate Cancer. Prostate, 45, 158-166.

Schally A.V., Halmos G., Rekasi Z. and Arencibia J.M. (2001b). The actions of LHRH agonists, antagonists, and cytotoxic analogs on the LHRH receptors on the pituitary and tumors. In Infertil Reprod Med Clin N Am, 12, 17-44.

Schally A.V., Kastin A.J. and Arimura A. (1971c). Hypothalamic FSH and LH-regulating hormone, structure, physiology, and clinical studies. Fertil Steril, 22, 703-721.

Schally A.V. and Nagy A. (1999). Cancer chemotherapy based on targeting of cytotoxic peptide conjugates to their receptors on tumors. Eur J Endocrinol, 141, 1-14.

Shriver S.P., Bourdeau H.A., Gubish C.T., Tirpak D.L., Davis A.L., Luketich J.D. and Siegfried J.M. (2000). Sex-specific expression of gastrin-releasing peptide receptor: relationship to smoking history and risk of lung cancer. J Natl Cancer Inst, 92, 24-33.

Sun B., Halmos G., Schally A.V., Wang X. and Martinez M. (2000). The presence of receptors for bombesin/gastrin-releasing peptide and mRNA for three receptor subtypes in human prostate cancers. Prostate, 42, 295-303.

Sunday M.E., Kaplan L.M., Motoyama E., Chin W.W. and Spindel E.R. (1988). Gastrin-releasing peptide (mammalian bombesin) gene expression in health and disease. Lab Invest, 59, 5-24.

Szepeshazi K., Schally A.V., Halmos G., Armatis P., Hebert F., Sun B., Feil A., Kiaris H. and Nagy A. (2002). Targeted cytotoxic somatostatin analogue an-238 inhibits somatostatin receptor-positive experimental colon cancers independently of their *p53* status. Cancer Res, 62, 781-788.

Szepeshazi K., Schally A.V., Halmos G., Sun B., Hebert F., Csernus B. and Nagy A. (2001). Targeting of cytotoxic somatostatin analog AN-238 to somatostatin receptor subtypes 5 and/or 3 in experimental pancreatic cancer. Clin Cancer Res, 7, 2854-2861.

Szereday Z., Schally A.V., Nagy A., Plonowski A., Bajo A.M., Halmos G., Szepeshazi K. and Groot K. (2002). Effective treatment of experimental U-87MG human glioblastoma in nude mice with a targeted cytotoxic bombesin analogue, AN-215. Br J Cancer, 86, 1322-1327.

Tolis G., Ackman D., Stellos A., Mehta A., Labrie F., Fazekas A.T., Comaru-Schally A.M. and Schally A.V. (1982). Tumor growth inhibition in patients with prostatic carcinoma treated with luteinizing hormone-releasing hormone agonists. Proc Natl Acad Sci USA, 79, 1658-1662.

CHAPTER 2

Analogs of Luteinizing Hormone-releasing Hormone in Benign Prostatic Hyperplasia and Advanced Renal Cell Carcinoma

A.M. COMARU-SCHALLY

Benign Prostatic Hyperplasia

Background

Benign prostatic hyperplasia (BPH) is a significant health problem all over the world. This condition will affect most men should they live long enough and can lead to serious complications, such as acute or chronic urinary retention, renal insufficiency, urinary tract infection and sexual dysfunction (Oesterling, 1996; Isaacs, 1990). Symptomatic BPH causes morbidity and can lower the quality of life (QoL) (Hoznek and Abben, 2001; Hegarty et al., 2001). We investigated whether short-term administration of the LHRH antagonist cetrorelix could provide a new treatment for men with BPH (Comaru-Schally et al., 1998).

Participants and Methods

Thirteen men aged 57-75 years with moderate to severe symptomatic BPH participated in this open phase I/II study, which was approved by the local institutional review board. Each patient gave written informed consent to this study. To qualify for enrollment, all participants had to have: a total International Prostate Symptom Score (IPSS) of ≥ 18; an enlarged prostate per rectal exam (DRE) and transrectal ultrasound (TRUS); serum prostatic antigen (PSA) < 10 ng/ml; peak urine flow rate (2 max) < 15 cc/s by uroflowmetry and a postvoid residual volume (PVR) < 300 cc estimated by bladder scan. Qualified subjects also had clinical and laboratory evaluations 1-2 weeks before the initiation of cetrorelix therapy to establish baseline values. All the men answered three patient self-administered questionnaires at baseline and during the study before each clinic visit for the assessment of urinary symptoms (IPSS), QoL due to urinary symptoms and sexual function. The IPSS includes seven questions that assess urinary symptoms (Barry and Roenborn, 1997). The total score can be in the range 0-35. The severity of the urinary symptoms was estimated according to the American Urological Association Symptom Index: scores of 1-7, mild; 8-19, moderate; and 20-35, severe. The questionnaire recommended by the international consensus committee was used to assess QoL (Barry and Roenborn, 1997). Sexual function was assessed based on a self-administered questionnaire developed by Reynolds et al. (1998).

Laboratory Evaluations

Studies consisted of determinations of hematology, chemistry (SMAI6), urinalysis, serum levels of PSA, LH, FSH, testosterone (T), DHT, cetrorelix, and growth factors [insulin-like growth factors (IGF-1 and IGF-2), transforming growth factor ($TGF\beta_2$), and basic fibroblast growth factor (bFGF)]. LHRH antagonist cetrorelix was provided by ASTA Medica (Frankfurt am Main, Germany). The initial dose of cetrorelix was 5 mg, sub-cutaneous (s.c.), twice daily, for 2 days (loading dose), followed by a maintenance dose of 1 mg/day, s.c., for 2 months. Clinical, laboratory and radiological re-evaluations were carried out on all subjects during maintenance therapy and up to 18 months after the completion of treatment. Clinical evaluations were performed at weeks 1, 4, 8, 12, 16 and 20 and periodically thereafter.

Results

Figs 1, 2 and 3 illustrate the long-term effects of administration of cetrorelix on total IPSS, QoL score and prostate volume determined by TRUS. Treatment with cetrorelix produced a decline of 52.9% in IPSS, a 46% improvement in

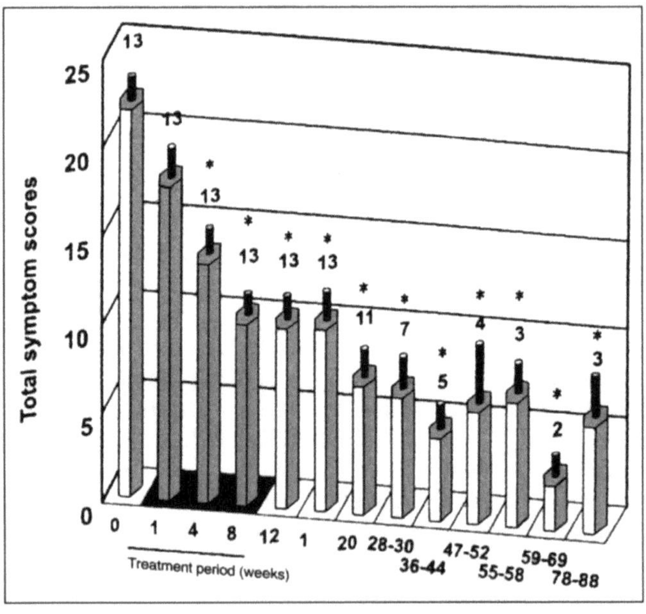

Fig. 1. Mean IPSS values in men with symptomatic BPH before, during and after treatment with cetrorelix. Error bars indicate the S.E.M. The numbers above the error bars show the number of evaluable patients. Asterisks designate statistically significant decrease as compared with the baseline (student's two-tailed *t*-test, $p < 0.05$). During the follow-up, some evaluations were performed in the combined range of weeks, as indicated. Reprinted by permission from Comaru-Schally et al. (1998). © 1998, The Endocrine Society

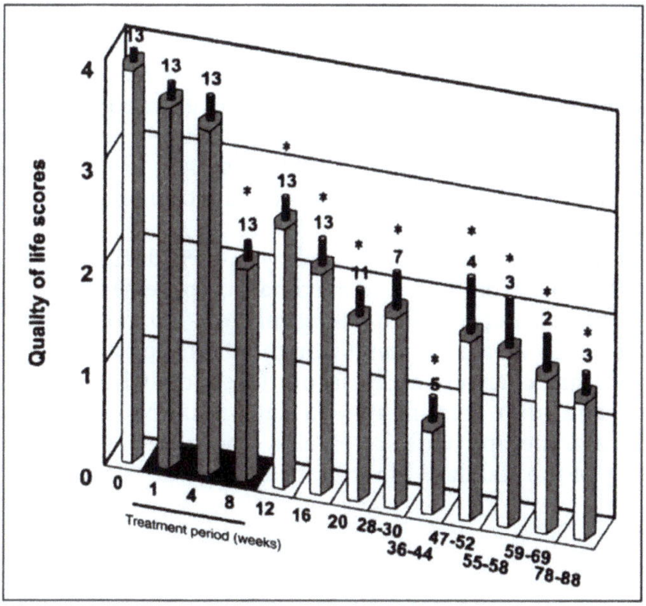

Fig. 2. Mean QoL scores in men with symptomatic BPH before, during, and after treatment with cetrorelix. Other designations are explained in Figure 1. Reprinted by permission from Comaru-Schally et al. (1998). © 1998, The Endocrine Society

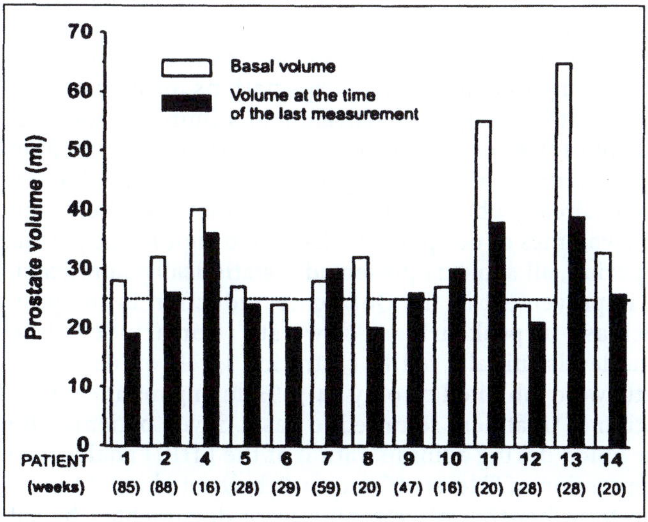

Fig. 3. Individual PVs estimated by TRUS at baseline and at the time of the last evaluation of 13 men with symptomatic BPH treated with cetrorelix. The dashed line represents the normal prostatic volume. The time of the last evaluation is indicated in brackets. Reprinted by permission from Comaru-Schally et al. (1998). © 1998, The Endocrine Society

the QoL score, a rapid reduction of 27% in prostatic volume (PV), and an increase in peak urinary flow rates by 2.86 ml/s. Serum testosterone (T) fell to castration levels on day 2, but was inhibited by only 64-74% during maintenance therapy and after cessation of treatment returned to normal. During long-term follow-up, most patients continued to show a progressive improvement in urinary symptoms (decline in IPSS from 67% to 72% at weeks 20 and 85, respectively), an enhancement in sexual function, and prostatic volume remained normal.

Serum levels of FSH and LH decreased by 54-59% during therapy, but later returned to normal. Serum PSA was maximally suppressed at week 8 of treatment when the levels decreased to 0.8 ng/ml from a basal mean of 1.6 ng/ml. PSA continued below basal values throughout the follow up period. There were no significant changes in the serum levels of IGF-1, IGF-2, TGF-β_2 or bFGF during and after treatment with cetrorelix. No serious side effects occurred during therapy with cetrorelix, and there were no significant changes in any of the standard blood tests during this trial.

Comments

The etiology of BPH and the mechanism of progression from pathological to clinical BPH are incompletely understood (Oesterling, 1996; Shapiro and Lepor, 1995). The natural history of BPH is variable, but the disease can lead to severe complications, such as acute or chronic urine retention, renal insufficiency and infection. Improvement in the QoL of patients suffering from BPH is an important issue in the management of this condition (Comaru-Schally et al., 1998; Hoznek and Abbou, 2001). Medical and surgical treatment of BPH and minimally invasive procedures can affect erectile function, ejaculation and sexual satisfaction (Hegarty et al., 2001). For a selection of therapy, baseline sexual function and patient expectations must be considered.

The results of this study demonstrate that administration of cetrorelix for 2 months is well-tolerated and rapidly alleviated urinary symptoms, irrespective of prostate size (Comaru-Schally et al., 1998). The rapid onset of action of cetrorelix was already observed by week 4 of therapy, when symptom scores and prostate volumes of our patients decreased significantly. At the end of the treatment period, all subjects presented a statistically significant decrease in total IPSS, improvement in the QoL score, reduction in the prostate volume and an increase in peak urinary flow rate (Comaru-Schally et al., 1998). Testosterone levels initially fell to castration levels on day 2 of therapy, but subsequently were inhibited by only 64-74% during maintenance therapy and after cessation of treatment returned to basal. Seven patients who temporarily lost their libido during administration of the LHRH analog were those with greater suppression of T levels (Comaru-Schally et al., 1998).

The long-term benefits of cetrorelix were documented by subjective and objective parameters (Comaru-Schally et al., 1998). During long-term follow-up, most patients continued to show a progressive improvement in urinary symptoms and in QoL scores and prostate volumes were maintained below basal values in 10 of 13 men. Three patients had a mild enlargement of prostate at the end of the study (Comaru-Schally et al., 1998).

The improvement in sexual function of some of our patients after completion of therapy was notable and it is likely that the relief of urinary symptoms can have a major impact on the quality of sexual life (Comaru-Schally et al., 1998).

Currently the great majority of patients with symptomatic BPH elect medical therapy because of the probability of clinical improvement and concern about surgery or other invasive treatments. Inhibitors of 5α-reductase or α_1-adrenergic receptor antagonists do not offer long-term remission of urinary symptoms after discontinuation and should be used only in a selected population of patients (McKiernan and Lowe, 1997; Wise and Ostad, 2001; Lepor et al., 1996). Finasteride requires long-term therapy to achieve a clinical response and causes significant sexual dysfunction (Wise and Ostad, 2001; Nickel et al., 1996). The best patients for finasteride might be those with a large prostate > 50 g, modest lower urinary symptoms, little interest in sexual function and no immediate need for pharmacolgic relief of symptoms (Wise and Ostad, 2001). Treatment with α-blockers rapidly alleviates urinary symptoms in patients with a moderate or very large prostate, but needs to be applied chronically and can cause orthostatic hypotension and syncope (Comaru-Schally et al., 1998; Wise and Ostad, 2001). The outcome of trials with agonistic analogs of LHRH, nafarelin or leuprolide for 4-6 months in men with BPH was disappointing (Peters and Walsh, 1987; Gabrilove et al., 1989). Medical castration induced by prolonged administration of these analogs caused a reduction in prostate size and improved urinary symptoms, but after the cessation of therapy these beneficial effects were abolished.

The mechanism of action of cetrorelix responsible for the improvement in clinical BPH is not clear. Previously, we had demonstrated that therapy with cetrorelix caused improvement in prostatism and a reduction of 44% in prostate volume in BPH patients with a mean basal PV of 67.8 ml (Gonzalez-Barcena et al., 1994). In the present study, subjects with a relatively small prostate had a prolonged therapeutic response to cetrorelix, although the reduction in PV was smaller (Comaru-Schally et al., 1998).

The transient suppression of T levels can only account in part for the beneficial effects of cetrorelix. Various peptide growth factors may be involved in the pathogenesis of BPH (De Bellis et al., 1996; Steiner, 1995; Culig et al., 1996; Cohen et al., 1994; Begun et al., 1995). In the present study we found no changes in serum levels of IGF-1, IGF-2, TGF-β_2 or bFGF in patients treated with cetrorelix (Comaru-Schally et al., 1998). It is possible that alterations in growth factors during therapy with cetrorelix occur only in hyperplastic prostate tissue and not in serum. In future studies, needle biopsies of prostate might determine possible changes in growth factors. It is of importance that cetrorelix was previously shown to inhibit the growth of human prostatic, mammary, ovarian and other cancers xenografted into nude mice, with the induction of apoptosis (Schally and Comaru-Schally, 1997a, 1997b, 2000). This tumor growth suppression was invariably linked to a major reduction in the levels of epidermal growth factor receptor tumors (Schally and Comaru Schally, 1997b). Cetrorelix can also interfere with the growth-stimulating effects of IGFs in mammary and endometrial cancer cells (Schally and Comaru Schally, 1997a). Low doses of cetrorelix cause only a temporary submaximal suppression of T, but may provide clinical benefits by induction of apoptosis and inhibition of prostatic growth factors (Comaru-Schally et al., 1998). Phase II/III double-blind placebo-controled studies are in progress to extend these preliminary findings.

Renal Cell Carcinoma

Renal cell carcinoma (RCC) is the most common renal tumor and its estimated worldwide incidence is about 150,000 cases yearly (Godley and Kim, 2002; Jemal et al., 2002; Richie et al., 1997; Motzer et al., 1996; Sokoloff et al., 1996). The American Cancer Society projects that in the year 2002 approximately 32,000 patients in the USA will be diagnosed with this neoplasm, with an expected 12,000 deaths (Jemal et al., 2002). About 30% of patients with RCC have evidence of metastatic disease at the initial presentation and the 2 year survival rate in this group is poor, ranging from 10% to 20% (Motzer et al., 1996; Papadopoulos, 1996). For the advanced stages of RCC, no effective therapy is available. Chemotherapeutic agents or radiotherapy are of no benefit. Immunotherapy based on administration of interferon-α, interleukin-2 or combinations of these cytokines has only a marginal efficacy and is associated with significant clinical toxicity (Dutcher et al., 1997; Henriksson et al., 1998). The etiology of RCC and the mechanisms of progression from an early stage to advanced disease are incompletely understood. Various growth factors and sex steroids appear to be involved in RCC (Jungwirth et al., 1998; Schally et al., 2001). An increased expression of growth factors or their receptors may enhance cellular replication in renal cell carcinoma. The overexpression of the receptor for epidermal growth factor (EGF), its ligands (EGF, TGF-α), and IGF receptors has been reported in RCC (Aoyagi et al., 1996; Jungwirth et al., 1998). Thus, one strategy to treat patients with advanced RCC could be based on the inhibition of growth factors or their receptors, which might be implicated in this malignancy. Receptors for LHRH are also present on RCC (Sion-Vardi et al., 1992). One of the agents we are using in phase II clinical trials is the LHRH antagonist cetrorelix. This is based on the finding that LHRH antagonist cetrorelix effectively inhibits the growth of human renal adenocarcinomas in nude mice (Jungwirth et al., 1998). Clinical trials with cetrorelix in patients with advanced renal cell carcinoma are in progress in New Orleans.

References

Aoyagi T., Takishima K., Hayakawa M. and Nakamura H. (1996). Gene expression of TGF-α, EGF and IL-6 in cultured renal tubular cells and renal cell carcinoma. Int J Urol, 3, 392-396.

Barry M. and Roehrborn C. (1997). Management of benign prostatic hyperplasia. Annu Rev Med, 48, 177-189.

Begun F.P., Story M.T., Hopp K.A., Shapiro E. and Lawson R.K. (1995). Regional concentration of basic fibroblast growth factor in normal and benign hyperplastic human prostates. J Urol, 153, 839-843.

Cohen P., Peehl D.M., Baker B., Liu F., Hintz R.L. and Rosenfeld R.G. (1994). Insulin-like growth factor axis abnormalities in prostatic stromal cells from patients with benign prostatic hyperplasia. J Clin Endocrinol Metab, 79, 1410-1415.

Comaru-Schally A.M., Brannan W., Schally A.V., Colcolough M. and Monga M. (1998). Efficacy and safety of LHRH antagonist cetrorelix in the treatment of symptomatic benign prostatic hyperplasia. J Clin Endocrinol Metab, 83, 3826-3831.

Culig Z., Hobisch A., Cronauer M.V., Radmayr C., Hittmair A., Zhang J., Thurnher M., Bartsch G. and Klocker H. (1996). Regulation of prostatic growth and function by peptide growth factors. Prostate, 28, 392-405.

De Bellis A., Ghiandi P., Comerci A., Fiorelli G., Grappone C., Milani S., Salerno R., Marra F. and Serio M. (1996). Epidermal growth factor, epidermal growth factor receptor, and transforming growth factor-alpha in human hyperplastic prostate tissue: expression and cellular localization. J Clin Endocrinol Metab, 81, 4148-4154.

Dutcher J.P., Fisher R.I., Weiss G., Aronson F., Margolin K., Louie A., Mier J., Caliendo G., Sosman J.A., Eckardt J.R., Ernest M.L., Doroshow J. and Atkins M. (1997). Outpatient subcutaneous interleukin-2 and interferon-α for metastatic renal cell cancer: 5-year follow-up of the Cytokine Working Group Study. Cancer J Sci Am, 3, 157-162.

Gabrilove J.L., Levine A.C., Kirschenbaum A., Droller M. (1989). Effect of long-acting gonadotropin-releasing hormone analog (leuprolide) therapy on prostatic size and symptoms in 15 men with benign prostatic hypertrophy. J Clin Endocrinol Metab, 69, 629-632.

Godley P. and Kim S.W. (2002). Renal cell carcinoma. Curr Opin Oncol, 14, 280-285.

Gonzalez-Barcena D., Vadillo-Buenfil M., Gomez-Orta F., Fuentes Garcia M., Cardenas-Cornejo I., Graef-Sanchez A., Comaru-Schally A.M. and Schally A.V. (1994). Responses to the antagonistic analog of LHRH (SB-75, Cetrorelix) in patients with benign prostatic hyperplasia and prostatic cancer. Prostate, 24, 84-92.

Hegarty P.K., Hegarty N.J., Fitzpatrick J.M. (2001). Sexual function in patients with benign prostatic hyperplasia. Curr Urol Rep, 2, 292-296.

Henriksson R., Nilsson S., Colleen S., Wersall P., Helsing M., Zimmerman R. and Engman K. (1998). Survival in renal cell carcinoma-a randomized evaluation of tamoxifen vs. interleukin 2, α-interferon (leucocyte) and tamoxifen. Br J Cancer, 77, 1311-1317.

Hoznek A. and Abbou C.C. (2001). Impact of interventional therapy for benign prostatic hyperplasia on quality of life and sexual function. Curr Urol Rep, 2, 311-317.

Isaacs J.T. (1990). Importance of the natural history of benign prostatic hyperplasia in the evaluation of pharmacologic intervention. Prostate, 3, 1-7.

Jemal A., Thomas A., Murray T. and Thun M. Cancer statistics. (2002). CA Cancer J Clin, 52, 23-47.

Jungwirth A., Schally A.V., Halmos G., Groot K., Szepeshazi K., Pinski J. and Armatis P. (1998). Inhibition of the growth of Caki-I human renal adenocarcinoma in vivo by LHRH antagonists Cetrorelix, somatostatin analog RC-160 and bombesin antagonist RC-3940-II. Cancer, 82, 909-917.

Lepor H., Williford W.O., Barry M.J., Brawer M.K., Dixon C.M., Gormley G., Haakenson C., Machi M., Narayan P. and Padley R.J. (1996). The efficacy of terazosin, finasteride, or both in benign prostatic hyperplasia. Veterans Affairs Cooperative Studies Benign Prostatic Hyperplasia Study Group. N Engl J Med, 335, 533-539.

McKiernan J.M. and Lowe F.C. (1997). Side effects of terazosin in the treatment of symptomatic benign prostatic hyperplasia. South Med J, 90, 509-513.

Motzer R.J., Bander N.H., Nanus D.M. Renal-cell carcinoma. N Engl J Med, 1996, 335, 865-875.

Nickel J.C., Fradet Y., Boake R.C., Pommerville P.J., Perreault J.P., Afridi S.K. and Elhilali M.M. (1996). Efficacy and safety of finasteride therapy for benign prostatic hyperplasia: results of a 2-year randomized controlled trial (the PROSPECT study). PROscar Safety Plus Efficacy Canadian Two year Study. Can Med Assoc J, 155, 1251-1259.

Oesterling J.E. (1996). Benign prostatic hyperplasia: a review of its histogenesis and natural history. Prostate, 6, 67-73.

Papadopoulos I., Rudolph P., Weichert-Jacobsen K., Thiemann O. and Papadopoulou D. (1996). Prognostic indicators for response to therapy and survival in patients with metastatic renal cell cancer treated with interferon-$\alpha_{2\beta}$ and vinblastine. Urology, 48, 373-378.
Peters C.A. and Walsh P.C. (1987). The effect of nafarelin acetate, a luteinizing-hormone-releasing hormone agonist, on benign prostatic hyperplasia. N Engl J Med, 317, 599-604.
Reynolds C.F. III, Frank E., Thase M.E., Houck P.R., Jennings J.R., Howell J.R., Lilienfeld S.O. and Kupfer D.J. (1988). Assessment of sexual function in depressed, impotent, and healthy men: factor analysis of a Brief Sexual Function Questionnaire for men. Psychiat Res, 24, 231-250.
Richie J.P., Kantoff P.W. and Shapiro C.L. (1997). Renal cell carcinoma. In Cancer Medicine, 4th edn, eds, Holland J.F., Frei E. III, Bast R.C. Jr, Kufe D.W., Morton D.L. and Weichselbaum R.R., pp. 2085-2096. Baltimore, MD, Williams & Wilkins.
Schally A.V. and Comaru-Schally A.M. (1997a). Hypothalamic and other peptide hormones. In Cancer Medicine, 4th edn, eds, Holland J.F., Frei E. III, Bast R.C. Jr, Kufe D.W., Morton D.L. and Weichselbaum R.R., pp. 1067-1086. Baltimore, MD, Williams & Wilkins.
Schally A.V. and Comaru-Schally A.M. (1997b). Rational use of agonists and antagonists of luteinizing hormone-releasing hormone (LHRH) in the treatment of hormone-sensitive neoplasms and gynecologic conditions. Adv Drug Deliv Rev, 28, 157-169.
Schally A.V. and Comaru-Schally A.M. (2000). Hypothalamic and other peptide hormones. In Cancer Medicine, 4th edn, eds, Holland J.F., Frei E. III, Bast R.C. Jr, Kufe D.W., Morton D.L. and Weichselbaum R.R., pp.715-729 Hamilton, Ontario, B.C. Dekker.
Schally A.V., Comaru-Schally A.M., Nagy A., Kovacs M., Szepeshazi K., Plonowski A., Varga J.L. and Halmos G. (2001). Hypothalamic Hormones and cancer. Front Neuroendocrinol, 22, 248-291.
Shapiro E. and Lepor H. (1995). Pathophysiology of clinical benign prostatic hyperplasia. Urol Clin North Am, 22, 285-290.
Sion-Vardi N., Kaneti J., Segal-Abramson T., Giat J., Levy J. and Sharoni Y. (1992). Gonadotropin-releasing hormone specific binding sites in normal and malignant renal tissue. J Urol, 148, 1568-1570.
Sokoloff M.H., deKernion J.B., Figlin R.A. and Belldegrun A. (1996). Current management of renal cell carcinoma. CA Cancer J Clin, 46, 284-302.
Steiner M.S. (1995). Review of peptide growth factors in benign prostatic hyperplasia and urological malignancy. J Urol, 153, 1085-1096.
Wise G.J. and Ostad E. (2001). Hormonal treatment of patients with benign prostatic hyperplasia: pros and cons. Curr Urol Rep, 2, 285-291.

CHAPTER 3

Luteinizing Hormone-releasing Hormone Antagonists in Gynecology

J.B. ENGEL AND K. DIEDRICH

Mechanism of Action

The elucidation of the structure of LHRH in 1971 (Schally et al., 1971), a major breakthrough in endocrinology, was soon followed by the synthesis of LHRH superagonists (Karten and Rivier, 1986), which were more stable to cleavage and showed greater affinity to the LHRH receptor, mainly through amino acid substitutions at positions 6 and 10 of the native LHRH (Koch et al., 1977). These analogs were originally synthesized to mimic the action of LHRH but it was soon discovered that the compounds, after a flare-up of FSH and LH, led to pharmacological hypophysectomy via LHRH receptor depletion of the pituitary (Emons and Schally, 1994).

Thus, LHRH agonists such as Decapeptyl (triptorelin), Lupron (leuprolide), Zoladex (goserelin) and Suprefact (buserelin) have been commercially available since the 1980s. They are clinically applied when ablation of sex steroids is desired.

Early on, some of the synthetic LHRH analogs were found to exert competitive antagonistic activity at the receptor and they are now considered as a separate class of compounds, referred to as "LHRH antagonists". As the first- and second-generation LHRH antagonists led to histamine liberation via mast cell degranulation (Morgan et al., 1986) and represented certain pharmaceutical problems due to their hydrophobicity, their development lagged some ten years behind the agonists.

Further amino acid substitutions, notably with amino acids in the unnatural D-configuration, finally led to the third-generation antagonists, devoid of major histamine liberating potential (Bajusz et al., 1988).

Recently two third-generation antagonists (cetrorelix, Cetrotide, Serono Int., Geneva, Switzerland; ganirelix, Orgalutran/Antagon, Organon, Oss, The Netherlands) became available on the market. Unlike the agonists, which after a flare-up of the gonadotrophins only achieve a hypogonadotrophic state within several weeks, LHRH antagonists lead to an immediate suppression of FSH and LH after the first application (Leroy et al., 1994). Recently, Schally et al. demonstrated that high doses of cetrorelix led to pituitary LHRH-receptor depletion and decrease in the m-RNA level for LHRH receptors (Pinski et al., 1996; Kovacs et al., 2001).

In gynecology a hypogonadotrophic state is desired in several conditions: in hormone dependent diseases such as endometriosis or uterine fibroma, in controlled ovarian hyperstimulation for assisted reproduction and in hormone-dependent malignant tumors, such as breast cancer. As a certain percentage of human breast and ovarian cancer cells are known to carry receptors for LHRH, direct antitumor effects have also been postulated for LHRH antagonists such as cetrorelix (Emons and Schally, 1994).

LHRH Antagonists in Assisted Reproduction

LHRH agonists were introduced in to the field of reproductive medicine (in vitro fertilization; IVF) about 20 years ago. They have been demonstrated to be safe and effective in preventing a premature LH surge, which leads to premature luteinization of the follicles, thus diminishing oocyte quality, fertilization and pregnancy rate in IVF. The stimulation protocol mostly used worldwide is the so-called long protocol. The LHRH agonist is applied in the luteal phase of the cycle; ovarian stimulation is initiated when pituitary desensitation is achieved.

LHRH antagonists, due to their dose-dependent competitive receptor blockade, allow the application of simpler and shorter stimulation protocols. LHRH antagonists can be administered in the course of ovarian stimulation, thus avoiding hormonal withdrawal symptoms associated with the use of the agonists. Two stimulation protocols using antagonists have been established so far, a single- and a multiple-dose protocol.

In the single-dose protocol (only introduced with cetrorelix), 3 mg of the compound is administered on stimulation day 8; when ovulation is not triggered within 96 h 0.25 mg cetrorelix are injected daily until ovulation is induced (Frydman et al., 1991; Olivennes et al., 1995). In the multiple-dose protocol (established first with cetrorelix and later with ganirelix), 0.25 mg are injected daily from stimulation day 6 up to the day of ovulation induction (Diedrich et al., 1994). Both antagonist protocols have been demonstrated to be safe and effective, preventing the premature LH surge in several phase II and III studies (Olivennes et al., 1998, 2000; Albano et al., 2000; Felberbaum et al., 2000; Hamm et al., 2001).

They seem to be equivalent in terms of pregnancy rate. So far no large prospective randomized study has been performed comparing the two regimens. The single-dose protocol seems to be more convenient for the patient.

Compared with the long agonist protocol, antagonist protocols offer numerous advantages, such as shorter duration of treatment, no ovarian cyst formation due to the flare-up effect, no hormonal withdrawal symptoms, lower cumulative doses of gonadotrophins needed for ovarian stimulation, lower rate of hyperstimulation syndrome (Ludwig et al., 2000), and ovulation can be induced with native LHRH or LHRH agonist. However, in all five agonist controlled phase III studies performed with both antagonists the pregnancy rate was slightly, but never significantly, lower in the antagonist arm.

- A cetrorelix single-dose study (Olivennes et al., 2000) was performed, triptorelin-controlled, in 148 patients and reports a clinical pregnancy rate per attempt of 22.6% (cetrorelix) vs. 28.2% (triptorelin). The rate of ovarian hyperstimulation syndrome (OHSS) was 1.7% vs 5.6%.
- A cetrorelix multiple-dose study was buserelin-controlled and performed in 273 patients. The clinical pregnancy rate per attempt was 22.3% for

cetrorelix and 25.9% for buserelin. The rate of OHSS was 1.1% vs. 6.5% (Albano et al., 2000).

- The European ganirelix multiple-dose study included 672 patients, was buserelin-controlled and yielded pregnancy rates of 21.8% (ganirelix) vs. 28.2% (buserelin) (The European Orgalutran Study Group, 2000). The rate of OHSS was 1.0 vs. 2.9.
- The North American ganirelix multiple-dose study (n = 313) was leuprolide-controlled and resulted in pregnancy rates of 35.4% for ganirelix vs. 38.4% for leuprolide (The North American Ganirelix Study Group, 2001). The rate of OHSS was 6.0 vs. 2.0 in favour of leuprolide.
- The European and Middle East ganirelix multiple-dose study included 337 patients and used triptorelin as an LHRH agonist for the control group. Pregnancy rates were 35.8% (ganirelix) vs. 41.7% (triptorelin). The rate of OHSS was 1.8 vs. 0.9 in favour of the agonist (The European and Middle East Orgalutran Study Group, 2001).

So far, three meta-analyses comparing the clinical outcome of the long with the antagonist protocols have been performed. Ludwig et al. (2001) analysed the data for both antagonists separately and found a statistically significantly lower pregnancy rate in the patient group treated with ganirelix, while in the cetrorelix group no such difference was observed. The same analysis also detected a significant reduction of OHSS compared to the long protocol only after treatment with cetrorelix.

The second meta-analysis did not compare the clinical outcome for each antagonist separately in spite of potential differences in the two compounds (Al-Inani and Aboulghar, 2002). This study observed a significant difference between the pregnancy rate in favour of the long agonist protocol and no significant difference between the rate of OHSS.

The third meta-analysis using an intention to treat approach suggests similar pregnancy rates for antagonist and agonist IVF cycles (Daya, 2003).

It was stated that body weight adjustment of the ganirelix dose led to a better pregnancy rate (de Greef et al., 2001). A recent analysis of cetrorelix-controlled IVF cycles of 1881 patients did not observe body-weight dependency of the pregnancy rate (Engel et al., 2003a). These differences in clinical outcome between the two antagonists could be explained by their different pharmacokinetic parameters (Duijker et al., 1998; Oberyé et al., 1999a, 1999b; Erb et al., 2001).

Thus, in spite of the same mechanism of action, the two LHRH antagonists could be to some extent different and their clinical data should be analysed separately in order to avoid misleading conclusions.

The trend towards a lower pregnancy rate obtained in antagonist cycles should not lead to drawing hasty conclusions, as there is a learning curve inherent to the use of any new treatment scheme.

Large comparative studies would be required to answer this still open question, but a comparative study designed to assess a 5% difference for pregnancy rate in the region of 20% would require over 1200 patients in each treatment group (Olivennes et al., 2002).

As in antagonist-controlled IVF, there is still a functional pituitary-ovary axis in the beginning of the cycle, and innovative stimulation protocols could be established using clomiphene pretreatment before gonadotrophin stimulation and antagonist application. This should permit less aggressive stimulation protocols, using a smaller amount of gonadotrophin. So far the results are preliminary. Using a multiple-dose application of the antagonist, in spite of an acceptable pregnancy rate, the increased incidence of premature LH surges remains a major drawback (Engel et al., 2002). Clomiphene upregulates the GnRH receptors at pituitary level (Schally et al., 1970; Engel et al., 2002). Thus, the use of higher antagonist doses seems the more logical approach. A pilot study performed in 10 patients with clomiphene pretreatment, subsequent gonadotrophin stimulation and single-dose application of 3 mg cetrorelix yielded a pregnancy rate of 30%, with no premature LH surge (Engel et al., 2003b). In both studies the amount of gonadotrophins could be reduced but not yet be lowered to the desired extent. More studies with protocol adjustments are required for optimizing this promising approach.

The definition of "poor responder" is heterogeneous and has caused an important bias in published studies. The rationale for utilizing antagonist protocols in poor responders is that LHRH antagonists do not suppress endogenous gonadotrophin secretion in the beginning of ovarian stimulation.

A trial in 42 patients compared the cetrorelix multiple-dose schedule (partly with clomiphene pretreatment) with the long protocol. A trend regarding pregnancy rate in favour of the antagonist protocol was observed (14.3% vs. 9.5%), although the difference was not statistically significant (Nikolettos et al., 2000). Another study (n = 48) comparing multiple-dose antagonist to agonist short protocol showed similar pregnancy rates, with a trend in favour of the agonist (21.1 vs. 16.6) (Akman et al., 2001). Larger randomized trials are needed to clarify the situation.

LHRH Antagonists for Treatment of Uterine Fibroids

Uterine fibroids represent the most common solid pelvic tumors and are associated with abnormal uterine bleeding and infertility. They occur in 25-30% of women during the reproductive years and often require hysterectomy (Buttram and Reiter, 1981; Cramer et al., 1985). Myomas are estrogen-dependent and rarely arise before puberty. Their progression stops after menopause. LHRH agonists lead to shrinkage of the fibroids by reversible induction of menopause (Filicori et al., 1983; Schally, 1989; Ayala et al., 1995). As regrowth of myomas occurs rapidly after the cessation of therapy (Lumsden et al., 1987), these compounds are mostly used to faciliate surgery by shrinkage of the fibroids if a uterus-conserving operation or vaginal hysterectomy is desired. However, a relevant reduction of uterine volume is only achieved after at least 8 or more weeks of treatment (Healy et al., 1984; Letterie et al., 1989). A 3-6 month treatment with LHRH-agonists prior to surgery is a well-established therapy. LHRH antagonists act more rapidly than the agonists, without producing an initial flare-up of the gonadotrophins and thus seem a more promising therapeutic approach.

Shrinkage rates of over 50% within the first 4 weeks were obtained with the daily subcutaneous application of the LHRH antagonist Nal-Glu (Kettel et al., 1993). The fast reduction in size was attributed to the avoidance of any flare-up.

Four clinical trials have been carried out so far using cetrorelix. The first investigation was an open and non-controlled study (Gonzalez-Barcena et al., 1997). The dosing scheme of cetrorelix was 5 mg b.i.d. for the first 2 days, followed by daily injection of 0.8 mg of the antagonist for at least 3 months. The mean treatment duration was 4.4 months. Uterine volume was determined by ultrasonography. In total, 16 out of 18 patients showed a regression in uterine size. The mean volume in the whole group ($n = 18$) decreased from a value of 395.4 ± 69.2 to 238.5 ± 47.1 after 3 months of treatment ($p < 0.001$). After treatment, 12 patients underwent surgical myomectomy and after follow-up for 25 months only one patient showed regrowth of fibroma. One of the patients who had a myomectomy subsequently became pregnant. In three patients who responded well to treatment, no surgery was performed. The first patient became pregnant within 2 months, the second had a stable uterine volume for the period of follow-up (25 months) and the third showed regrowth after 21 months. In three patients, total hysterectomy was necessary. In the other 15 patients, normal menstrual function started 1 month after the end of treatment.

In the second open and randomized study (Felberbaum et al., 1998), cetrorelix was administered by intramuscular injection of an "early" pamoate depot formulation. On day 2 of the menstrual cycle, a total of 20 patients with symptomatic uterine fibroids were treated with 60 mg cetrorelix pamoate. The patients were randomized for receiving a second dose of either 60 or 30 mg cetrorelix pamoate. The second dose was to be administered on day 21 after the first, if the estradiol serum concentration surpassed 50 pg/ml. If the estradiol serum concentration was below this threshold, the second dose was to be injected on day 28. Surgery was performed after 6-8 weeks, depending on the second cetrorelix administration. Uterus and fibroid volume were assessed by transvaginal ultrasound and magnetic resonance imaging (MRI). Four patients were withdrawn from the study because of insufficient estradiol suppression 14 days after the first dose. In the 16 remaining patients, a mean fibroid shrinkage of 33.5% was observed at the end of treatment; 31.3% of fibroid shrinkage had already occurred 14 days after the first injection. No statistical significant difference in size reduction could be observed between the low-dose and high-dose groups.

In a Japanese open, randomized multicenter dose-finding study (Yano et al., 2001), a total of 48 patients were treated with weekly s.c. doses of 1, 3 or 5 mg cetrorelix acetate for 8 weeks. Myoma volumes were reduced to 50%, 63% or 74% of the pretreatment size at 5, 3 and 1 mg respectively. Thus it was concluded that the weekly administration of 3 or 5 mg cetrorelix could be an effective therapeutic approach for uterine fibroids.

Another group (Felberbaum et al., 2001) suggested a short-term treatment with four injections of 3 mg cetrorelix acetate every 4 days, starting on the first day of the menstrual cycle. In six out of 10 premenopausal women, mean reduction of fibroid size (determined by MRI) of 31% after only 16 days of treatment could be obtained. In nine patients laparoscopic myomectomy was performed, while in one patient laparotomy was necessary.

These data show that GnRH antagonists are a fast, safe and effective therapy for uterine fibroids. However, for optimizing the dosing schedule, larger prospective randomized studies are required.

LHRH Antagonists for the Treatment of Endometriosis

Endometriosis is one of the most commom benign diseases in gynecology and is associated with dysmenorrhea and infertility. While surgery still remains the treatment of choice for endometriosis, LHRH analogues are known to alleviate pelvic pain and to decrease the size of endometrial implants (Adamson and Pasta, 1994; Hughes et al., 1993). Thus, these compounds are most frequently used for down-staging and reduction of the activity of the disease prior to surgery.

However, the development of medical treatment schedules is important as reinduction therapy in cases of repeated occurrence or as a long-term strategy to avoid multiple surgical interventions. The threshold theory of Barbieri (1992) postulates that growth of endometriotic lesions requires an estradiol concentration of > 40 pg/ml over a longer period of time. In accordance with this theory, long-term agonist treatment with low-dose estradiol add-back has been proposed, to reduce the risk of bone loss and avoid vasomotor symptoms. Most of the studies, using different steroidal and non-steroidal agents combined with LHRH agonist treatment, could demonstrate no decrease of effectivity by the addition of hormonal replacement therapy (Leather et al., 1993; Edmonds, 1996; Franke et al., 2000).

As LHRH antagonists act via a dose-dependent receptor blockade, a fine-tuning of the suppression of estradiol should be possible with these compounds and it can be speculated that hormonal replacement could be avoided.

So far, only one trial in 15 patients with histologically confirmed endometriosis has been carried out, with 3 mg cetrorelix injected once a week over a peroid of 8 weeks (Küpker et al., 2002). Before and after treatment a laparoscopy was performed to evaluate the number and size of endometriotic lesions. All patients were free of symptoms of endometriosis. Occasional bleeding in the later stages of treatment occurred in three patients. Mood changes, vaginal dryness, hot flushes, loss of libido or other estrogen withdrawal symptoms were not observed. Serum estradiol levels were about 50 pg/ml throughout the treatment. Morphological improvement of the endometriotic lesions occurred in 70% of the patients, confirmed by second-look laparoscopy.

Larger studies are required to elucidate whether long-term or intermittent treatment with LHRH antagonists is a promising therapeutic approach.

LHRH Antagonists for the Treatment of Gynecological Cancers

There is ample experimental evidence for the efficacy of cetrorelix in endometrial, ovarian and breast cancer via endocrine and paracrine mechanisms of action (reviewed by Schally, 1999). So far, only one clinical study with cetrorelix has been performed in 17 patients with chemotherapy-resistant ovarian cancer. Three patients showed partial remission and four showed stabilization of the disease (Emons et al., 1999).

Conclusions

As the reviewed data demonstrate, LHRH antagonists are already well established in the field of assisted reproduction. They will contribute to facilitation of stimulation protocols for both patients' and physicians' convenience and lower the rate of side effects, notably of OHSS, the most hazardous condition in assisted reproduction. Furthermore, they will lead to lowering the consumption of gonadotropins used for stimulation. For cetrorelix, so far no prospective randomized study has shown significantly lower pregnancy rates associated with either the single- or the multiple-dose antagonist protocol compared to the standard treatment, the long agonist protocol. Taking into account the learning curve present with every new treatment, pregnancy rates may increase in the future.

In uterine leiomyoma and endometriosis, clinical experience is limited but remains promising. In uterine fibroma it has been demonstrated that, using LHRH antagonists, fibroid shrinkage can be obtained after only 2-4 weeks of treatment, thus facilitating preoperative management.

In endometriosis, LHRH antagonists have been shown to be efficacious with respect to endometriotic pain without any symptoms of hypoestrogenism; however, the patient sample was small and the treatment period was only 8 weeks.

In gynecological cancer, clinical evidence is limited to the treatment of chemotherapy-resistant ovarian carcinoma, where satisfying results were obtained in a small patient sample.

References

Adamson G.D. and Pasta D.J. (1994). Surgical treatment of endometriosis-associated infertility: a meta-analysis compared with survival analysis. Am J Obstet Gynecol, 171, 1488-1505.

Akman M.A., Erden H.F., Tosun S.B. et al. (2001). Comparison of agonistic flare-up-protocol and antagonistic multiple dose protocol in ovarian stimulation of poor responders: results of a prospective randomized trial. Hum Reprod, 16, 868-870.

Al-Inany H. and Aboulghar M. (2002). GnRH antagonist in assisted reproduction: a Cochrane review. Hum Reprod, 17, 874-885.

Albano C., Felberbaum R.E., Smitz J. et al. (2000). Ovarian stimulation with HMG: results of a prospective randomised phase III European study comparing the luteinizing-releasing hormone (LHRH)-antagonist cetrorelix and the LHRH-agonist buserelin. Hum Reprod, 15, 526-531.

Ayala R.A., Meza E., Cervera A.R. et al. (1995). Effect of insulfated nafarelin (D-Nal-GnRH) upon uterine leiomyomata. Arch Med Res, 26, 523-526.

Barbieri R.L. (1992). Hormonal therapy of endometriosis: the estrogen threshold hypothesis. Am J Obstet Gynecol, 166, 740-745.

Bajusz S., Kovacs M., Gazdag M., Bokser L., Karashima T., Csernus V.J., Janaky T., Guoth J. and Schally A.V. (1988). Highly potent antagonists of luteinizing hormone-releasing hormone free of edematogenic effects. Proc Natl Acad Sci, USA, 85, 1637-1641.

Buttram V.C. Jr and Reiter R.C. (1981). Uterine leiomyomata: etiology, symptomatology and management. Fertil Steril, 36, 433-435.

Cramer S.F., Robertson A.L. Jr, Ziats N.P. et al. (1985). Growth potential of humane uterine leiomyomas: some in vitro observations and their implications. Obstet Gynecol, 66, 36-41.

Daya S. (2003). A comparison of clinical pregnancy rates in the efficacy evaluation of GnRH agonist verus antagonist use for assisted reproduction – a meta-analysis using an intention-to-treat approach. 7th International Symposium on GnRH analogues in Cancer and Human Reproduction, Abstract 086, 44.

De Greef H., Mannaerts B. and Orleman E. (2001). Gonadotropin releasing hormone antagonist. Patent application WO 01/00227.

Diedrich K., Diedrich C., Santos E. et al. (1994). Suppression of the endogenous LH surge by the GnRH antagonist cetrorelix during ovarian stimulation. Hum Reprod, 9, 788-791.

Duijker I.-J., Klipping C., Willremsen W.-N. et al. (1998). Single- and multiple-dose pharmacokinetics and pharmacodynamics of the gonadotrophin-releasing hormone antagonist cetrorelix in healthy female volunteers. Hum Reprod, 23, 92-98.

Edmonds D.K. (1996). Add-back therapy in the treatment of endometriosis: the European experience. Br J Obstet Gynecol, 103 (suppl 14), 10-14.

Emons G., Westphalen S., Schulz K.-D. et al. (1999). First results of the GnRH antagonist cetrorelix in patients with ovarian cancer. Gynecol Endocrinol, 13, 064.

Emons G., Schally A.V. (1994). The use of luteinizing hormone-releasing hormone agonists and antagonists in gynecological cancers. Hum Reprod, 9, 1364-1379.

Engel J.B. (2002). Clomiphene-induced LH surges and cetrorelix. RBM Online, 5, 109-111.

Engel J.B., Ludwig M., Felberbaum R. et al. (2002). Use of cetrorelix in combination with clomiphene citrate and gonadotrophins: a suitable approach to 'friendly IVF'? Hum Reprod, 17, 2022-2026.

Engel J.B., Ludwig M., Junge K. et al. (2003a). No influence of body weight on the pregnancy rate in patients treated with cetrorelix according to the single and multiple-dose protocol. Reprod BioMed Online, 6.

Engel J.B., Olivennes F., Fanchin R. et al. (2003b). Single dose application of cetrorelix in combination with clomiphene for friendly IVF: results of a feasibility study. Reprod BioMed Online, 6, 444-447.

Erb K., Klipping C., Duijker I.-J. et al. (2001). Pharmakodynamic effects and plasma pharmacokinetics of single doses of cetrorelix acetate in healthy premenopausal women. Fertil Steril, 75, 316-323.

Felberbaum R.E., Germer U., Ludwig M. et al. (1998). Treatment of uterine fibroids with a slow-release formulation of the gonadotrophin releasing hormone antagonist cetrorelix. Hum Reprod, 13, 1660-1668.

Felberbaum R.E., Albano C., Ludwig M. et al. (2000). Ovarian stimulation for assisted reproduction with HMG and concomitant midcycle administration of GnRH-antagonist cetrorelix according to the multiple dose protocol: a prospective uncontrolled phase III study. Hum Reprod, 15, 1015-1020.

Felberbaum R.E., Kuepker W., Krapp M. et al. (2001). Preoperative reduction of uterine fibroids in only 16 days by administration of a gonadotrophin-releasing hormone antagonist (Cetrotide). Reprod BioMed Online, 3, 14-18.

Filicori M., Hall D.A., Loughlin J.S. et al. (1983). A conservative approach to the management of uterine leimyoma: pituitary desensitization by a luteinizing hormone-releasing hormone analogue. Am J Obstet Gynecol, 7, 726-727.

Franke H.R., van der Weijer P.H.M., Pennings T.M.M. et al. (2000). Gonadotropin-releasing hormone agonist plus "add-back" hormone replacement therapy for treatment of endometriosis: a prospective, randomized, placebo-controlled, double-blind trial. Fertil Steril, 74, 534-539.

Frydman R., Cornel C., de Ziegler D. et al. (1991). Prevention of premature luteinizing hormone and progesterone rise with a GnRH antagonist Nal-Glu in controlled ovarian hyperstimulation. Fertil Steril. 56, 923-927.

Gonzalez-Barcena D., Banuelos Alvarez R., Pere Ochoa E. et al. (1997). Treatment of uterine leiomyomas with luteinizing hormone-releasing hormone antagonist cetrorelix. Hum Reprod, 9, 2028-2035.

Hamm W.J. (2001). Broad experience with Cetrotide® (cetrorelix)-Results of a large multinational phase IIIB study. VIth International Symposium on GnRH Analogs in Cancer and Human Reproduction, Geneva, 2001.

Healy D.L., Fraser H.M. and Lawson S.L. (1984). Shrinkage of a uterine fibroid after a subcutaneous infusion of LH-RH agonist. Br Med J, 289, 1267-1268.

Hughes E.G., Fedorkow D.M., Collins J.A. et al. (1993). A quantitative overview of controlled trials in endometriosis associated infertility. Fertil Steril, 59, 963-970.

Karten M.J. and Rivier J.E. (1986). Gonoadotropin-releasing hormone analog design. Structure-function studies toward the development of agonists and antagonists: rationale and perspective. Endocr Rev, 7, 44-66.

Kettel L.M., Murphy A.A., Morales A.J. et al. (1993). Rapid regression of uterine leiomyomas in response to daily administration of gonadotrophin-releasing hormone antagonist. Fertil Steril, 60, 642-646.

Koch Y., Baram T., Hazum E. et al. (1977). Resistance to enzymatic degradation of LHRH analogs possessing increased biological activity. Biochem Biophys Res Commun, 74, 488-492.

Kovacs M., Schally A.V., Csernus B. et al. (2001). Luteinizing hormone-releasinig hormone (LHRH) antagonist cetrorelix down regulates the mRNA expression of pituitary receptors for LHRH by counteracting the stimulatory effect of endogenous LHRH. Proc Natl Acad Sci, 98, 1829-1834.

Küpker W., Felberbaum R.E., Krapp M. et al. (2002). Use of GnRH antagonists in the treatment of endometriosis. Reprod BioMed Online, 5, 12-16.

Leroy I., Dacrémont M.F., Brailly-Trabard S. et al. (1994). A single injection of a gonadotrophin-releasing hormone antagonist (cetrorelix) postpones the luteinizing hormone (LH) surge: further evidence for the role of GnRH during the LH surge. Fertil Steril, 62, 461-467.

Leather A.T., Studd J.W.W., Watso N.R. et al. (1993). The prevention of bone loss in young women treated with GnRH analogues with "add-back" estrogen therapy. Obstet Gynecol, 81, 104-107.

Letterie G.S., Coddington C.C. and Winkel C.A. (1989). Efficacy of a gonadotropin-releasing hormone agonist in the treatment of uterine leiomyomata: a long-term follow-up. Fertil Steril, 51, 951-956.

Ludwig M., Felberbaum R.E., Devroey P. et al. (2000). Significant reduction of the incidence of ovarian hyperstimulation syndrome (OHSS) by using the LHRH antagonist cetrorelix (Cetrotide) in controlled ovarian stimulation for assisted reproduction. Arch Gynecol Obstet, 264, 29-32.

Ludwig M., Katalinic A. and Diedrich K, (2001). Use of GnRH antagonists in ovarian stimulation for ART compared to the long protocol: a meta-analysis. Arch Gynecol Obstet, 265, 175-182.

Lumsden M.A., West C.P. and Baird D.T. (1987). Goserelin therapy before surgery for uterine fibroids. Lancet, I, 36-37.

Morgan J.E., O'Neill C.E., Coy D.H. et al. (1986). Antagonist analogs of luteinizing hormone-releasing hormone are mast cell secretagogues. Int Arch Allergy Appl Immun, 80, 70-75.

Nikolettos N., Al-Hasani S., Felberbaum R. et al. (2000). Gonadotrophin-releasing hormone antagonist protocol: a novel method of ovarian stimulation in poor responders. Eur J Obstet Gynecol Rerod Biol, 97, 202-207.

Oberyé J.J.J., Mannaerts B.M.J.L., Kleijn H.J. et al. (1999a). Pharmacokinetic and pharmacodynamic characteristics of ganirelix (Orgalutran). Part I. Absolute bioavailability of 0.25 mg ganirelix after single subcutaneous injection in healthy female volunteers. Fertil Steril, 72, 1001-1005.

Oberyé J.J.L., Mannaerts B.M.J.L., Huisman C.J. et al. (1999b). Pharmacokinetic and pharmacodynamic characteristics of ganirelix (Antagon/Orgalutran). Part II. Dose-proportionality and gonadotropin suppression after multiple doses of ganirelix in healthy female volunteers. Fertil Steril, 72, 1006-1012.

Olivennes F., Fanchin R., Bouchard P. et al. (1995). Scheduled administration of GnRH antagonist (cetrorelix) on day 8 of in vitro fertilization cycles: a pilot study. Hum Reprod, 10, 1382-1386.
Olivennes F., Alvarez S., Bouchard P., Fanchin R., Salat-Baroux J. and Frydman R. (1998). The use of a GnRH-antagonist (cetrorelix) in a single-dose protocol in IVF-embryo transfer: a dose-finding study of 3 vs. 2 mg. Hum Reprod, 13, 2411-2414.
Olivennes F., Belaisch-Allart J., Emperaire J.C. et al. (2000). Prospective, randomised, controlled study of in vitro fertilization embryo transfer with a single dose of luteinizing hormone-releasing hormone (LHRH)-antagonist (cetrorelix) or a depot formula of a LHRH agonist (triptorelin). Fertil Steril, 73, 314-320.
Olivennes F., Cunha-Filho J.S., Fanchin R. et al. (2002). The use of GnRH antagonist in human reproduction. Hum Reprod Update, 8, 279-290.
Pinski J., Lamharzi M., Halmos G. et al. (1996). Chronic administration of luteinizing hormone-releasing hormone (LHRH) antagonist cetrorelix decreases gonadotrope responsiveness and pituitary LHRH receptor messenger ribonucleic acid levels in rats. Endocrinology, 137, 3430-3436.
Schally A.V., Arimura A., Baba Y. et al. (1971). Isolation and properties of the FSH and LH-releasing hormone. Biophys Res Commun, 43, 393-399.
Schally A.V., Carter W.H., Parlow A.F. et al. (1970). Alteration of LH- and FSH-release in rats treated with clomiphene or its isomers. Am J Obstet Gynecol 107, 1156-1167.
Schally A.V. (1989). The use of LH-RH analogs in gynecology and tumor therapy. In Advances in Gynecology and Obstetrics: eds Belfort P., Pinotti J.A., Eskes T.K.A.B.. General Gynecology, Vol 6, pp 3-20, Carnforth, Parthenon.
Schally A.V. (1999). LHRH analogues: their impact on the control of tumorigenesis. Peptides, 20, 1247-1262.
The European and Middle East Orgalutran Study Group (2001). Comparable clinical outcome using the GnRH antagonist ganirelix or a long protocol of the GnRH agonist triptorelin for the prevention of premature LH surges. Hum Reprod, 16, 644-651.
The European Orgalutran Study Group (2000). Treatment with the gonadotrophin releasing hormone antagonist ganirelix in women undergoing ovarian stimulation with recombinant follicle stimulating hormone is effective, safe and convenient: results of a controlled, randomized multicentre trial. Hum Reprod, 15, 1490-1498.
The North American Ganirelix Study Group (2001). Efficacy and safety of ganirelix acetate vs. leuprolide acetate in women undergoing controlled ovarian hyperstimulation. Fertil Steril, 75, 38-45.
Yano T., Minaguchi H., Taketani Y. et al. (2001). Cetrorelix in the treatment of uterine leiomyomas. VIth International Symposium on GnRH Analogues in Cancer and Human Reproduction. Geneva, 2001.

CHAPTER 4

Physiology and Pharmacology of Somatostatin and Its Receptors

J. EPELBAUM

Somatostatin is an "old" neuropeptide, discovered 30 years ago as a hypothalamic neurohormone for its ability to inhibit growth hormone secretion (Brazeau et al., 1972). Later, it was found to be widely distributed in other brain regions, in which it fulfills a neuromodulatory role. It is also located in several organs of the gastrointestinal tract, where it can act as a paracrine factor or as a true circulating factor (Fig. 1).

In mammals, two molecules of 14 (somatostatin 14) and 28 (somatostatin 28) amino acids are the only biologically active peptides alternatively cleaved in different tissues from the C-terminal portion of a single prohormone. The somatostatins are strongly conserved over evolution. However, in fishes and lower vertebrates, a second gene encodes for less conserved peptides related

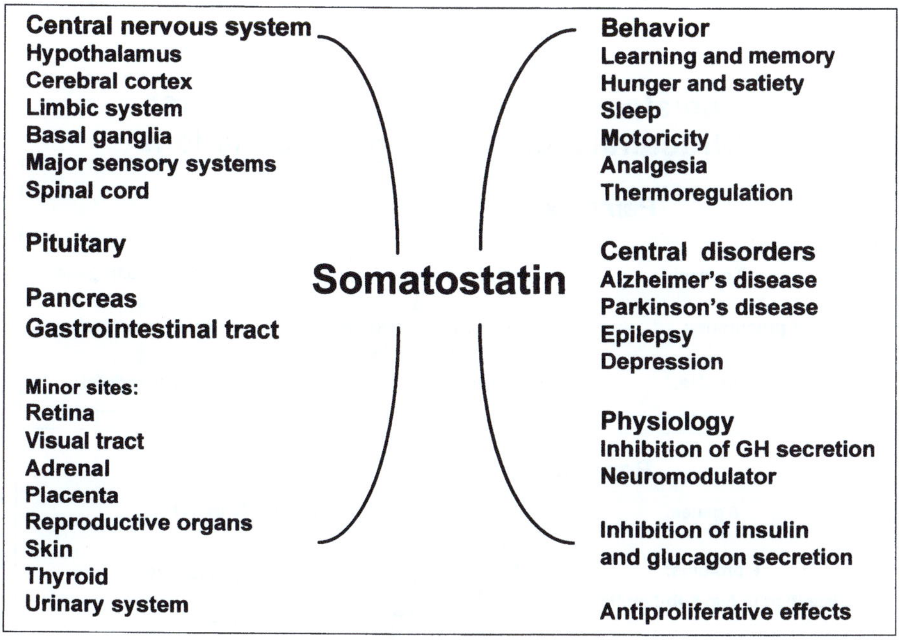

Fig. 1. Summary of the ubiquitous localization of somatostatin, its functional diversity, and the clinical implications. Somatostatin may be considered as a good example of the family of brain-gut peptides, being widely distributed both in many parts of the nervous system as well as the gastrointestinal tract

to somatostatins, and it is mostly expressed in gut tissues. Very recently, a second mammalian gene has also been found but, in contrast to the case in fishes, the expression of the new peptide cortistatin seems to be restricted to brain cortex and hippocampus (de Lecea et al., 1996).

On the basis of earlier pharmacological characterizations, the various actions of somatostatin were thought to be mediated by two different receptor subtypes (for review, see Reisine and Bell, 1995). However, between January and December 1992, our understanding of the biological role of somatostatin was greatly modified by the cloning of five different somatostatin receptor (SST1-5) genes and a shorter splice variant of SST2A, SST2B (for review, see Reisine and Bell, 1995) (Fig. 2).

The SST receptors consist of single polypeptide chains of 345 to 428 amino acids in length and belong to the heptahelical receptors that are coupled to G-proteins. By sequence comparisons and by comparing their pharmacological properties, SST1 and 4 on the one hand and SST2A & B, 3 and 5 on the other are seen to form two receptor subfamilies (Hoyer et al., 1995). When individual receptors were expressed in mammalian cell lines, it was observed that SST1 and SST4 (members of the type 2 subfamily) were much less prone to agonist-induced internalization by the endosomal recycling pathway than were SST2, SST3, and SST5 receptors (members of the type 1 subfamily) (Csaba and Dournaud, 2001). Moreover, agonists used in clinical practice such as octreotide (Novartis) and lanreotide (Ipsen-Biomeasure) are relatively selective ligands for subtypes 2 and 5 (for review, see Hoyer et al., 1995). Nowadays, relatively selective agonists are also available for SST1 (Liapakis et

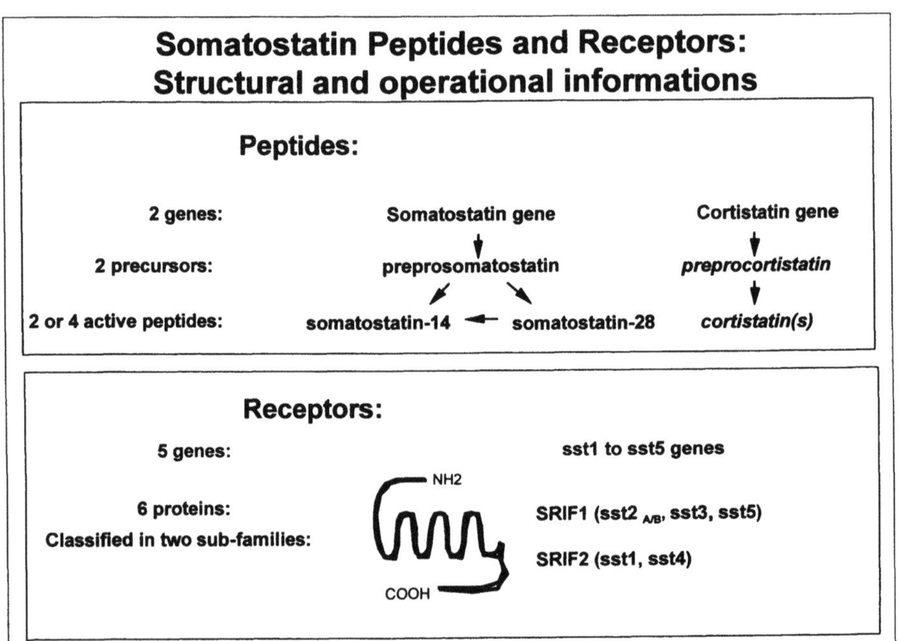

Fig. 2. Somatostatin peptides and receptors: structural and operational information

al., 1996; Rivier et al., 2001), SST2, SST3, and SST4 (Rohrer et al., 1998), and semiselective antagonists for SST2 (Bass et al., 1996, 1997; Hocart et al., 1999; Tulipano et al., 2002) and SST3 (Reubi et al., 2000). All SST subtypes can inhibit adenylate cyclase activity (Patel et al., 1994). Furthermore, SST subtypes are coupled to several protein phosphotyrosine phosphatase activities (Buscail et al., 1994; Florio et al., 2001) and to the inositol phosphate pathway (Akbar et al., 1994). The SST2 receptors can inhibit high-voltage-activated calcium channels (Fujii et al., 1994) and SST4 receptors induce arachidonate release and the activation of the mitogen-stimulated protein kinase cascade (Bito et al., 1994). Somatostatin receptors do not only interact with G-proteins but can physically bind, through their C-terminal domain, to a class of proteins displaying anchoring and scaffolding functions (Kreienkamp et al., 2002). Such proteins may be involved in the targeting of somatostatin receptors to the cell surface. However, whether the signal transduction pathways or binding proteins to which recombinant SST subtypes are coupled in vitro are relevant to the in vivo situation remains an open question. In any case these studies, though far from complete, have added unsuspected levels of complexity to the pharmacology of somatostatin and its receptors.

Anti-receptor-subtype antibodies have been used to define the localization of somatostatin receptors, mostly in the brain (for review, see Dournaud et al., 2000; Schulz et al., 2000) and neuroendocrine tumors (Kulaksiz et al., 2002). Immunohistochemistry with subtype-specific antibodies could be used in clinical routine work to analyse somatostatin receptor expression patterns for each patient before treatment in order to optimize individual therapy. In mammalian brain, SST2A is the most widely distributed receptor subtype, and its localization at the regional level corresponds closely to radioligand binding studies. In contrast, SST1 immunoreactivity appears restricted to the hypothalamus (Helboe et al., 1998) and SST4 immunoreactivity is prominent in the hippocampus CA1 (Schreff et al., 2000; Viollet et al., 2000). Surprisingly, SST3 immunoreactivity appears localized in a subcellular compartment corresponding to ciliae and not targeted to perisynaptic locations (Handel et al., 1999). When expressed in human embryonic kidney 293 cells (Pfeiffer et al., 2001), SST2A and SST3 subtypes exist as homodimers at the plasma membrane. Heterodimerization of SST2A and SST3 can result in a new receptor with a pharmacological and functional profile resembling that of the SST2A receptor, but with a greater resistance to agonist-induced desensitization. Thus, inactivation of SST3 receptor by heterodimerization with SST2A or possibly other G-protein-coupled receptors such as μ-opioid receptors (Pfeiffer et al., 2002) may explain some of the difficulties in detecting SST3-specific binding and signaling in mammalian tissues. In similar experiments, SST5 receptors appear also able to dimerize with SST1 (Rocheville et al., 2000a) and dopaminergic D2 receptors (Rocheville et al., 2000b). However, in mammals, SST5 expression is very low in most tissues, with the noticeable exception of the pituitary and pancreatic islets, where it mediates some of the inhibitory functions of somatostatin on hormonal secretions (Strowski et al., 2000, 2002).

According to a thorough literature survey (Myers, 1994) somatostatin was one of the few neuropeptides which had not yet attained a steady state of publication 21 years after its discovery (Fig. 3). This was certainly due to the fact

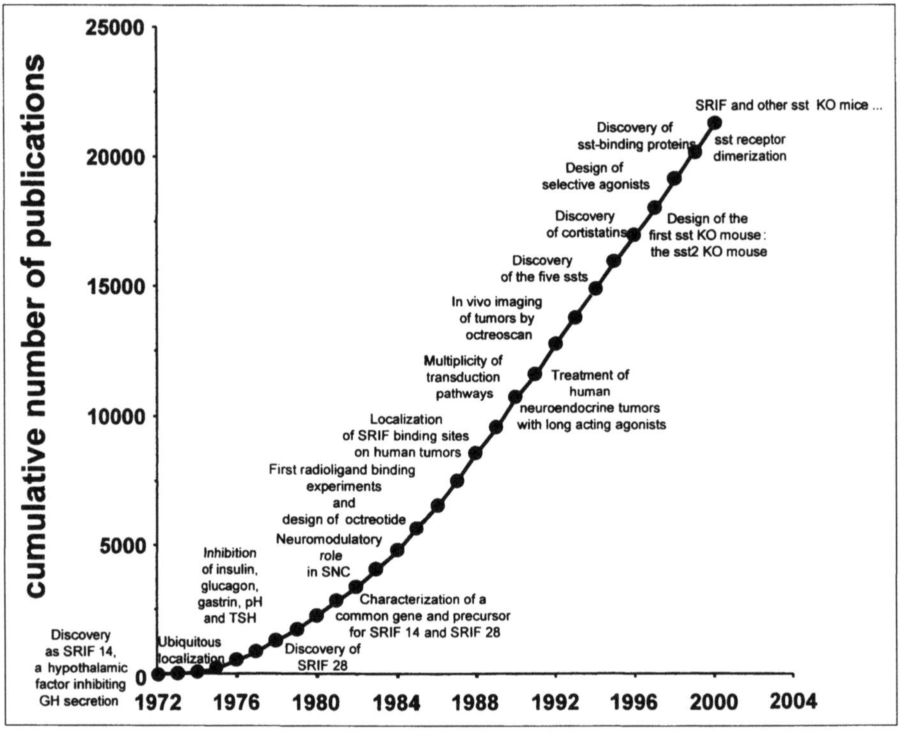

Fig. 3. Cumulative number of publications on somatostatin as a function of time

that somatostatin had acquired a therapeutic value. Long-acting agonists are currently used in the treatment of acromegaly and the management of gastrointestinal tract tumors. Moreover, radioactively labeled somatostatin agonists are helpful in the visualization of many tumors and their metastases (de Herder and Lamberts, 2002; Hofland and Lamberts, 2003).

Genetically engineered knockout (KO) mice for preprosomatostatin (Low et al., 2001; Zeyda et al., 2001), SST1- (Kreienkamp et al., 1999), and SST2-receptor genes (Zheng et al., 1997) are now available, and SST3-5 KO mice are well under way (Strowski et al., 2003). Though all these mice display minor endocrine or behavioral phenotypes, they can now be used to approach the specific biological functions of somatostatin and its five individual receptors during brain development and adulthood and their clinical implications in neurology (epilepsy, neurodegenerative diseases) and oncology (neuroendocrine tumors, gliomas).

References

Akbar M., Okajima F., Tomura H., Majid M.A., Yamada Y., Seino S. and Kondo Y. (1994). Phospholipase C activation and Ca^{2+} mobilization by cloned human somatostatin receptor subtypes 1-5, in transfected COS-7 cells. FEBS Lett, 348, 192-196.

Bass R.T., Buckwalter B.L., Patel B.P., Pausch M.H., Price L.A., Strnadt J. and Hadcock J.R. (1996). Identification and characterization of novel somatostatin antagonists. Mol Pharmacol, 50, 709-715.
Bass R.T., Buckwalter B.L., Patel B.P., Pausch M.H., Price L.A., Strnadt J. and Hadcock J.R. (1997). Erratum. Mol Pharmacol, 51, 170.
Bito H., Mori M., Sakanaka C., Takano T., Honda Z., Gotoh Y., Nishida E. and Shimizu T. (1994). Functional coupling of SSTR4, a major hippocampal somatostatin receptor, to adenylate cyclase inhibition, arachidonate release and activation of the mitogen-activated protein kinase cascade. J Biol Chem, 269, 12722-12730.
Brazeau P., Vale W., Burgus R., Ling N., Rivier J. and Guillemin R. (1972). Hypothalamic polypeptide that inhibits the secretion of immunoreactive pituitary growth hormone. Science, 129, 77-79.
Buscail L., Delesque N., Esteve J.P., Saint-Laurent N., Prats H., Clerc P., Robberecht P., Bell G.I., Liebow C., Schally A.V. et al. (1994). Stimulation of tyrosine phosphatase and inhibition of cell proliferation by somatostatin analogues: mediation by human somatostatin receptor subtypes SSTR1 and SSTR2. Proc Natl Acad Sci USA, 91, 2315-2319.
Csaba Z. and Dournaud P. (2001). Cellular biology of somatostatin receptors. Neuropeptides, 35, 1-23.
de Herder W.W. and Lamberts S.W. (2002). Somatostatin and somatostatin analogues: diagnostic and therapeutic uses. Curr Opin Oncol, 14, 53-57.
de Lecea L., Criado J.R., Prospero-Garcia O., Gautvik K.M., Schweitzer P., Danielson P.E., Dunlop C.L., Siggins G.R., Henriksen S.J. and Sutcliffe J.G. (1996). A cortical neuropeptide with neuronal depressant and sleep-modulating properties. Nature, 381, 242-245.
Dournaud P., Slama A., Beaudet A. and Epelbaum J. (2000). Somatostatin receptors. In Handbook of Chemical Neuroanatomy, vol 16, part I, eds. Bjorklund A., Hökfelt T. and Quirion R. Elsevier, Amsterdam, pp. 1-44.
Florio T., Arena S., Thellung S., Iuliano R., Corsaro A., Massa A., Pattarozzi A., Bajetto A., Trapasso F., Fusco A. and Schettini G. (2001). The activation of the phosphotyrosine phosphatase eta (r-PTP eta) is responsible for the somatostatin inhibition of PC Cl3 thyroid cell proliferation. Mol Endocrinol, 15, 1838-1852.
Fujii Y., Gonoi T., Yamada Y., Chihara K., Inagaki N. and Seino S. (1994). Somatostatin receptor subtype SSTR2 mediates the inhibition of high-voltage-activated calcium channels by somatostatin and its analogue SMS 201-995. FEBS Lett, 355, 117-120.
Handel M., Schulz S., Stanarius A., Schreff M., Erdtmann-Vourliotis M., Schmidt H., Wolf G. and Hollt V. (1999). Selective targeting of somatostatin receptor 3 to neuronal cilia. Neuroscience, 89, 909-926.
Helboe L., Stidsen C.E. and Moller M. (1998). Immunohistochemical and cytochemical localization of the somatostatin receptor subtype sst1 in the somatostatinergic parvocellular neuronal system of the rat hypothalamus. J Neurosci, 18, 4938-4945.
Hocart S.J., Jain R., Murphy W.A., Taylor J.E. and Coy D.H. (1999). Highly potent cyclic disulfide antagonists of somatostatin. J Med Chem, 42, 1863-1871.
Hofland L.J. and Lamberts S.W. (2003). The pathophysiological consequences of somatostatin receptor internalization and resistance. Endocr Rev, 24, 28-47.
Hoyer D., Bell G.I., Berelowitz M., Epelbaum J., Feniuk W., Humphrey P.P., O'Carroll A.M., Patel Y.C., Schonbrunn A., Taylor J.E. et al. (1995). Classification and nomenclature of somatostatin receptors. Trends Pharmacol Sci, 16, 86-88.
Kreienkamp H.J., Akgun E., Baumeister H., Meyerhof W. and Richter D. (1999). Somatostatin receptor subtype 1 modulates basal inhibition of growth hormone release in somatotrophs. FEBS Lett, 462, 464-466.
Kreienkamp H.J., Soltau M., Richter D. and Bockers T. (2002). Interaction of G-protein-coupled receptors with synaptic scaffolding proteins. Biochem Soc Trans, 30, 464-468.
Kulaksiz H., Eissele R., Rossler D., Schulz S., Hollt V., Cetin Y. and Arnold R. (2002). Identification of somatostatin receptor subtypes 1, 2A, 3, and 5 in neuroendocrine tumours with subtype specific antibodies. Gut, 50, 52-60.

Liapakis G., Hoeger C., Rivier J. and Reisine T. (1996). Development of a selective agonist at the somatostatin receptor subtype sstr1. J Pharmacol Exp Ther, 276, 1089-1094.
Low M.J., Otero-Corchon V., Parlow A.F., Ramirez J.L., Kumar U., Patel Y.C. and Rubinstein M. (2001). Somatostatin is required for masculinization of growth hormone-regulated hepatic gene expression but not of somatic growth. J Clin Invest, 107, 1571-1580.
Myers R.D. (1994). Neuroactive peptides: unique phases in research on mammalian brain over three decades. Peptides, 15, 367-381.
Patel Y.C., Greenwood M.T., Warszynska A., Panetta R. and Srikant C.B. (1994). All five cloned human somatostatin receptors (hSSTR1-5) are functionally coupled to adenylyl cyclase. Biochem Biophys Res Commun, 198, 605-612.
Pfeiffer M., Koch T., Schroder H., Klutzny M., Kirscht S., Kreienkamp H.J., Hollt V. and Schulz S. (2001). Homo- and heterodimerization of somatostatin receptor subtypes. Inactivation of sst(3) receptor function by heterodimerization with sst(2A). J Biol Chem, 276, 14027-14036.
Pfeiffer M., Koch T., Schroder H., Laugsch M., Hollt V. and Schulz S. (2002). Heterodimerization of somatostatin and opioid receptors cross-modulates phosphorylation, internalization, and desensitization. J Biol Chem, 277, 19762-19772.
Reisine T., Bell G.I. (1995). Molecular biology of somatostatin receptors. Endocr Rev, 427-442.
Reubi J.C., Schaer J.C., Wenger S., Hoeger C., Erchegyi J., Waser B. and Rivier J. (2000). SST3-selective potent peptidic somatostatin receptor antagonists. Proc Natl Acad Sci USA, 97, 13973-13978.
Rivier J.E., Hoeger C., Erchegyi J., Gulyas J., DeBoard R., Craig A.G., Koerber S.C., Wenger S., Waser B., Schaer J.C. and Reubi J.C. (2001). Potent somatostatin undecapeptide agonists selective for somatostatin receptor 1 (sst1). J Med Chem, 44, 2238-2246.
Rocheville M., Lange D.C., Kumar U., Sasi R., Patel R.C., Patel Y.C. (2000a). Subtypes of the somatostatin receptor assemble as functional homo- and heterodimers. J Biol Chem, 275, 7862-7869.
Rocheville M., Lange D.C., Kumar U., Patel S.C., Patel R.C. and Patel Y.C. (2000b). Receptors for dopamine and somatostatin: formation of hetero-oligomers with enhanced functional activity. Science, 288, 154-157.
Rohrer S.P., Birzin E.T., Mosley R.T., Berk S.C., Hutchins S.M., Shen D.M., Xiong Y., Hayes E.C., Parmar R.M., Foor F., Mitra S.W., Degrado S.J., Shu M., Klopp J.M., Cai S.J., Blake A., Chan W.W., Pasternak A., Yang L., Patchett A.A., Smith R.G., Chapman K.T. and Schaeffer J.M. (1998). Rapid identification of subtype-selective agonists of the somatostatin receptor through combinatorial chemistry. Science, 282, 737-740.
Schulz S., Handel M., Schreff M., Schmidt H. and Hollt V. (2000). Localization of five somatostatin receptors in the rat central nervous system using subtype-specific antibodies. J Physiol Paris, 94, 259-264.
Schreff M., Schulz S., Handel M., Keilhoff G., Braun H., Pereira G., Klutzny M., Schmidt H., Wolf G. and Hollt V. (2000). Distribution, targeting, and internalization of the sst4 somatostatin receptor in rat brain. J Neurosci, 20, 3785-3797.
Strowski M.Z., Parmar R.M., Blake A.D. and Schaeffer J.M. (2000). Somatostatin inhibits insulin and glucagon secretion via two receptors subtypes: an in vitro study of pancreatic islets from somatostatin receptor 2 knockout mice. Endocrinology, 141, 111-117.
Strowski M.Z., Dashkevicz M.P., Parmar R.M., Wilkinson H., Kohler M., Schaeffer J.M. and Blake A.D. (2002). Somatostatin receptor subtypes 2 and 5 inhibit corticotropin-releasing hormone-stimulated adrenocorticotropin secretion from AtT-20 cells. Neuroendocrinology, 75, 339-346.
Strowski M.Z., Kohler M., Chen H.Y., Trumbauer M.E., Li Z., Szalkowski D., Gopal-Truter S., Fisher J.K., Schaeffer J.M., Blake A.D., Zhang B.B. and Wilkinson H.A. (2003). Somatostatin receptor subtype 5 regulates insulin secretion and glucose homeostasis. Mol Endocrinol, 17, 93-106.

Tulipano G., Soldi D., Bagnasco M., Culler M.D., Taylor J.E., Cocchi D. and Giustina A. (2002). Characterization of new selective somatostatin receptor subtype-2 (sst2) antagonists, BIM-23627 and BIM-23454. Effects of BIM-23627 on GH release in anesthetized male rats after short-term high-dose dexamethasone treatment. Endocrinology, 143, 1218-1224.
Viollet C., Vaillend C., Videau C., Bluet-Pajot M.T., Ungerer A., L'Heritier A., Kopp C., Potier B., Billard J., Schaeffer J., Smith R.G., Rohrer S.P., Wilkinson H., Zheng H. and Epelbaum J. (2000). Involvement of sst2 somatostatin receptor in locomotor, exploratory activity and emotional reactivity in mice. Eur J Neurosci, 12, 3761-3770.
Zeyda T., Diehl N., Paylor R., Brennan M.B. and Hochgeschwender U. (2001). Impairment in motor learning of somatostatin null mutant mice. Brain Res, 906, 107-114.
Zheng H., Bailey A., Jiang M.H., Honda K., Chen H.Y., Trumbauer M.E., Van der Ploeg L.H., Schaeffer J.M., Leng G. and Smith R.G. (1997). Somatostatin receptor subtype 2 knockout mice are refractory to growth hormone-negative feedback on arcuate neurons. Mol Endocrinol, 11, 1709-1717.

Chapter 5

Investigation of LHRH Receptor Involvement in Melanoma Growth and Progression

M. Montagnani Marelli, R.M. Moretti and P. Limonta

Luteinizing Hormone-Releasing Hormone

The hypothalamic decapeptide luteinizing hormone-releasing hormone (LHRH) is the prime controller of reproductive function (Fink, 1988). It performs this function, after being secreted from the hypothalamus into the hypophysial portal circulation, by binding and activating specific receptors on gonadotrophs (Stojilkovic et al., 1994).

The neurohormone stimulates the synthesis and the release of the two gonadotropins LH and FSH (follicle stimulating hormone), and for this reason, it is also called GnRH (gonadotropin-releasing hormone) (Stojilkovic and Catt, 1995).

Hypothalamic neurosecretory cells release LHRH in a pulsatile way, and LHRH pulses are critical for the maintenance of gonadotropin gene expression and for the physiological pattern of secretion of LH and FSH (Kalra, 1993). The two gonadotropins are themselves secreted in a pulsatile way in the systemic circulation and act on the gonads to regulate gametogenesis and steroid synthesis (Kalra, 1993). Pulsatile administration of LHRH in patients with hypothalamic dysfunction has been shown to induce a regular pattern of gonadotropin secretion, thus restoring the fertility (Conn and Crowley, 1994; Schally, 1994). On the other hand, chronic applications of LHRH or LHRH analogues lead to complete suppression of the reproductive function, due to LHRH receptor down-regulation and desensitization (Stojilkovic and Catt, 1995; Schally, 1994). This mechanism of action has provided the rationale for the wide and successful use of LHRH agonists in the treatment of hormone-dependent tumors (e.g., prostate and breast carcinoma; Schally, 1994).

The human pituitary LHRH receptor (LHRH-r) has been cloned and characterized (Kakar et al., 1992). It encodes a 328-amino-acid protein belonging to the superfamily of seven transmembrane domain receptors. Recently, LHRH and LHRH-r have been consistently shown to be expressed in the brain and in a variety of peripheral organs, both normal and tumoral, where the peptide probably sets in an autocrine/paracrine fashion (Limonta et al., 1992, 1993; Dondi et al., 1994; Imai et al.,1994; Chatzaki et al., 1996). In our laboratory we investigated whether this LHRH-based system might also be present in prostate cancer, and whether it might be involved in the control of tumor growth. These studies were performed in human prostate cancer cell lines, either androgen-dependent (LNCaP) or androgen-independent (DU 145). Our data demonstrated that, in either androgen-dependent or androgen-independent prostate cancer, a local LHRH system is present and might act as a paracrine/autocrine negative regulator of tumor growth (Limonta et al., 1992;

Dondi et al., 1994, 1998). These observations are in agreement with those reported for tumors of the female reproductive tract, such as breast (Kakar et al., 1994; Kottler et al., 1997), endometrial (Imai et al., 1994; Chatzaki et al., 1996), and ovarian cancer (Emons et al., 1993, 2000).

These data seem to suggest that, when utilized for the treatment of hormone-related tumors, LHRH agonists might exert an additional and more direct inhibitory action at the level of the tumor tissue. Moreover, LHRH analogues might also be considered for a possible treatment of prostate cancer in its androgen-independent stage.

LHRH in Melanoma

In a recent paper, it has been reported that binding sites for LHRH are expressed in glioblastoma biopsies; this finding suggests that LHRH receptors might represent a diagnostic marker, and possibly a new therapeutic target, for tumors of the nervous system (van Groeninghen et al., 1998). Since both glial cells and melanocytes share the same neuroectodermal origin, we reasoned that a LHRH-based system (LHRH and LHRH-r), similar to that present in tumors of the reproductive tract, might also be expressed in melanoma cells.

Cutaneous melanoma is one of the most frequent malignant tumors in younger people and is characterized by uncontrollable growth and the ability to give rise to metastases (MacKie, 1998). The incidence of this tumor is increasing dramatically (Parkin et al., 1999) and, although its prognosis has improved in the past 10 or 20 years, particularly due to early diagnosis, the prognosis remains very poor in advanced cases, when tumor cells acquire a strong potential to disseminate metastases (MacKie, 1998). Moreover, advanced melanoma is a multistep process, which starts from the initial transformation of normal melanocytes or from potential precursor lesions such as atypical melanocytes or dysplastic or congenital nevi (Herlyn et al., 1987; Albino et al., 1997). The pathology then goes through a radial growth phase, eventually progressing to the vertical growth phase (Lazar-Molnar et al., 2000). It is particularly in this phase that tumor cells start giving rise to metastases (Shih and Herlyn, 1993). Prevention of metastasis is the main goal in melanoma treatment. In current practice, however, this can be achieved only by early detection and excision (Breslow, 1978). A recently introduced new chemotherapeutic drug for metastasized melanoma, temozolomide, failed to offer a significant mean survival improvement compared to the treatment with the traditional cytostatic drug DTCI (decarbazine) (Danny and Wilson, 2000; Hwu, 2000). Both the chemotherapeutics mentioned have thrombocytopenia as the classical side-effect.

The experiments here described were performed to clarify whether an LHRH-based system (LHRH and the respective receptors) is expressed in melanoma cells. We also investigated whether the activation of this system might affect the proliferative rate and the metastatic properties of this tumor. For these studies we used the human melanoma cell line BLM (kindly provided by Dr. Van Muijen, Department of Pathology, University Hospital Nijmegen, The Netherlands). LHRH receptor activation was achieved using a potent LHRH agonist (Zoladex, LHRH-A; provided by AstraZeneca Pharmaceuticals, Divisione Farmaceutici, Milan, Italy).

Expression of LHRH and LHRH Receptors

The expression of both LHRH and LHRH-r in melanoma cells was investigated by reverse transcription polymerase chain reaction (RT-PCR). With regard to the expression of LHRH, according to the sequence of the oligonucleotide primers used, the predicted fragment of 228 bp was observed in BLM cells. After Southern blotting, the cDNA fragments hybridized with the ^{32}P-labeled oligonucleotide probe specific for the LHRH cDNA (Oikawa et al., 1990) (Fig.1). In the case of the expression of the LHRH-r mRNA, the results obtained demonstrate that the predicted 885-bp cDNA fragment is present in BLM cells; this band hybridized with the ^{32}P-labeled probe specific for the LHRH-r cDNA (Kakar et al., 1994) (Fig. 2A). The presence of LHRH-r in melanoma cells has been further investigated at the protein level, by Western blot and by using the specific F1G4 antibody raised against the human pituitary receptor (Karande et al., 1995) (Fig. 2B). The results obtained demonstrate that a protein of approximately 64 kDa

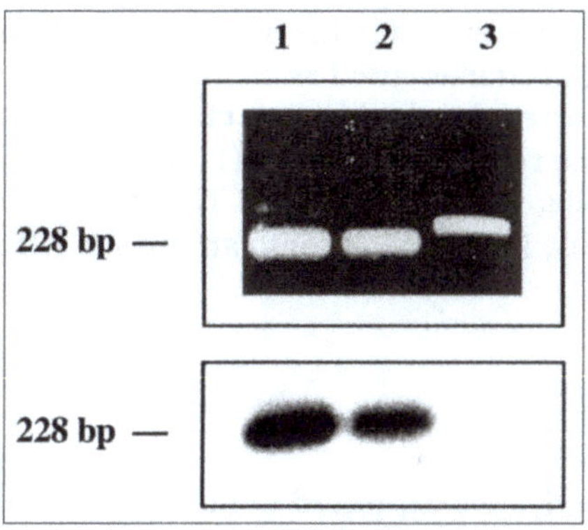

Fig. 1. RT-PCR analysis of the expression of LHRH in BLM cells. *Top panel*, Ethidium bromide-stained agarose gel of the amplified cDNAs. *Bottom panel*, Autoradiograph of the Southern blot obtained from the gel shown in the top panel after hybridization with a 32P-labeled oligonucleotide LHRH cDNA probe. *Lane 1*, BLM cells; *lane 2*, prostate cancer cells; *lane 3*, RT-PCR control

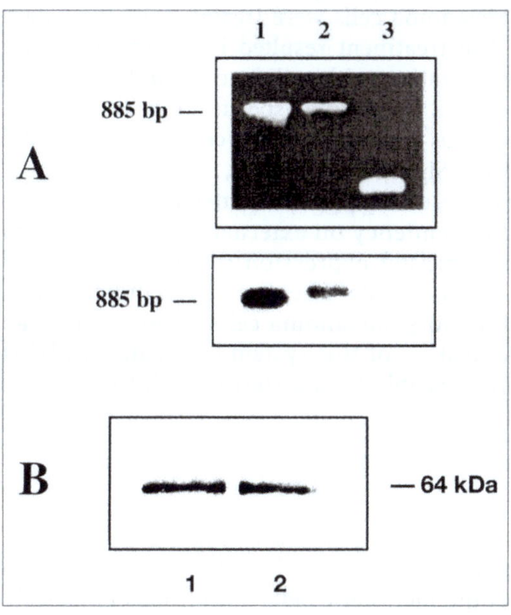

Fig. 2. **A** RT-PCR analysis of the expression of LHRH receptor in BLM cells. *Top*, Ethidium bromide-stained agarose gel of the amplified cDNAs. *Bottom*, Autoradiograph of the Southern blot obtained from the gel shown in the top panel after hybridization with a ^{32}P-labeled oligonucleotide LHRH receptor cDNA probe. *Lane 1*, BLM cells; *lane 2*, prostate cancer cells; *lane 3*, RT-PCR control. **B** Western blot analysis of solubilized membrane proteins from BLM cells (*lane 1*) and prostate cancer cells (*lane 2*), probed with the F1G4 monoclonal antibody raised against the human pituitary LHRH receptor

Table 1. Characteristics of 125I-labeled LHRH-A binding to human melanoma cell membrane

	Dissociation constant (K_d) (nM)	^{125}I-LHRH-A binding capacity (fmol/mg protein)
BLM cells	0.7-1.1	150-200
Rat pituitaries	1.5-2.0	70-100

molecular mass is present in membrane preparations from BLM cells. This molecular weight corresponds to that previously reported for the human pituitary receptor (Wormald et al., 1985). Finally, LHRH receptors in melanoma cells were also analyzed in terms of binding parameters. Radioreceptor assays were performed by using ^{125}I-labeled LHRH-A as the specific ligand (Limonta et al., 1992; Dondi et al., 1994). The assays demonstrated that binding sites for ^{125}I-labeled LHRH-A are present on the membranes of BLM cells. Computer analysis of the data obtained from displacement curves indicated the presence of a single class of high-affinity binding sites (dissociation constant Kd in the nanomolar range) in the melanoma cell line, as well as in rat pituitaries, used as controls (Table 1).

So far, divergent results have been reported for the binding characteristics of LHRH receptors in cancers related to the reproductive tract (Limonta et al., 1992; Emons et al., 1993; Dondi et al., 1994; Imai et al., 1994). The data here described indicate that, in melanoma cells, LHRH receptors can bind LHRH analogues with a high affinity.

Antiproliferative Activity of LHRH

The observation that both LHRH and LHRH-r are expressed in melanoma cells prompted us to investigate the possible role played by this LHRH-based system in the control of melanoma growth. Melanoma cells were treated daily for 7 days with LHRH-A ($10^{-11}$to 10^{-6} mol/l). The treatment resulted in a significant and dose-dependent inhibition of cell proliferation, with an EC_{50} dose in the nanomolar range. This antimitogenic activity was found to be specific since it was completely counteracted by the simultaneous treatment of the cells with an LHRH antagonist antide (Ant; purchased from Sigma Chemical Co, St. Louis, Mo.).

As in the case of other tumors, the development of melanoma has been found to be related to a decreased dependency on external mitogenic stimuli (Halaban, 1996) as well as to an increased expression of locally produced growth factors (Shih and Herlyn, 1994). The data here reported indicate that, in addition to stimulatory growth factors, melanoma cells might express an LHRH-based inhibitory system. Activation of this system by means of LHRH agonists may reduce tumor growth, possibly by interfering with the positive effect of the mitogenic stimuli.

Antimetastatic Activity of LHRH

Experiments were performed to verify whether the activation of locally expressed LHRH-r might also affect the metastatic behavior of melanoma cells.

In a first series of experiments, we evaluated the effects of LHRH-A on the ability of BLM cells to migrate towards a chemoattractant (fetal bovine serum 5%), using the Boyden's chamber technique. We found that treatment of BLM cells with LHRH-A (10^{-6} mol/l for 5 days) significantly reduced the ability of the cells to migrate in response to the chemoattractant (Fig. 3A). We then analyzed the effects of LHRH-A (10^{-6} mol/l) on the ability of melanoma cells to invade a reconstituted basement membrane (Matrigel). BLM cells spontaneously form cell aggregates when prepared by the hanging-drop technique. For these experiments, the aggregates in Matrigel were covered with culture medium in the absence or in the presence of LHRH-A (10^{-6} mol/l) for 4, 8, or 12 days. The results obtained show that BLM cells actively leave the aggregate by degrading the Matrigel preparation. The treatment of the cells with LHRH-A completely counteracted the migration of the cells at all the time intervals considered (Fig. 3B).

Taken together, these data indicate that the activation of locally expressed LHRH receptors significantly reduces the ability of melanoma cells to migrate in response to a chemotactic stimulus and to degrade extracellular matrix components. To the authors' knowledge, this is the first report of a

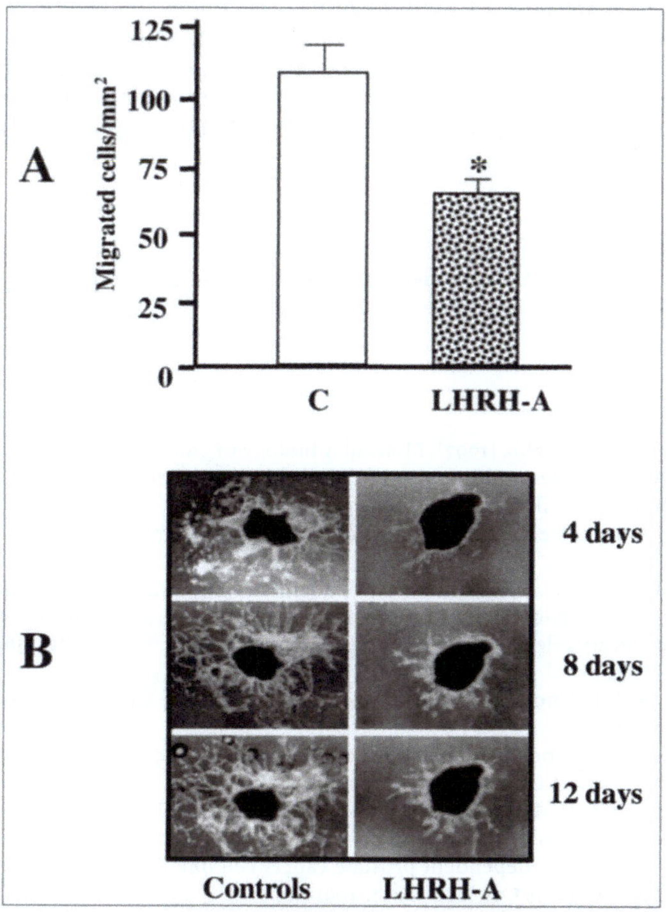

Fig. 3. Effects of the LHRH agonist LHRH-A (Zoladex) on **A** the migratory (Chemomigration assay) and **B** the invasive (Matrigel assay) properties of melanoma cells. * $p < 0.05$ vs controls

possible antimetastatic activity of LHRH in tumors. Preliminary data obtained in our laboratory seem to indicate that LHRH exerts this antimetastatic activity by reducing the expression of cell adhesion molecules (integrins) as well as the expression and the activity of enzymes able to degrade the extracellular matrix (matrix metalloproteinases, MMPs). Both integrins and MMPs have been shown to play a crucial role in the molecular mechanisms leading to melanoma progression (Natali et al., 1993; Hofmann et al., 2000).

As pointed out above, the clinical options for advanced melanoma are still limited, due to the intrinsic resistance of the tumor to standard chemotherapy, but also to its ability to give rise to metastases (Meyer and Hart, 1998). The data reported here seem to suggest that LHRH agonists might reduce not only the proliferation rate, but also the metastatic potential of melanoma cells.

Conclusions

LHRH and LHRH receptors are also expressed in tumors that are not classically related to the endocrine system, such as melanoma. In melanoma cells, the locally expressed LHRH-based system negatively regulates the proliferation of the cells as well as their ability to migrate towards chemotactic stimuli and to invade a reconstituted basement membrane. Therefore, in melanoma, the activation of LHRH receptors might reduce not only tumor growth but also its metastatic potential. Moreover, the LHRH receptor might represent a new diagnostic (and possibly prognostic) marker for the detection of skin tumors.

Acknowledgements. This work was supported by AIRC (Associazione Italiana per la Ricerca sul Cancro), by MURST (Ministero dell'Università e della Ricerca Scientifica e Tecnologica), and by the Center for Endocrinological Oncology.

References

Albino A.P., Reed J.A. and McNutt N.S. (1997). Molecular biology of cutaneous malignant melanoma. In Cancer Principles and Practice of Oncology, 5th edn, eds. De Vita V.T., Hellman S., Rosenberg S.A. Philadelphia, Lippincott-Raven.

Breslow A. (1978). The surgical treatment of stage I cutaneous melanoma. Cancer Treat Rev, 5, 195-198.

Chatzaki E., Bax C.M.R., Eidne K.A., Anderson L., Grudzinskas J.G. and Gallagher C.J. (1996). The expression of gonadotropin releasing hormone and its receptor in endometrial cancer and its relevance as an autocrine growth factor. Cancer Res, 56, 2055-2065.

Conn P.M. and Crowley W.F. Jr. (1994). Gonadotropin-releasing hormone and its analogs. Ann Rev Med, 45, 391-405.

Danny W.A. and Wilson W.R. (2000). Tirapazamine: a bioreductive anticancer drug that exploit tumor hypoxia. Expert Opin Investig Drug, 9, 2889-2901.

Dondi D., Limonta P., Moretti R.M., Montagnani Marelli M., Garattini E. and Motta M. (1994). Antiproliferative effects of luteinizing hormone-releasing hormone (LHRH) agonists on human androgen-independent prostate cancer cell line DU 145: evidence for an autocrine-inhibitory loop. Cancer Res, 54, 4091-4095.

Dondi D., Moretti R.M., Montagnani Marelli M., Pratesi G., Polizzi D., Milani M., Motta M. and Limonta P. (1998). Growth inhibitory effects of luteinizing hormone-releasing hormone (LHRH) agonists on xenografts of the DU 145 human androgen-independent prostate cancer cell line in nude mice. Int J Cancer, 76, 506-511.

Emons G. and Schally A.V. (1994). The use of luteinizing hormone releasing hormone agonists and antagonists in gynaecological cancers. Hum Reprod, 9, 1364-1379.

Emons G., Ortmann O., Becker M., Irmer G., Springer B., Laun R., Holzel F., Schulz K.D. and Schally A.V. (1993). High affinity binding and direct antiproliferative effects of LHRH analogues in human ovarian cancer cell lines. Cancer Res, 54, 5439-5446.

Emons G., Weiss S., Ortmann O., Grundker C. and Schulz K.D. (2000). LHRH might act as a negative autocrine regulator of proliferation of human ovarian cancer. Eur J Endocrinol, 142, 665-670.

Fink G. (1988). Gonadotropin secretion and its control. In The Physiology of Reproduction, eds. Knobil E. and Kneill J.D., pp. 1349-1377. New York, Raven Press.

Halaban R. (1996). Growth factors and melanoma. Semin Oncol, 23, 673-681.

Herlyn M., Clark W.H., Rodeck U., Mancianti M.L., Jambrosic J. and Koprowski H. (1987). Biology of tumor progression in human melanocytes. Lab Invest, 56, 461-474.

Hofmann U.B., Westphal J.R., van Muijen G.N.P. and Ruiter D.J. (2000). Matrix metalloproteinases in human melanoma. J Invest Dermatol, 115, 337-344.

Hwu W.J. (2000). New approaches in the treatment of metastatic melanoma: thalidomide and temozolomide. Oncology, 14, 25-28.

Imai A., Ohno T., Iida K., Fuseya T., Furui T. and Tamaya T. (1994). Gonadotropin-releasing hormone receptors in gynecological tumors. Cancer, 74, 2555-2561.

Kakar S.S., Musgrove L.C., Devor D.C., Sellers J.C. and Neill J.D. (1992). Cloning, sequencing and expression of human gonadotropin-releasing hormone (GnRH) receptor. Biochem Biophys Res Commun, 189, 289-295.

Kakar S.S., Grizzle W.E. and Neill J.D. (1994). The nucleotide sequences of human GnRH receptors in breast and ovarian tumors are identical with that found in pituitary. Mol Cell Endocrinol, 106, 145-149.

Kalra S.P. (1993). Mandatory neuropeptide-steroid signaling for the preovulatory luteinizing hormone-releasing hormone discharge. Endocr Rev, 14, 507-538.

Karande A.A., Rajeshwari K., Schol D.J. and Hilgers J.H.M. (1995). Establishment of immunological probes to study human gonadotropin-releasing hormone receptors. Mol Cell Endocrinol, 114, 51-56.

Kottler M.L., Starzec A., Carre M.C., Lagarde J.P., Martin A. and Counis R. (1997). The genes for gonadotropin-releasing hormone and its receptor are expressed in human breast with fibrocystic disease and cancer. Int J Cancer, 71, 595-599.

Lazar-Molnar E., Hegyesi H., Toth S. and Falus A. (2000). Autocrine and paracrine regulation by cytokines and growth factors in melanoma. Cytokine, 12, 547-554.

Limonta P., Dondi D., Moretti R.M., Maggi R. and Motta M. (1992). Antiproliferative effects of luteinizing hormone-releasing hormone agonists on the human prostatic cancer cell line LNCaP. J Clin Endocrinol Metab, 75, 207-212.

Limonta P., Dondi D., Moretti R.M., Fermo D., Garattini E. and Motta M. (1993). Expression of luteinizing hormone-releasing hormone mRNA in the human prostatic cancer cell line LNCaP. J Clin Endocrinol Metab, 76, 797-800.

Lu C. and Kerbel R.S. (1994). Cytokines, growth factors and the loss of negative growth controls in the progression of human cutaneous malignant melanoma. Curr Opin Oncol, 6, 212-220.

Mackie R.M. (1998) Incidence, risk factors and prevention of melanoma. Eur J Cancer, 34 (Suppl 3), S3-S6.

Meyer T. and Hart I.R. (1998). Mechanisms of tumor metastasis. Eur J Cancer, 34, 214-221.

Natali P.G., Nicotra M.R., Bartolazzi A., Cavaliere R. and Bigotti A. (1993). Integrin expression in cutaneous malignant melanoma: association of the $\alpha 3/\beta 1$ heterodimer with tumor progression. Int J Cancer, 54, 68-72.

Oikawa M., Dargan C., Ny T. and Hsueh A.J.W. (1990). Expression of gonadotropin-releasing hormone and prothymosin-α messenger ribonucleic acid in the ovary. Endocrinology 127, 2350-2356.
Parkin D.M., Pisani P. and Ferlay J. (1999). Global cancer statistics. CA Cancer J Clin, 49, 33-64.
Schally A.V. (1994). Hypothalamic hormones from neuroendocrinology to cancer therapy. Anticancer Drugs, 5, 115-130.
Shih I.M. and Herlyn M. (1993). Role of growth factors and their receptors in the development and progression of melanoma. J Invest Dermatol, 100, S196-S203.
Shih I.M. and Herlyn M. (1994). Autocrine and paracrine roles for growth factors in melanoma. In Vivo, 8, 113-123.
Stojilkovic S.S., Reinhart J. and Catt K.J. (1994). Gonadotropin-releasing hormone receptors. Structure and signal transduction pathways. Endocr Rev, 15, 462-499.
Stojilkovic S.S. and Catt K.J. (1995). Expression and signal transduction pathways of gonadotropin releasing hormone receptors. Recent Prog Horm Res, 30, 161-205.
van Groeninghen JC, Kiesel L, Winkler D and Zwirner M (1998). Effects of luteinizing hormone-releasing hormone on nervous-system tumours. Lancet, 352, 372-373.
Wormald PJ, Eidne KA and Millar RP (1985). Gonadotropin-releasing hormone receptors in human pituitary: ligand structural requirements, molecular size, cationic effects. J Clin Endocrinol and Metab, 61, 1190-1194.

SOMATOSTATIN/GHRH/GH

Chapter 6

Cortistatin: Not Simply a Natural Somatostatin Analogue

R. Deghenghi, F. Broglio, F. Prodam, C. Gottero, M. Papotti, G. Muccioli
and E. Ghigo

Introduction

Cortistatin (CST) is a recently described peptide mostly expressed in cerebral cortex and hippocampus, but also in peripheral tissues such as fetal heart and lung, prostate, colon and the immune system (de Lecea et al., 1997a,b; Fukusumi et al., 1997; Spier and de Lecea, 2000; Dalm et al., 2003). Pre-pro-CST shows high structural homology with pre-pro-somatostatin (pre-pro-SST), particularly in the carboxyl terminus from which SST-14 and SST-28 are enzymatically processed (Spier and de Lecea, 2000). Interestingly, rat pre-pro-CST may also be cleaved to pro-CST from which the two mature products CST-14 and CST-29 can be generated in rats (de Lecea et al., 1996; Spier and de Lecea 2000) and CST-17 and CST-29 in humans (de Lecea et al., 1997a; Fukusumi et al., 1997; Spier and de Lecea, 2000). CST-14 shares 11 of the 14 amino acid residues with SST-14, although these peptides are encoded by distinct genes (de Lecea et al., 1996; Spier and de Lecea, 2000).

SST exerts its biological effects via membrane-bound receptors, the so-called SST receptors (SST-R), of which five subtypes (SST-R 1-5) have been cloned (Reichlin, 1998; Kreienkamp, 1999). The SST-R are expressed in the brain and periphery (Reichlin, 1998; Kreienkamp, 1999) and mediate multiple SST activities including neurotransmission, neuromodulation, regulation of endocrine and exocrine secretions, and also the inhibition of tumor growth (Reichlin, 1998; Kreienkamp, 1999).

CST binds to all SST-R subtypes with an affinity (1-2 nM) quite close to that of SST and therefore is expected to have similar biological activities (Fukusumi et al., 1997; Siehler et al., 1998; Spier and de Lecea, 2000). However, the existence of specific receptors which selectively bind SST or CST has been hypothesized (Siehler et al., 1998; Spier and de Lecea, 2000), and, in fact, CST possesses central activities which are not shared by SST (Vasilaki et al., 1999; Sanchez-Alavez et al., 2000; Spier and de Lecea, 2000). For instance, CST, unlike SST, reduces locomotor activity and induces slow-wave sleep (de Lecea et al., 1996; Spier and de Lecea, 2000). Moreover, CST and SST are often coexpressed in the same neurons but are regulated by different stimuli (de Lecea et al., 1997b; Calbet et al., 1999; Spier and de Lecea, 2000). Interestingly, we have recently found that CST but not SST also binds GH secretagogue (GHS) receptors (GHS-R) (Deghenghi et al., 2001a; Muccioli et al., 2001).

Cortistatin, Somatostatin and Ghrelin Interactions

Ghrelin is a 28-aminoacid peptide that has been discovered as a natural ligand of the orphan GHS-R type 1a that, in turn, had been shown to be specific for synthetic GHS (Smith et al, 1997; Kojima et al., 2001a). Like synthetic GHS, ghrelin is endowed with a potent GH-releasing effect in both humans and animals provided that the molecule is acylated in serine 3 (Kojima et al., 1999; Muccioli et al., 2002; Broglio et al., 2003). Ghrelin is produced predominantly by the stomach but also in bowel, pancreas, kidneys, gonads, placenta, pituitary, and hypothalamus (Kojima et al, 1999, 2001b; Gnanapavan et al., 2002; Muccioli et al., 2002).

GHS-R have been postulated to mediate a major role in the control of GH secretion, in addition to GHRH-R and SST-R (Casanueva, 1992; Smith et al., 1997; Ghigo et al., 1999, 2001; Bluet-Pajot et al., 2001). As anticipated, the GHS-R were cloned following the evidence that synthetic peptidyl and nonpeptidyl molecules, named GHS, show strong GH-releasing activity acting at the pituitary and, especially at the hypothalamic levels where specific receptors are present (Smith et al., 1997; Muccioli et al., 1998; Ghigo et al., 2001; Bluet-Pajot et al., 2001). Recent reports demonstrated that GHS-R are also present in some extrahypothalamic brain areas and even in several peripheral organs, suggesting that these binding sites could be involved in mediating various GH-independent activities of GHS, such as metabolic, cardioprotective, antiproliferative and orexigenic effects (Casanueva, 1992; Muccioli et al., 1998; Ong et al., 1998; Ghigo et al., 1999, 2001; Bluet-Pajot et al., 2001; Muccioli et al., 2000; Papotti et al., 2000; Cassoni et al., 2001).

Regarding GH secretion, ghrelin as well as GHS and GHRH have a synergic effect, indicating that they act, at least partially, via different mechanisms (Smith et al., 1997; Bluet-Pajot et al., 2001; Ghigo et al., 2001; Tannenbaum and Bowers, 2001). Nevertheless, GHS need GHRH activity to fully express their GH-releasing effect, and it has been recently reported that in vitro ghrelin induces a significant stimulation of GHRH release from hypothalamic explants (Smith et al., 1997; Bluet-Pajot et al., 2001; Ghigo et al., 2001; Tannenbaum and Bowers, 2001; Wren et al., 2002). On the other hand, infusion of GHRH induces a significant increase in pituitary gene expression of both ghrelin and its receptors (Kamegai et al., 2000; Yoshihara et al., 2002). Moreover, to further underline the close relationship between GHRH and ghrelin system, it has been recently demonstrated that coactivation of the GHS and GHRH receptors selectively potentiate the GHRH-induced activation of the intracellular cAMP signaling pathway (Cunha and Mayo, 2002).

In humans the GH response to GHS is strongly inhibited, though not abolished, by a GHRH receptor antagonist as well as by hypothalamus-pituitary disconnection (Popovic et al., 1995; Pandya et al., 1998), which is in agreement with the assumption that the most important action of GHS takes place at the hypothalamic level (Smith et al., 1997; Bluet-Pajot et al., 2001; Ghigo et al., 2001). Moreover, patients with GHRH-receptor deficiency show no GH response to GHS, which maintain their stimulatory effect on prolactin (PRL), adenocorticotropin hormone (ACTH), and cortisol secretion (Maheshwari et al., 1999).

Both ghrelin and synthetic GHS have been reported to be ineffective in modifying hypothalamic SST release, but there are data indicating that ghrelin and GHS might act as functional SST antagonists at the pituitary and the hypothalamic level (Goth et al., 1992; Ghigo et al., 2001; Tannenbaum and Bowers, 2001; Wren et al., 2002). In humans the GH response to both natural and synthetic GHS is not modified by substances acting via SST inhibition (such as acetylcholine receptor agonists and arginine) which, in turn, truly potentiate the GHRH-induced GH rise (Ghigo et al., 2001). Moreover, the GH-releasing activity of ghrelin and synthetic GHS is partially refractory to the inhibitory effect of substances acting via stimulation of hypothalamic SST (such as acetylcholine receptor antagonists, β-adrenoceptor agonists and glucose) which, in turn, almost abolish somatotroph responsiveness to GHRH (Ghigo et al., 2001). Indeed both ghrelin and GHS are partially refractory to the inhibition of substances acting on somatotroph cells such as free fatty acids, and even to exogenous SST. GHS are also partially refractory to the negative GH autofeedback (Ghigo et al., 2001) and show peculiar sensitivity to the negative insulin-like growth factor 1 (IGF-1) feedback action (Ghigo et al., 2001).

More recently, another endogenous ligand for the GHS-R type 1a, as the result of an alternative splicing of the ghrelin gene, has been isolated from the stomach (Hosoda et al., 2000). It has been named Des-Gln14-ghrelin, being homologous to ghrelin except for one missing glutamine, has the same acylation in serine 3, and possesses the same activity as ghrelin (Kojima et al., 1999; Hosoda et al., 2000). GHS-R are also bound by other molecules such as adenosine, which, however, is not able to activate the receptor (Smith et al., 2000; Tullin et al., 2000). Interestingly, although native SST does not bind GHS-R, it has surprisingly been observed that some synthetic SST octapeptide agonists (mainly lanreotide, octreotide, and vapreotide) displace ^{125}I-Tyr-Ala-hexarelin from pituitary binding sites (Deghenghi et al., 2001a,b).

This evidence suggested the working hypothesis that an endogenous factor related to SST might exist and interact with the GHS-R, thus representing another natural ligand of these receptors. To clarify this hypothesis, the ability of different SST-like peptides such as various SST fragments (SRIH3-14, SRIH7-14, SRIH7-10, SRIH2-9) and of CST-14 and CST-17 to compete with ^{125}I-Tyr-Ala-hexarelin binding sites of human pituitary gland in comparison with hexarelin and ghrelin has been investigated and recently described in rat and human brains (Deghenghi et al., 2001a-c). The different SST fragments were chosen as potential metabolites (Deghenghi et al., 2001b), whereas CST was chosen because, although it shares high structural homology with SST (de Lecea et al., 1996; Fukusumi et al., 1997; Spier and de Lecea, 2000) and binds all five SST-R subtypes (Siehler et al., 1998; Deghenghi et al., 2001b), it possesses several effects that do not parallel those of SST and might therefore be related to the activation of another SST-unrelated receptor (Spier and de Lecea, 2000). First results showed that CST, like hexarelin and ghrelin, but not various fragments of native SST, displaces ^{125}I-Tyr- Ala-hexarelin from its pituitary receptors. Later on it was demonstrated that CST-17 and CST-14, as well as some SST analogues, but not native SST, inhibit the binding of labeled acyl-ghrelin to human hypothalamus-pituitary tissues (Deghenghi et al., 2001a; Muccioli et al., 2001). Evidence that CST, like natural and synthetic

GHS, but differently from SST, binds the GHS-R, suggested that this peptide could represent another endogenous GHS ligand. This hypothesis could, in turn, imply that GHS-R is another specific receptor for CST. It is interesting to note that CST displaces radio-iodinated natural and synthetic peptidyl GHS from pituitary binding sites with an IC_{50} value about 50-fold higher (Deghenghi et al., 2001a; Muccioli et al., 2001) than that required to inhibit the binding of radiolabeled SST to SST-R (Siehler et al., 1998; Spier and de Lecea, 2000).

Endocrine Activities of Cortistatin: Differences from and Similarities with Somatostatin

Animal Studies

Following the results coming from binding studies, in vivo animal studies have been performed in order to verify whether the endocrine effect of CST and its specific binding to the GHS-R might induce some peculiar effects not related to the activation of the SST-R subtypes.

Preliminary studies show that CST-14 is active in vivo to induce a dose-related inhibition of GH secretion in normal male anesthetized rats (Deghenghi et al., 2001c). Comparison with the inhibitory effect evoked by graded doses of native SST-14 in the same experimental conditions indicate that both neuropeptides share an overlapping GH-reducing activity, probably mediated by an action at the five cloned SST-R receptor subtypes (Deghenghi et al., 2001c).

Human Studies

The effects of CST-14 on GH, insulin, glucose, and ghrelin secretion as well as on the somatotroph responsiveness to either GHRH or ghrelin in normal young volunteers have been evaluated. The effects of CST were compared with those of the same dose of SST-14. The effects of ghrelin both alone and during infusion of either CST or SST on PRL, ACTH, cortisol, insulin and glucose levels were also evaluated (Broglio et al., 2002a,b).

These studies showed that CST, similarly to SST, remarkably inhibits GH, insulin, and spontaneous ghrelin secretion in humans. The inhibitory effect (approximately 55%) of CST and SST on circulating ghrelin levels followed that on GH and insulin secretion. At the end of CST or SST infusion, GH and insulin secretion almost immediately recovered despite persistent inhibition of ghrelin levels (Broglio et al., 2002a,b).

Anyway, CST inhibited both the GHRH and the ghrelin-stimulated GH secretion in humans to the same extent as SST. In comparison to GHRH, the GH-releasing activity of ghrelin was partially refractory to the inhibitory effect of either CST or SST (Broglio et al., 2002a). Neither CST nor SST modified the lactotroph and corticotroph responsiveness to ghrelin; this finding agrees with previous studies showing that SST does not influence the lactotroph and corticotroph response to synthetic GHS (Massoud et al., 1997; Broglio et al., 2002a). CST and SST also shared the same inhibitory effect on insulin secretion, and their effect was not modified by the acute administration of ghrelin, which, in turn, has an inhibitory effect on insulin secretion (Broglio et al., 2002a).

Evidence that ghrelin does not modify CST- or SST-induced insulin inhibition would indicate that ghrelin negatively influences β-cell secretion via an SST-mediated mechanism. This hypothesis agrees with the observation that either hypothalamic or pancreatic SST release is enhanced after exposure to natural or synthetic GHS (Arosio et al., 2003).

Conclusions

CST is a neuropeptide with high structural homology to SST which also exerts some activities that are not shared by SST. CST binds all five SST-R subtypes but, unlike SST, it is also able to bind GHS-R. Based on these data suggesting that CST may represent a new putative endogenous ligand of the GHS-R, in vivo studies (in animal and in human) have been performed in order to verify whether CST may exert some endocrine effect and whether the specific binding to the GHS-R might reveal some peculiar activities not related to the activation of the SST-R. However, at present, CST and SST seem to possess the same endocrine activities, suggesting that CST binding to SST-R probably overrides other potential endocrine activities of this neuropeptide. CST analogues able to bind the GHS-R only might probably clarify other potential endocrine "ghrelin-linked" activities of this neuropeptide. The search for analogues with selective activity on GHS-R led to the octapeptide Pro-c[Cys-Phe-D-Trp-Lys-Thr-Cys]-Lys-NH_2 (named CST-8), which does not displace SST from its receptors but has high affinity on the ghrelin receptor (Muccioli, 2002). This compound is currently under investigation.

Acknowledgements. The authors wish to thank Drs. A. Benso, P. Cassoni, F. Catapano, C. Ghè, S. Destefanis, and M. Volante for their participation to the studies described in the present review. The authors' studies reported in this review were supported by Eureka (Peptido Project 1923), MURST (Ministero dell'Università e della Ricerca Scientifica e Tecnologica), Cofin 2002, University of Turin, Europeptides, and the SMEM (Studio Malattie Endocrine e Metaboliche) Foundation.

References

Arosio M., Ronchi C.L., Gebbia C., Cappiello V., Beck-Peccoz P. and Peracchi M. (2003). Stimulatory effects of ghrelin on circulating somatostatin and pancreatic polypeptide levels. J Clin Endocrinol Metab, 88, 701-704.

Bluet-Pajot M.T., Tolle V., Zizzari P., Robert C., Hammond C., Mitchell V., Beauvillain J.C., Viollet C., Epelbaum J. and Kordon C. (2001). Growth hormone secretagogues and hypothalamic networks. Endocrine, 14, 1-8.

Broglio F., Arvat E., Benso A., Gottero C., Prodam F., Grottoli S., Papotti M., Muccioli G., van der Lely A.J., Deghenghi R. and Ghigo E. (2002a). Endocrine activities of cortistatin-14 and its interaction with GHRH and ghrelin in humans. J Clin Endocrinol Metab, 87, 3783-3790.
Broglio F., Van Koetsveld P., Benso A., Gottero C., Prodam F., Papotti M., Muccioli G., Gauna C., Hofland L., Deghenghi R., Arvat E., van der Lely A.J. and Ghigo E. (2002b). Ghrelin secretion is inhibited by either somatostatin or cortistatin in humans. J Clin Endocrinol Metab, 87, 4829-4832.
Broglio F., Benso A., Gottero C., Prodam F., Gauna C., Filtri L., Arvat E., van der Lely A.J., Deghenghi R. and Ghigo E. (2003). Non-acylated-ghrelin does not possess the pituitaric and pancreatic endocrine activity of acylated ghrelin. J Endocrinol Invest, 26, 192-196.
Calbet M., Guadano-Ferraz A., Spier A.D., Maj M., Sutcliffe J.G., Przewlocki R. and de Lecea L. (1999). Cortistatin and somatostatin mRNAs are differentially regulated in response to kainate. Brain Res Mol Brain Res, 72, 55-64.
Casanueva F.F. (1992). Physiology of growth hormone secretion and action. In Endocrinology and Metabolism Clinics of North America, ed. Melmed S., pp. 483-517. Philadelphia, Saunders.
Cassoni P., Papotti M., Ghe C., Catapano F., Sapino A., Graziani A., Deghenghi R., Reissmann T., Ghigo E. and Muccioli G. (2001). Identification, characterization, and biological activity of specific receptors for natural (ghrelin) and synthetic growth hormone secretagogues and analogs in human breast carcinomas and cell lines. J Clin Endocrinol Metab, 86, 1738-1745.
Cunha S.R., Mayo K.E. (2002). Ghrelin and growth hormone (GH) secretagogues potentiate GH-releasing hormone (GHRH)-induced cyclic adenosine 3', 5'-monophosphate production in cells expressing transfected GHRH and GH secretagogue receptors. Endocrinology, 143, 4570-4582.
Dalm V.A., van Hagen P.M., van Koetsveld P.M., Langerak A.W., van der Lely A.J., Lamberts S.W. and Hofland L.J. (2003). Cortistatin rather than somatostatin as a potential endogenous ligand for somatostatin receptors in the human immune system. J Clin Endocrinol Metabol, 88, 270-276.
de Lecea L., Criado J.R., Prospero-Garcia O., Gautvik K.M., Schweitzer P., Danielson P.E., Dunlop C.L., Siggins G.R., Henriksen S.J. and Sutcliffe J.G. (1996). A cortical neuropeptide with neuronal depressant and sleep-modulating properties. Nature, 381, 242-245.
de Lecea L., Ruiz-Lozano P., Danielson P.E., Peelle-Kirley J., Foye P.E., Frankel W.N. and Sutcliffe J.G. (1997a). Cloning, mRNA expression, and chromosomal mapping of mouse and human preprocortistatin. Genomics, 42, 499-506.
de Lecea L., del Rio J.A., Criado J.R., Alcantara S., Morales M., Danielson P.E., Henriksen S.J., Soriano E. and Sutcliffe J.G. (1997b). Cortistatin is expressed in a distinct subset of cortical interneurons. J Neurosci, 17, 5868-5880.
Deghenghi R., Papotti M., Ghigo E. and Muccioli G. (2001a). Cortistatin, but not somatostatin, binds to growth hormone secretagogue (GHS) receptors of human pituitary gland. J Endocrinol Invest, 24, RC1-RC3.
Deghenghi R., Papotti M., Ghigo E., Muccioli G. and Locatelli V. (2001b). Somatostatin octapeptides (lanreotide, octreotide, vapreotide, and their analogs) share the growth hormone-releasing peptide receptor in the human pituitary gland. Endocrine, 14, 29-33.
Deghenghi R., Avallone R., Torsello A., Muccioli G., Ghigo E. and Locatelli V. (2001c). Growth hormone-inhibiting activity of cortistatin in the rat. J Endocrinol Invest, 24, RC31-RC33.
Fukusumi S., Kitada C., Takekawa S., Kizawa H., Sakamoto J., Miyamoto M., Hinuma S., Kitano K. and Fujino M. (1997). Identification and characterization of a novel human cortistatin-like peptide. Biochem Biophys Res Commun, 232, 157-163.
Ghigo E., Arvat E., Gianotti L., Maccario M. and Camanni F. (1999). The regulation of

growth hormone secretion. In The Endocrine Response to Acute Illness, eds. Jenkins R.C. and Ross R.J.M., Frontiers of Hormone Research, pp. 152-175. Basel, Karger.
Ghigo E., Arvat E., Giordano R., Broglio F., Gianotti L., Maccario M., Bisi G., Graziani A., Papotti M., Muccioli G., Deghenghi R. and Camanni F. (2001). Biologic activities of growth hormone secretagogues in humans. Endocrine, 14, 87-93.
Gnanapavan S., Kola B., Bustin S.A., Morris D.G., McGee P., Fairclough P., Bhattacharya S., Carpenter R., Grossman A.B. and Korbonits M. (2002). The tissue distribution of the mRNA of ghrelin and subtypes of its receptor, GHS-R, in humans. J Clin Endocrinol Metab, 87, 2988-2991.
Goth M.I., Lyons C.E., Canny B.J. and Thorner M.O. (1992). Pituitary adenylate cyclase activating polypeptide, growth hormone (GH)-releasing peptide and GH-releasing hormone stimulate GH release through distinct pituitary receptors. Endocrinology, 130, 939-944.
Hosoda H., Kojima M., Matsuo H. and Kangawa K. (2000). Purification and characterization of rat des-Gln14-Ghrelin, a second endogenous ligand for the growth hormone secretagogue receptor. J Biol Chem, 275, 1995-2000.
Kamegai J., Tamura H., Shimizu T., Ishii S., Sugihara H. and Wakabayashi I. (2000). Central effect of ghrelin, an endogenous growth hormone secretagogue, on hypothalamic peptide gene expression. Endocrinology, 141, 4797-4800.
Kojima M., Hosoda H., Date Y., Nakazato M., Matsuo H. and Kangawa K. (1999). Ghrelin is a growth-hormone-releasing acylated peptide from stomach. Nature, 402, 656-660.
Kojima M., Hosoda H., Matsuo H. and Kangawa K. (2001a). Ghrelin: discovery of the natural endogenous ligand for the growth hormone secretagogue receptor. Trends Endocrinol Metab, 12, 118-122.
Kojima M., Hosoda H. and Kangawa K. (2001b). Purification and distribution of ghrelin: the natural endogenous ligand for the growth hormone secretagogue receptor. Hormone Res, 56, 93-97.
Kreienkamp H.J. (1999). Molecular biology of the receptors for somatostatin and cortistatin. Results Probl Cell Differ, 26, 215-237.
Maheshwari H.G., Rahim A., Shalet S.M. and Baumann G. (1999). Selective lack of growth hormone (GH) response to the GH-releasing peptide hexarelin in patients with GH-releasing hormone receptor deficiency. J Clin Endocrinol Metab, 84, 956-959.
Massoud A.F., Hindmarsh P.C. and Brook C.G. (1997). Interaction of the growth hormone releasing peptide hexarelin with somatostatin. Clin Endocrinol, 47, 537-547.
Muccioli G., Ghe C., Ghigo M.C., Papotti M., Arvat E., Boghen M.F., Nilsson M.H., Deghenghi R., Ong H. and Ghigo E. (1998). Specific receptors for synthetic GH secretagogues in the human brain and pituitary gland. J Endocrinol, 157, 99-106.
Muccioli G., Broglio F., Valetto M.R., Ghe C., Catapano F., Graziani A., Papotti M., Bisi G., Deghenghi R. and Ghigo E. (2000). Growth hormone-releasing peptides and the cardiovascular system. Ann Endocrinol, 61, 27-31.
Muccioli G., Papotti M., Locatelli V., Ghigo E. and Deghenghi R. (2001). Binding of ^{125}I-labeled ghrelin to membranes from human hypothalamus and pituitary gland. J Endocrinol Invest, 24, RC7-RC9.
Muccioli G., Tschop M., Papotti M., Deghenghi R., Heiman M. and Ghigo E. (2002a). Neuroendocrine and peripheral activities of ghrelin: implications in metabolism and obesity. Eur J Pharmacol, 440, 235-254.
Muccioli G. (2002b). Interplay between ghrelin, somatostatin and cortistatin. In Hormones. Body Composition and Physical Performances, pp. 51 (abstract). Turin, Italy, 15-17 November 2002.
Ong H., Bodart V., McNicoll N., Lamontagne D. and Bouchard J.F. (1998). Binding sites for growth hormone-releasing peptide. Growth Horm IGF Res, 8, 137-140.
Pandya N., DeMott-Friberg R., Bowers C.Y., Barkan A.L. and Jaffe C.A. (1998). Growth hormone (GH)-releasing peptide-6 requires endogenous hypothalamic GH-releasing hormone for maximal GH stimulation. J Clin Endocrinol Metab, 83, 1186-1189.

Papotti M., Ghe C., Cassoni P., Catapano F., Deghenghi R., Ghigo E. and Muccioli G. (2000). Growth hormone secretagogue binding sites in peripheral human tissues. J Clin Endocrinol Metab, 85, 3803-3807.
Popovic V., Damjanovic S., Micic D., Djurovic M., Dieguez C. and Casanueva F.F. (1995). Blocked growth hormone-releasing peptide (GHRP-6)-induced GH secretion and absence of the synergic action of GHRP-6 plus GH-releasing hormone in patients with hypothalamopituitary disconnection: evidence that GHRP-6 main action is exerted at the hypothalamic level. J Clin Endocrinol Metab, 80, 942-947.
Reichlin S. (1998). Neuroendocrinology. In: Williams Textbook of Endocrinology, 9th edn, ed. Wilson J.D., pp. 165-248. Philadelphia, Saunders.
Sanchez-Alavez M., Gomez-Chavarin M., Navarro L., Jimenez-Anguiano A., Murillo-Rodriguez E., Prado-Alcala R.A., Drucker-Colin R. and Prospero-Garcia O. (2000). Cortistatin modulates memory processes in rats. Brain Res, 858, 78-83.
Siehler S., Seuwen K. and Hoyer D. (1998). [125I]Tyr10-cortistatin14 labels all five somatostatin receptors. Naunyn Schmiedebergs Arch Pharmacol, 357, 483-489.
Smith R.G., Van der Ploeg L.H., Howard A.D., Feighner S.D., Cheng K., Hickey G.J., Wyvratt M.J. Jr., Fisher M.H., Nargund R.P. and Patchett A.A. (1997). Peptidomimetic regulation of growth hormone secretion. Endocrine Rev, 18, 621-645.
Smith R.G., Griffin P.R., Xu Y., Smith A.G., Liu K., Calacay J., Feighner S.D., Pong C., Leong D., Pomes A., Cheng K., Van der Ploeg L.H., Howard A.D., Schaeffer J. and Leonard R.J. (2000). Adenosine: a partial agonist of the growth hormone secretagogue receptor. Biochem Biophys Res Commun, 276, 1306-1313.
Spier A.D. and de Lecea L. (2000). Cortistatin: a member of the somatostatin neuropeptide family with distinct physiological functions. Brain Res Brain Res Rev, 33, 228-241.
Tannenbaum G.S. and Bowers C.Y. (2001). Interactions of growth hormone secretagogues and growth hormone-releasing hormone/somatostatin. Endocrine, 14, 21-27.
Tullin S., Hansen B.S., Ankersen M., Moller J., Von Cappelen K.A. and Thim L. (2000). Adenosine is an agonist of the growth hormone secretagogue receptor. Endocrinology, 141, 3397-3402.
Vasilaki A., Lanneau C., Dournaud P., de Lecea L., Gardette R. and Epelbaum J. (1999). Cortistatin affects glutamate sensitivity in mouse hypothalamic neurons through activation of sst2 somatostatin receptor subtype. Neuroscience, 88, 359-364.
Wren A.M., Small C.J., Fribbens C.V., Neary N.M., Ward H.L., Seal L.J., Ghatei M.A. and Bloom S.R. (2002). The hypothalamic mechanisms of the hypophysiotropic action of ghrelin. Neuroendocrinology, 76, 316-324.
Yoshihara F., Kojima M., Hosoda H., Nakazato M. and Kangawa K. (2002). Ghrelin: a novel peptide for growth hormone release and feeding regulation. Curr Opin Clin Nutr Metab Care, 5, 391-395.

CHAPTER 7

Antineoplastic and Antiangiogenic Actions of Somatostatin Analogs

L. BUSCAIL

Introduction

Somatostatin is a tetradecapeptide which participates in a variety of biological processes, including inhibition of exocrine and hormonal secretions and cell proliferation (Lamberts, 1991; Pollak and Schally, 1998). These properties are used for the treatment of hormone-producing pituitary or gastroenteropancreatic tumors by stable somatostatin analogs. Thus, hormonal suppression is produced in patients with acromegaly, or with neuroendocrine tumors such as insulinoma, glucagonoma, gastrinoma, vipoma or carcinoid syndrome. In some patients analog therapy leads to an inhibition of tumor growth. Somatostatin exerts an antiproliferative effect, either by indirectly inhibiting hormone and growth factor release, or by an inhibition of angiogenesis, or by acting directly on neoplastic cells. Somatostatin exerts its biological effects by interacting with specific receptors, which have been detected by binding assay or autoradiography in various human tumors and normal tissues. These proteins are expressed in a tissue-specific manner. A total of five somatostatin receptor subtypes (sst_1-sst_5) and one splice variant have been cloned from human, mouse and rat (Bell and Reisine, 1993; Hoyer et al., 1995). After expression of sst_1-sst_5 gene clones in mammalian cell lines we and others demonstrated a distinct profile for binding of clinically employed somatostatin analogs, such as SMS 201-995 (octreotide), BIM 23014 (lanreotide) and RC-160 (vapreotide). These analogs bind with high affinity to sst_2 and sst_5 (IC_{50}, 0.1-1 nM, $sst_2 > sst_5$), moderate affinity to sst_3 (IC_{50}, 22-25 nM). They do not bind (or display a low affinity to) sst_1 and sst_4 (IC_{50}, 200-1000 μM) (Hoyer et al., 1995, Buscail et al., 1995). They are differentially regulated and intracellular pathways coupled to each receptor have been found to be common or distinct, depending on cell type and/or G protein equipment (Table 1). The biological functions mediated by the five sst receptors has not been yet completely established. Many studies have been conducted in vitro using transfected cells, and in vivo using various somatostatin analogs that do not always display full selectivity for a given receptor subtype. However, it seems that individual sst receptors may mediate different functions. Table 2 details the main physiological functions attributed to different sst subtypes, based on studies conducted in transfected cells, animals (including sst_2 KO mice) or isolated organs.

Table 1. Transduction signal pathways coupled to somatostatin receptor subtypes

	sst_1	sst_2	sst_3	sst_4	sst_5
G Protein	G_{i3}	G_{i1}, G_{i3}, G_{o2}	G_{i1}	G_i ?	G_{i3}, G_q
Adenylate cyclase activity	↓	↓	↓	↓	↓
Tyrosine phosphatase activity	↑	↑	↑	↑	–
Calcium channels	↓	↓			↓
Potassium channels	–	↑	↑	↑	↑
Na^+/H^+ antiport	↑	–	–	–	–
Phospholipase C activity	↑	↑	↑	↑	↑↓
Phospholipase A2 activity	–	–	–	↑	–
MAPK (ERK) activity	↑	–	–	↑	↓

↑, positive regulation; ↓, negative regulation

Table 2. Biological effects coupled to the somatostatin receptor subtypes

	sst_2	sst_3	sst_5
Pituitary	↓ GH secretion	–	–
Stomach	↓ Gastrin secretion ↓ Gastric acid secretion	↓ Smooth muscle relaxation	–
Pancreas	↓ Glucagon secretion ↓ Insuline secretion	–	↓ Amylase secretion ↓ Insulin secretion
Colon	↓ Chloride secretion	–	–

Antiproliferative Effects of Somatostatin Analogs

Somatostatin and its analogs exert their antiproliferative effect through different mechanisms.

Indirect Effect

Inhibition of hormone and growth factor release, e.g. insulin, GH, gastrin, CCK- and IGF-1 may participate to this indirect antiproliferative effect. Sst_5 and sst_1 receptors would be more precisely implicated in this effect, as they can mediate the inhibition of hormone release in rodent and human. Somatostatin and analogs are also known to inhibit the local tissue production of growth factors such as IGF-1, EGF, FGF, TGFα, bombesin and VEGF.

Antiangiogenic Effect

The presence of somatostatin receptors on tumor and peritumoral vessels may suggest an effect of the peptide on neovascularization, such as inhibition of vascular cell proliferation or anoxic vasoactive effect. Inhibition of angiogenesis has been observed in many models established in vitro and in vivo, such as chicken chorioallantoic membrane, retinal vessels, human placental vein, vascular endothelial cells in culture (HUVEC) or Kaposi tumors implanted in nude mice (Danesi et al., 1997, Albini et al., 1999). Several mechanisms are possible: inhibition of vascular endothelial or myointimal cell proliferation, inhibition of cell monocyte migration and chemotaxis, and inhibition of VEGF and bFGF effects. Sst_1, sst_2, sst_3 and sst_5 have been successively implicated in these effects without a precise selectivity for a given subtype.

Immunomodulatory Effect

The Immune system is highly implicated in tumor processes. Somatostatin receptors (sst_2-sst_5) have been detected in lymphocytes and macrophagic mononuclear cells and, through these receptors, somatostatin and its anlogs may inhibit lymphocyte proliferation and IL-6, IL-2 or IFNγ release, as well as modulate NK activity. Some of these effects may thus interfere with tumor growth and progression behavior (Lichtenauer-Kaligis et al., 2000).

Direct Antiproliferative Effect

This effect have been demonstrated in many studies conducted especially on rodent and human cancer cells. After stable expression of sst(s) in NIH 3T3 and CHO cells, we demonstrated that only sst_1, sst_2 and sst_5 mediated the antiproliferative effect of the somatostatin analog RC-160. However, these receptor subtypes are coupled to distinct signal transduction pathways. Sst_1 and sst_2, mediated the stimulation of a tyrosine phosphatase activity, which is involved in the antiproliferative effect of the analogs (Buscail et al., 1994, 1995). We demonstrated that the sst_2 receptor mediated this antiproliferative effect through the association and stimulation of tyrosine phosphatase SHP-1 activity, then nNOS activation and the subsequent arrest of cells in G_0/G_1 phase of cell cycle in response to an upregulation of CDKI $p27^{KIP1}$ expression and an increase in hypophosphorylated retinoblastoma protein level (Table 3);

Table 3. Antiproliferative effect (inhibition of cell proliferation and/or cell cycle blockade and/or apoptosis) mediated by somatostatin receptor subtypes

	sst_1	sst_2	sst_3	sst_4	sst_5
Cell cycle G_0/G_1 blockade	+	+	–	+	+
Apoptosis	–	+	+	–	–
Coupling	PTP (SHP2) MAPK $p21^{WAF1}$	PTP (SHP1) nNOS $p27^{KIP1}$	?	?	cGMP

PTP, phosphoprotein tyrosine phosphatase; MAPK, mitogen activity protein kinase; nNOS, neuronal nitric oxide synthase.
+, presence of the effect; –, absence of effect; ?, unknown

(Lopez et al., 1997). For sst_5, we demonstrated a negative coupling with the GMPc/guanylate cyclase systems (Cordelier, 1997), while for sst_1 others suggested the implication of SHP2 and $p21^{WAF1}$ protein activation. Finally, sst_2 and sst_3 have been implicated in the induction of apoptosis in normal and tumor cells (Rochaix et al., 1999; Vernejoul et al., 2002).

Antioncogenic Effect of sst_2 Receptor in Human Pancreatic Cancer Cells and Pancreatic Cancer Models

Endocrine Tumors

Somatostatin analog administration is now considered an accepted treatment for neuroendocrine tumors of the gut (with stabilization and sometimes regression of tumor volumes). The dissociation observed clinically between a frequent antisecretory response and an inconstant antitumor effect after administration of somatostatin analogs may reflect in these tumors an absence of expression or coupling of the receptor(s) involved in antiproliferative effect. Moreover, a desensitization or mutation of these receptors may also occur in tumors (Aparicio et al., 2001; Arnold et al., 2000).

Non-endocrine Tumors

It is still unclear whether analog therapy is effective against non-endocrine pancreatic cancers. Clinical studies have revealed that somatostatin analog therapy does not produce an adequate clinical response in patients suffering from advanced tumor stages of pancreatic carcinoma cancer. We and others have demonstrated in this way that a specific loss of sst_2 gene expression occurs in human pancreatic adenocarcinomas and in most derived cell lines. These results correlate well with studies revealing that somatostatin binding sites are undetected or poorly detected in pancreatic adenocarcinomas using both in vitro binding assay and in vivo scintigraphy or immunohistochemistry. We postulated that the loss of sst_2 expression in pancreatic cancer could represent a growth advantage in these tumors. This conclusion was subsequently strengthened by the correction of the sst_2 defect in the human pancreatic cancer cell lines BxPC-3 and Capan-1. Stable transfection of these cells with human sst_2 cDNA resulted in the induction of a negative autocrine loop with secretion of endogenous ligand that constitutively activated the recombinant sst_2 receptor (Delesque et al., 1997). In vitro cell growth and both in vitro and in vivo tumorigenicity were significantly reduced in sst_2-expressing cells. Experiments conducted in athymic mice demonstrated a dramatic decrease in tumor growth, as well as both local and distant antitumor bystander effects. These results led us to conclude that: (a) human sst_2 acts as a tumor suppressor in pancreatic cancer; and (b) the transfer of sst_2 gene could represent a novel therapeutic approach to this adenocarcinoma.

We recently investigated the in vivo gene transfer of sst_2 in two transplantable models of primary and metastatic pancreatic carcinoma developed in hamsters.

Sst_2 was injected and expressed in exponentially growing pancreatic primary tumors or hepatic metastases by means of two different delivery agents: an adenoviral vector and a synthetic polycationic carrier (linear polyethylenimine PEI). Both adenoviral and PEI vector-based sst_2 gene transfer resulted in significant reduction of pancreatic tumor growth. This effect is associated with a significant inhibition of the proliferative index and a significant increase of apoptosis, as possible mechanisms implicated in the antitumor bystander effect (Vernejoul et al., 2002). We concluded that a synthetic gene delivery system can achieve in vivo sst_2 gene transfer and results in a significant antitumor effect. This new strategy of gene therapy allows the restoration of expression of antioncogenic molecules and could be promising for the treatment of advanced pancreatic cancer.

Analog Targeting Antineoplastic Effects

Radiotherapy

Scintigraphy using a ^{111}In-labeled somatostatin analog, octreotide (Octeroscan), is the examination of choice for diagnosis of the spread of gastroenteropancreatic and carcinoid tumors, as it is often more sensitive than morphologic imaging techniques. It can also guide radiotherapy performed with the same pharmaceutical vector. ^{111} In can be replaced by ^{90}Y or ^{188}Re. A transient palliative effect is obtained for a variable number of tumors (usually large ones). Therapeutic trials with these agents for both endocrine and non-endocrine tumors are in progress but at the present time insufficient data exists to justify the indication of "first-line" therapy.

Cytotoxic Analogs

Recently, preclinical studies have been conducted demonstrating that somatostatin receptor-targeted chemotherapy caused inhibition of growth of primary tumors and their metastases. These results have been obtained after administration of the cytotoxic somatostatin analog AN-238 (2-pyrrolinodoxorubicin linked to carrier stable somatostatin analog RC-121) in mammary, brain, prostate, renal and ovarian cancer models expressing sst_2 and sst_5 receptors. The mechanism of action of AN-238 in cancer cells remains unknown but it probably binds to the tumor membrane receptor, such as sst_2 or sst_5 and this binding results in an accumulation of its cytotoxic radical, 2-pyrrolinodoxorubicine. AN-238 may thus provide a new treatment modality for patients with advanced non-endocrine carcinomas that express somatostatin receptors displaying high affinity for analogs (Plonowski et al., 2001; Szepashazi et al., 2001).

Sensitization of sst_2 Gene Transfer

In the transplantable model of pancreatic carcinoma in hamsters, sst_2 gene transfer in pancreatic cancer cells, in combination with targeted cytotoxic somatostatin analog treatment AN238, resulted in the inhibition of primary tumor growth and metastatic progression (Benali et al., 2000). Sst_2 gene transfer in pancreatic carcinomas may result in sensitization with a targeted cytotoxic somatostatin analog improving the outcome of systemic treatment of this malignancy. Another approach has been described in a model of lung tumor using in vivo sst_2 gene transfer (by means of an adenoviral vector) associated with in vivo [^{111}In]-DTPA-D-Phe(1)-octreotide injection. This a another model of targeted radiotherapy of cancer by means of in vivo sst_2 gene transfer (Rogers et al., 2002).

Conclusions

Somatostatin is a cyclic neuropeptide widely distributed in the nervous system and digestive tract. It negatively regulates a number of processes, such as epithelial cell proliferation, exocrine and endocrine secretions. Somatostatin and its stable analogs suppress the growth of various normal and cancer cells. Somatostatin exerts an antiproliferative effect, either by indirectly inhibiting hormone and growth factor release, or by an inhibition of angiogenesis, or by acting directly on neoplastic cells. This peptide exerts a direct antiproliferative effect mediated by specific cell surface receptors. Five subtypes of somatostatin receptors have been cloned from human, mouse and rat. Among them, the subtypes sst_1, sst_2 and sst_5 are responsible for the antiproliferative effect of somatostatin and its analogs in vitro. They can mediate the effects of clinically employed analogs and are the basis of future therapeutic development, such as gene therapy or cytotoxic analog or radionuclide-targeted therapy.

References

Albini A., Florio T. and Giunciuglio D. (1999). Somatostatin controls Kaposi's sarcoma tumor growth through inhibition of angiogenesis. FASEB J, 13, 647-655.

Aparicio T., Ducreux M. and Baudin E. (2001). Antitumour activity of somatostatin analogues in progressive metastatic neuroendocrine tumours. Eur J Cancer, 37, 1014-1019.

Arnold R., Simon B. and Wied M. (2000). Treatment of neuroendocrine GEP tumours with somatostatine analogues. Digestion, 62 (suppl 1), 84-91.

Bell G.I. and Reisine, T. (1993). Molecular biology of somatostatin receptors. Trends Neurosci, 16, 34-38.

Benali N., Cordelier P., Calise D., Pages P., Rochaix P., Nagy A., Esteve J. P., Pour P. M., Schally A.V., Vaysse N., Susini C. and Buscail L. (2000). Inhibition of growth and metastatic progression of pancreatic carcinoma in hamster after somatostatin receptor subtype 2 (sst_2) gene expression and administration of cytotoxic somatostatin analog AN-238. Proc Natl Acad Sci USA, 97, 9180-9185.

Buscail L., Delesque N., Esteve J.P., Saint-Laurent N., Prats H., Clerc P., Robberecht P., Bell G.I., Liebow C., Schally A.V., Vaysse N. and Susini C. (1994). Stimulation of tyrosine phosphatase and inhibition of cell proliferation by somatostatin analogues: mediation by human somatostatin receptor subtypes SSTR1 and SSTR2. Proc Natl Acad Sci USA, 91, 2315-2319.

Buscail L., Esteve J.P., Saint-Laurent N., Bertrand V., Reisine T., O'Carroll, A.M., Bell G.I., Schally A.V., Vaysse N. and Susini C. (1995). Inhibition of cell proliferation by the somatostatin analogue RC-160 is mediated by somatostatin receptor subtypes SSTR2 and SSTR5 through different mechanisms. Proc Natl Acad Sci USA, 92, 1580-1584.
Cordelier P., Estève J.P., Bousquet C., Delesque N., O'Carroll A.-M., Schally A.V., Vaysse N., Susini C. and Buscail L. (1997). Characterization of the antiproliferative signal mediated by the somatostatin receptor subtype sst5. Proc Nat Acad Sci USA, 94, 9343-9348.
Danesi R., Agen C. and Benelli U. (1997). Inhibition of experimental angiogenesis by the somatostatin octreotide acetate (SMS 201-995). Clin Cancer Res, 3, 265-272.
Delesque N., Buscail L., Esteve J.P., Saint-Laurent N., Muller C., Weckbecker G., Bruns C., Vaysse N. and Susini C. (1997). Sst_2 Somatostatin receptor expression reverses tumorigenicity of human pancreatic cancer cells. Cancer Res, 57, 956-962.
Hoyer D., Bell G.I., Berelowitz M., Epelbaum J., Feniuk W., Humphrey P.P., O'Carroll A.M., Patel Y.C., Schonbrunn A. and Taylor J.E. (1995). Classification and nomenclature of somatostatin receptors. Trends Pharmacol Sci, 16, 86-88.
Lamberts S.W., Krenning E.P. and Reubi J.C. (1991). The role of somatostatin and its analogs in the diagnosis and treatment of tumors. Endocr Rev, 12, 450-482.
Lichtenauer-Kaligis E.G., Van Hagen P.M., Lamberts S.W. and Hofland L.J. (2000). Somatostatin receptor subtypes in human immune cells. Eur J Endocrinol, 143 (suppl 1), S21-S25.
Lopez F., Esteve J.P., Buscail L., Delesque N., Saint-Laurent N., Theveniau M., Nahmias C., Vaysse N. and Susini C. (1997). The tyrosine phosphatase SHP-1 associates with the sst_2 somatostatin receptor and is an essential component of sst_2-mediated inhibitory growth signaling. J Biol Chem, 272, 24448-24454.
Plonowski A., Schally A.V., Koppan M., Nagy A., Arencibia J.M., Csernus B. and Halmos G. (2001). Inhibition of the UCI-107 human ovarian carcinoma cell line by a targeted cytotoxic analog of somatostatin, AN-238. Cancer, 92, 1168-1176.
Pollak M.N. and Schally A.V. (1998). Mechanisms of antineoplastic action of somatostatin analogs. Proc Soc Exp Biol Med, 217, 143-152.
Rochaix P., Delesque N., Esteve J. P., Saint-Laurent N., Voight J.J., Vaysse N., Susini C. and Buscail L. (1999). Gene therapy for pancreatic carcinoma: local and distant antitumor effects after somatostatin receptor sst_2 gene transfer. Hum Gene Ther, 10, 995-1008.
Rogers B.E., Zinn K.R., Lin C.Y., Chaudhuri T.R. and Buchsbaum D.J. (2002). Targeted radiotherapy with [(90)Y]-SMT 487 in mice bearing human non-small cell lung tumor xenografts induced to express human somatostatin receptor subtype 2 with an adenoviral vector. Cancer, 94 (suppl 4), 1298-1305.
Szepeshazi K., Schally A.V., Halmos G., Sun B., Hebert F., Csernus B. and Nagy A. (2001). Targeting of cytotoxic somatostatin analog AN-238 to somatostatin receptor subtypes 5 and/or 3 in experimental pancreatic cancers. Clin Cancer Res, 7, 2854-2861.
Vernejoul F., Faure P., Benali N., Calise D., Tiraby G., Pradayrol L., Susini C. and Buscail L. (2002). Antitumor effect of in vivo somatostatin receptor sst_2 gene transfer in primary and metastatic pancreatic cancer models. Cancer Res, 62, 6124-6131.

CHAPTER 8

Somatostatin in Clinical Endocrinology

W.W. DE HERDER AND S.W.J. LAMBERTS

Somatostatin and Its Receptor Subtypes

The small cyclic peptide hormone, somatostatin (ss), is present in the human body in two molecular forms: somatostatin-14 (consisting of 14 amino acids) and somatostatin-28 (28 amino acids). It exerts diverse biologic effects through interaction with specific somatostatin receptors (ssts) in its target tissues. Ss acts as an inhibitor of endocrine and exocrine secretory processes, neurotransmission and as an immune modulation (Lamberts et al., 1996). Ssts belong to the family of G-protein coupled receptors, which characteristically consist of a single polypeptide chain with seven transmembrane spanning domains: extracellular domains with ligand binding sites and intracellular domains with sites linked to the activation of second messengers. At present, five different human sst subtypes (sst_1, sst_2, sst_3, sst_4, and sst_5) have been cloned and characterised (Patel, 1999). Ssts are encoded by five different genes, each with a distinct chromosomal localization. Although the different sst subtypes are 40% to 60% structurally homologous, each sst subtype mediates different biologic actions of somatostatin. The inhibitory effects of somatostatin or its analogs, mediated via ssts, are linked with several intra-cellular systems: inhibition of adenylyl cyclase, resulting in a decrease in the intracellular cyclic AMP levels; reduction of Ca^{2+} influxes, resulting in reduced intracellular Ca^{2+} levels; and, in a number of tissues, stimulation of tyrosine phosphatase activity. Activation of sst_1 and sst_2, via the activation of tyrosine phosphatase, has been correlated with antimitotic activity of somatostatin analogs. Activation of sst_5, via reduction of intracellular Ca^{2+} levels, also results in inhibition of cell proliferation. Sst_3 mediates apoptosis (Sharma et al., 1996; Benali et al., 2000a; Patel, 1999; Bousquet et al., 2001). Although very preliminary, some specific physiologic regulatory roles might be attributed to these sst subtypes: in man sst_2 and sst_5 are involved in the control GH release; sst_5 seems of importance in the control of insulin, and possibly glucagon release.

A large variety of primary tumors and their metastases can express a high density of ssts. Pituitary tumors, endocrine pancreatic tumors, and carcinoids express multiple sst subtypes, but sst_2 predominance is found in 90% of carcinoids and 80% of endocrine pancreatic tumors. Sst_2 and sst_5 predominance is found in growth hormone-secreting pituitary tumors. It has also been demonstrated that the number and distribution of somatostatin receptors between primary tumors, but also between their tumor deposits, may vary. This receptor heterogeneity might explain differences in clinical responses to somatostatin analog treatment in the same class of tumors (Lamberts et al., 1996; Patel, 1999).

Somatostatin Analogs

Because of its half-life of less than 3 minutes, only continuous intravenous administration of somatostatin may produce therapeutic effects. However, the synthesized octapeptide analogs of somatostatin, octreotide and lanreotide, can be administered by multiple subcutaneous injections or by continuous subcutaneous infusion as well as by the intravenous route, either as a single injection or as a continuous infusion over many hours or days. The slow-release depot intramuscular formulation of octreotide (Sandostatin LAR) has to be administered once every 4 weeks and that of lanreotide (Lanreotide-PR) has to be administered once every 2 weeks. A new slow-release depot preparation of lanreotide, Lanreotide Autogel, has been introduced in a number of European countries. This drug has to be administered subcutaneously once every 4 weeks (Lamberts et al., 1996).

Both somatostatin-14 and somatostatin-28 bind with high affinities to all sst subtypes. Octreotide and lanreotide have comparable binding profiles and bind with a high affinity to sst_2 and sst_5, with only low affinity to sst_3, and with no affinity to sst_1 and sst_4 (Lamberts et al., 1996).

Using CHO-K_1 transfected cells, Patel's group demonstrated ligand-induced sst dimerization (Patel et al., 1999). Both natural SS and SS analogs can produce homo- or heterodimerization of sst_1 and sst_5 (Rocheville et al., 2000a, b). Such a ligand-induced dimerization process resulted in increased binding affinity and modified sst subtypes. This means that protein interaction between different members of the sst subfamiliy are involved in a molecular cross-talk, which induces new possibilities to regulate cellular hormonal sensitivity. This suggests that different sst subtypes in target organs and/or tumors operate in concert, rather than as individual members. The sst_2 and sst_5 bi-specific compound BIM 23244 suppresses GH and PRL release by primary cultures of acromegalic tumors synergistically (Saveanu et al., 2001). Unexpectedly, a sst_2 preferential agonist antagonized a sst_5-selective agonist on the growth of cultured medullary thyroid cancer cells, however (Zatelli et al., 2001). Also cross-talk between different related G-protein coupled receptor families resulting in enhanced functional activity was demonstrated: a SS-dopamine hybrid molecule, BIM 23A387 demonstrated in vitro an enhanced effect on PRL release by cultured rat pituitary cells (Ren et al., 2000). The simultaneous expression of multiple sst subtypes on the same cells in target organs, as well as most human sst expressing tumors indicates that a differential coupling via the 5 sst subtypes which activate simultaneously a variety of intracellular signaling systems are an essential part of SS function, which has to be further explored. The interactive, multireceptor responses which now include homo- and heterodimerization and cross-talk at the membrane level with other G-protein coupled systems is a tantalizing new concept for drug designers (Bruns et al., 2002).

Recently, following a rational drug design approach by synthesizing alanine-substituted SS-14 analogs, the importance of single amino acids in SS-14 for sst subtype binding was established (Bruns et al., 2002). The incorporation of structural elements of SS-14 in a stable cyclohexapeptide template in the form of modified unnatural amino acids resulted in the identification of the novel cyclohexapeptide SOM 230. SOM 230 binds with high affinity to sst_1,

sst_2, sst_3 and sst_5 and displays a 30- to 40- fold higher affinitiy for sst_1 and sst_5 that octreotide. In vivo SOM 230 showed a potent, long lasting inhibitory effect on GH and Insulin-like growth factor (IGF)-1 release, making it a promising development candidate for effective GH and IGF-1 inhibition (Bruns et al., 2002).

Somatostatin Analog Treatment

Expression of ssts by (neuro-) endocrine tumors is essential for the control of hormonal hypersecretion by the octapeptide somatostatin analogs. In sst_2- or sst_5-positive patients, clinical symptomatology can be controlled by the chronic administration of one of the currently available octapeptide somatostatin analogs. In sst_2- and sst_5-positive patients, these drugs may also exert some antiproliferative action. Several mechanisms might play a role in this effect: direct antimitotic effects, suppression of the production and biologic activity of IGF-1, regulation of the IGF-binding proteins, action through other tumor growth factors, action through inhibition of angiogenesis and tumor blood supply, regulation of the immune response, and induction of apoptosis (Bousquet et al., 2001; de Herder et al., 1996a, b; Öberg, 2001; Scarpignato and Pelosini, 2001).

Octreotide and lanreotide are registered in most European countries for the control of hormonal symptoms in patients with carcinoids and neuroendocrine pancreatic tumors and in patients with acromegaly.

Octreotide treatment (median dose, 100 μg tid sc) in patients with metastatic carcinoid tumors resulted in symptomatic improvement in more than 90% of patients, a biochemical response in 60% to 70% of patients, objective tumor regression in less than 10% of patients, and temporary stabilization of tumor growth in more than 80% of patients. Similar results have been obtained with subcutaneous lanreotide treatment (Kvols et al., 1986; Arnold et al., 2000; Caplin et al., 1998).

With the slow-release depot intramuscular formulations Sandostatin LAR and Lanreotide-PR, symptomatic improvement can be achieved in approximately 40% to 55% of patients, a biochemical response in 40% to 50%, objective tumor regression in less than 10%, and temporary stabilization of tumor growth in more than 80% (Ruszniewski et al., 1996; Wymenga et al., 1999). Although somatostatin analog treatment is not the primary treatment for patients with gastrinomas, they produce a significant reduction of serum gastrin and acid secretion, accompanied by a decrease of complaints related to gastric hypersecretion in more than 90% of patients. Approximately 50% of insulin-producing tumors do not express sst_2 and sst_5. In patients harbouring these tumors, somatostatin analog treatment may suppress hormones that counterregulate hypoglycaemia, such as growth hormone and IGF-1, and glucagon, which may eventually lead to more severe hypoglycaemias. In patients with VIPomas and glucagonomas, somatostatin analog treatment also produces significant biochemical responses in 80% and 60% of patients, respectively (de Herder et al., 1996; Öberg, 2001).

In primarily untreated patients with acromegaly as well as in patients primarily treated with surgery or radiotherapy, or both, octreotide treatment produces symptomatic relief, accompanied by normalization of pathologically elevated serum IGF-1 levels in 60% to 70% of patients and causes tumor stabilization or even reduction (Newman et al., 1998). With the slow-release depot intramuscular formulations Sandostatin LAR and Lanreotide-PR, similar results can be achieved (Verhelst et al., 2000; Chanson et al., 2000). Short- and long-acting somatostatin analogs also effectively control the excessive hormone production and tumor size in patients with thyroid-stimulating hormone-secreting pituitary tumors; in selected patients with clinically non-functioning pituitary adenomas who presented themselves with impairment of the visual system, clinical improvement has been observed (Beck-Peccoz et al., 1996; Warnet et al., 1997).

Preliminary data show that ultra-high doses of somatostatin analogs (1200 mg octreotide [Onco-LAR] per month, or 10-15 mg lanreotide per day) may induce apoptosis in some patients with metastatic carcinoids and pancreatic neuroendocrine tumors (Öberg, 2001).

Careful studies also suggest a temporary stabilization of (metastatic) tumor growth, during SS analog therapy in one third to two third of patients with carcinoids and islet cell tumors (Arnold et al., 2000). The observed prolonged survival in octreotide-treated patients with these metastasized gastroenteropancreatic (GEP) tumors seems related at least in part to this temporary inhibition of tumor growth, but might also be attributed to the improvement in the quality of life of these patients. The compliance of the use of SS analogs like octreotide and lanreotide has further improved as long-acting depot formulations of these compounds became available.

An important aspect of the long-term successful control of hormone secretion and tumor cell growth during SS analog treatment is tachyphylaxis (Lamberts et al., 2001). Whereas normal hormone secretion shows tachyphylaxis following continuous receptor activation within hours to days after the start of SS analog administration, hormone secretion by sst-positive NE tumors can be inhibited during prolonged periods. Octreotide controls hormone secretion effectively in most acromegalics for many years. "Escape" from therapy has not been observed. In striking contrast the initial rapid improvement of clinical symptomatology in the first weeks to months of SS analog therapy in patients with GEP tumors gradually "escapes", despite an increase in the dose administered. The potential mechanisms responsible for this loss of control, as well as for the considerable variability in the duration of the responses to octreotide are not known (Lamberts et al., 2001). The relative long time-frame of this "escape" suggests that mechanisms other that G-protein uncoupling or internalization are involved. Most probably this loss of sensitivity of NE cancers to octreotide is associated with the outgrowth of clones of tumor cells that lack, or that developed mutations in the sst (Lamberts et al., 2001).

Side Effects of Somatostatin Analog Treatment

Octapeptide somatostatin analogs are generally tolerated very well. Side effects are mild and include abdominal discomfort, flatulence, diarrhoea, steatorrhea, nausea, and formation of asymptomatic bile stones and gallbladder sludge in 20% to 50% of patients (Lamberts et al., 2001; Trendle et al., 1997).

Somatostatin Receptor Scintigraphy

Tumors and metastases that bear sst_2 or sst_5 can be visualised in vivo using gamma camera pictures obtained after injection of [^{111}In-DTPA0-D-Phe1]octreotide [111In-pentetreotide (OctreoScan)] or ^{111}In-DOTA-lanreotide (^{111}In-MAURITIUS) (Krenning et al., 1993; Kwekkeboom et al., 2000; Virgolini et al., 2000). A positive scintigram in a patient with a pancreatic neuroendocrine tumor or carcinoid tumor generally predicts a therapeutic effect of octapeptide analogs on hormonal hypersecretion by these tumors (Janson et al., 1994). False-negative scintigrams can be produced by tumors with low sst_2 and sst_5 density or tumors with high endogenous somatostatin production. False-positive results can be produced by non-neoplastic sst_2- and sst_5-positive tissues, binding to antibodies against chronically injected octreotide, and binding to sst_2 and sst_5 on the peritumoral vascular system and lymphocytes. ^{111}In-pentetreotide scintigraphy can also be useful in the follow-up of patients who have undergone curative surgery to detect tumor regrowth or new metastases at a very early stage. However, as already mentioned, this technique has a very high sensitivity for sst_2- and sst_5-positive tumors, but a low specificity. Somatostatin receptor scintigraphy has only limited value in the diagnosis and follow-up of patients with pituitary tumors (Kwekkeboom et al., 1999; de Herder and Lamberts, 1995).

Radiolabeled octapeptide analogs can also be used in combination with a hand-held radionuclide probe, assisting the surgeon as an intra-abdominal scanning device in the intraoperative search for sst_2- and sst_5-positive tumor deposits and allowing for complete removal (Benevento, 1998).

Tumor-Targeted Radioactive Somatostatin Analog Treatment and Chemotherapy

Most polypeptide hormones and neuropeptides are internalized after their binding to specific high affinity membrane receptors. A number of preclinical studies strongly support the concept that binding of SS to sst is followed by rapid internalization of the receptor-ligand complex (Lamberts et al., 2001). However the degree of internalization of SS may be cell type, as well as sst subtype specific. In CHO-K_1 cells stably expressing one of the five human sst subtypes it was found that sst_2, sst_3, sst_4 and sst_5 receptors displayed rapid agonist-dependent internalization of ^{125}I-SS28 ligand within minutes, with a maximum after 60 minutes (van Eijck et al., 1994; Ingle et al., 1999).

The demonstration of an efficient and considerable internalization of receptor-ligand complexes into sst-positive tumor cells formed the basis for the concept of targeted sst-mediated chemo- or radiotherapy of sst-expressing metastatic human cancer (Hofland et al., 1999; Jenkins et al., 2001). The process of internalization brings the cytotoxic SS analog or the radionucline-coupled analog into the cell closer to the nucleus and its DNA. This results in a prolonged cellular retention and exposure to radioactivity or the cytotoxic agent.

The wide spectrum of adverse reactions in patients with advanced, metastatic tumors treated with chemotherapeutic agents are caused by the severe toxicity of these agents to normal cells. The "magic bullet" approach by developing targeted hybrids directed against sst was extensively studied by Schally's group (Benali et al., 2000b). They synthesized two different cytotoxic SS analogs, codenamed AN-51 and AN-238 (consisting of methotrexate, and a metabolite of doxorubicin, respectively, coupled to the SS analog RC-121) which at low dose inhibit the growth of a number of experimental tumor models, including human pancreatic, breast, prostate and renal cancer. Sst-targeted chemotherapy is effective in these pre-clinical tumor models and is a highly promising approach to treat sst-positive human cancers. This approach using lower dosages of targeted chemotherapeutic agents causes lower toxicity. No clinical trials have reported so far with these new compounds.

A high uptake of radioactivity or the chemotherapeutic agent is necessary, as non-neoplastic tissues expressing ssts should not be exposed to the toxic effects of the radio-ligand or cytotoxic analog (Krenning et al., 1999). Currently, ^{111}In-pentetreotide, which emits Auger electrons (which have a tissue penetration of only 0.02-10 μm), as well as conversion electrons, has been used for radiotherapy of sst_2-and sst_5-positive advanced or metastatic endocrine tumors, such as carcinoids and pancreatic neuroendocrine tumors, pheochromocytomas, medullary thyroid carcinomas, and paragangliomas. However, depending on the homogeneity of sst expression patterns and tumor size, α-emitting radioligands such as [^{90}Y-DOTA0,Tyr3]-octreotide (OctreoTher), [^{177}Lu-DOTA0,Tyr^{3}]-octreotate and ^{90}Y-lanreotide may prove to be more effective for targeted-targeted radiotherapy in the near future (Smith et al., 2000; de Jong et al., 2001).

The effects of ^{177}Lu-octreotate therapy were studied in 35 patients with neuroendocrine gastro-entero-pancreatic tumors who underwent follow-up for 3-6 months after receiving their final dose (Kwekkeboom et al., 2003). Patients were treated with doses of 100, 150 or 200 mCi ^{177}Lu-octreotate, to a final cumulative dose of 600-800 mCi, with treatment intervals of 6-9 weeks. Nausea and vomiting within the first 24h after administration were present in 30% and 14% of the administrations, respectively. WHO toxicity grade 3 anemia, leucocytopenia, and thrombocytopenia occurred after 0%, 1% and 1% of the administrations, respectively. Serum creatinine and creatinine clearance did not change significantly. The effects of the therapy on tumor size were evaluable in 34 patients. Three months after the final administration, complete remission was found in one patient (3%), partial remission in 12 (35%), stable disease in 14 (41%) and progressive disease in seven (21%), including three patients who died during the treatment period. An example is given in Fig. 1. Tumor response correlated positively with a high uptake on the octreoscan, limited hepatic tumor mass and a high Karnofsky Performance Score (Kwekkeboom et al., 2003).

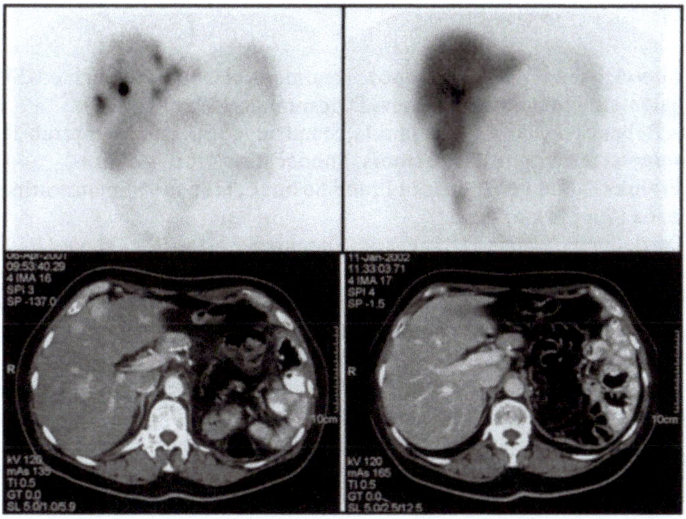

Fig. 1. Patient with liver metastases from a neuroendocrine tumor before (*lefthand images*) and 3 months after (*righthand images*) four cycles of 200 mCi [^{177}Lu-DOTA^0,Tyr^3]octreotate therapy. *Top row*: OcreoScans of the abdomen; *bottom row*: MRI of the abdomen. Note that the multiple liver metastases have completely disappeared after therapy. (Courtesy of Dr. D.J. Kwekkeboom)

Future Perspectives

Because every sst has distinct biologic functions, the development of new classes of sst subtype-selective analogs may provide valuable information for tumor diagnosis, prognosis, and prediction of somatostatin analog efficacy, not only in tumors that are sensitive to the currently available octapeptide analogs, but also in tumors that express ssts other than sst_2 and sst_5. Non-peptide compounds that can be administered via the oral route and display good bioavailability will give greater comfort to the patient. New compounds, which display higher plasma levels, greater distribution into sst-positive tissues, and a long stability in the body, will also contribute to better management of somatostatin-sensitive disorders. Powerful α- or β-emitting isotopes coupled to somatostatin (or analogs), in combination with drugs that stimulate their internalization and drugs that shorten accumulation of these radioligands in nontumorous tissues will potentially increase the therapeutic potential of tumor-targeted radiotherapy for metastatic sst-positive tumors. Also, as already alluded to, the concept of somatostatin analogs coupled to cytotoxic drugs is interesting and challenging. Although still at a very early stage, gene therapy may represent an exiting new treatment alternative for patients with advanced tumors. Transfer of genes that encode for the expression of sst_2 and sst_5 to sst-negative cancers may render these tumors responsive to the currently available (radiolabeled or cytotoxic) somatostatin analogs (Jenkins et al., 2001; Benali et al., 2000b).

References

Arnold R., Simon B. and Wied M. (2000). Treatment of neuroendocrine GEP tumours with somatostatin analogues: a review. Digestion, 62 (Suppl 1),84–91.

Beck-Peccoz P., Brucker-Davis F., Persani L., Smallridge R.C. and Weintraub B.D. (1996). Thyrotropin-secreting pituitary tumors. Endocr Rev, 17, 610–638.

Benali N., Ferjoux G., Puente E., Buscail L. and Susini C. (2000a). Somatostatin receptors. Digestion, 62 (Suppl 1), 27–32.

Benali N., Cordelier P., Calise D., Pages P., Rochaix P., Nagy A., Esteve J.P., Pour P.M., Schally A.V., Vaysse N., Susini C. and Buscail L. (2000b). Inhibition of growth and metastatic progression of pancreatic carcinoma in hamster after somatostatin receptor subtype 2 (sst_2) gene expression and administration of cytotoxic somatostatin analog AN-238. Proc Nat Acad Sci USA, 97, 9180–9185.

Benevento A., Dominioni L., Carcano G. and Dionigi R. (1998). Intraoperative localization of gut endocrine tumors with radiolabeled somatostatin analogs and a gamma-detecting probe. Semin Surg Oncol, 15, 239–244.

Bousquet C., Puente E., Buscail L., Vaysse N. and Susini C. (2001). Antiproliferative effect of somatostatin and analogs. Chemotherapy, 47 (Suppl 2), 30–39.

Bruns C., Lewis I., Briner U., Meno-Tetang G. and Weckbecker G. (2002). SOM230: a new somatostatin peptidomimetic with a broad SRIF receptor binding and a unique inhibitory profile. Eur J Endocrinol, 146, 707-716.

Caplin M.E., Buscombe J.R., Hilson A.J., Jones A.L., Watkinson A.F. and Burroughs A.K. (1998) Carcinoid tumour. Lancet, 352, 799–805.

Chanson P., Boerlin V., Ajzenberg C., Bachelot Y., Benito P., Bringer J., Caron P., Charbonnel B., Cortet C., Delemer B., Escobar-Jimenez F., Foubert L., Gaztambide S., Jockenhoevel F., Kuhn J.M., Leclere J., Lorcy Y., Perlemuter L., Prestele H., Roger P., Rohmer V., Santen R., Sassolas G., Scherbaum W.A., Schopohl J., Torres E., Varela C., Villamil F. and Webb S.M (2000). Comparison of octreotide acetate LAR and lanreotide SR in patients with acromegaly. Clin Endocrinol (Oxford), 53, 577–586.

de Herder W.W. and Lamberts S.W.J. (1995). Imaging of pituitary tumours. Baillieres Clin Endocrinol Metabolism, 9, 367–389.

de Herder W.W., van der Lely A.J. and Lamberts S.W.J. (1996). Somatostatin analogue treatment of neuroendocrine tumors. Postgrad Med J, 72, 403–408.

de Herder W.W., Hofland L.J., van der Lely A.J. and Lamberts S.W. (1996). Peptide receptors in gut endocrine tumours. Baillieres Clinical Gastroenterology, 10, 571–587.

de Jong M., Breeman W.A., Bernard B.F., Bakker W.H., Schaar M., van Gameren A., Bugaj J.E., Erion J., Schmidt M., Srinivasan A. and Krenning E.P. (2001). [^{177}Lu-DOTA(^{0}), Tyr^3] octreotate for somatostatin receptor-targeted radionuclide therapy. Int J Cancer, 92, 628–633.

Hofland L.J., Breeman W.A., Krenning E.P., de Jong M., Waaijers M., van Koetsveld P.M., Macke H.R. and Lamberts S.W. (1999). Internalization of [DOTA, ^{125}I-Tyr^3]Octreotide by somatostatin receptor-positive cells in vitro and in vivo: implications for somatostatin receptor-targeted radio-guided surgery. Proc Assoc Am Physician, 111, 63-69.

Ingle J.N., Suman V.J., Kardinal C.G., Krook J.E., Mailliard J.A., Veeder M.H., Loprinzi C.L., Dalton R.J., Hartmann L.C., Conover C.A. and Pollak M.N. (1999). A randomized trial of tamoxifen alone or combined with octreotide in the treatment of women with metastatic breast carcinoma. Cancer, 85, 1284-1292.

Jenkins S.A., Kynaston H.G., Davies N.D., Baxter J.N. and Nott D.M. (2001). Somatostatin analogs in oncology: a look to the future. Chemotherapy, 47 (Suppl 2), 162–196.

Krenning E.P., Kwekkeboom D.J., Bakker W.H., Breeman W.A., Kooij P.P., Oei H.Y., van Hagen M., Postema P.T., de Jong M. and Reubi J.C., (1993). Somatostatin receptor scintigraphy with [^{111}In-DTPA-D-Phe1]- and [^{123}I-Tyr^3]-octreotide: the Rotterdam experience with more than 1000 patients. Eur J Nucl Med, 20, 716–731.

Krenning E.P., de Jong M., Kooij P.P., Breeman W.A., Bakker W.H., de Herder W.W., van Eijck C.H., Kwekkeboom D.J., Jamar F., Pauwels S. and Valkema R. (1999). Radiolabelled somatostatin analogue(s) for peptide receptor scintigraphy and radionuclide therapy. Ann Oncol, 10 (Suppl 2), S23–S29.

Kvols L.K., Moertel C.G., O'Connell M.J., Schutt A.J., Rubin J. and Hahn R.G. (1986). Treatment of the malignant carcinoid syndrome: evaluation of a long-acting somatostatin analogue. New Engl J Med, 315, 663–666.

Kwekkeboom D.J., de Herder W.W. and Krenning E.P. (1999). Receptor imaging in the diagnosis and treatment of pituitary tumors. J Endocrinol Invest, 22, 80–88.

Kwekkeboom D., Krenning E.P. and de Jong M. (2000). Peptide receptor imaging and therapy. J Nucl Med, 41, 1704–1713.

Kwekkeboom D.J., Bakker W.H., Kam B.L., Teunissen J.J.M., Kooij P.P.M., Herder W.W., Feelders R.A., Eijck C.H.J., Jong M., Srinivasan A., Erion J.L. and Krenning E.P. (2003). Treatment of patients with gastro-entero-pancreatic (GEP) tumours with the novel radiolabelled somatostatin analogue [^{177}Lu-DOTA^{0},Tyr^{3}] octreotate. Eur J Nucl Med, 30, 417-422.

Lamberts S.W.J., van der Lely A.J., de Herder W.W. and Hofland L.J. (1996). Octreotide. New Engl J Med, 334, 246–254.

Lamberts S.W.J., Hofland L.J. and Nobels F.R. (2001) Neuroendocrine tumor markers. Frontiers Neuroendocrinology, 22, 309-339.

Newman CB, Melmed S, George A, Torigian D, Duhaney M, Snyder P, Young W, Klibanski A, Molitch ME, Gagel R, Sheeler L, Cook D, Malarkey W, Jackson I, Vance ML, Barkan A, Frohman L and Kleinberg DL. (1998). Octreotide as primary therapy for acromegaly. Journal of Clinical Endocrinology & Metabolism, 83, 3034–3040.

Öberg K. (2001). Established clinical use of octreotide and lanreotide in oncology. Chemotherapy, 47 (Suppl 2), 40–53.

Patel Y.C. (1999). Somatostatin and its receptor family. Frontiers Neuroendocrinology, 20, 157–198.

Ren, S., Culler M., Heany T. and Melmed S. (2000). Functional association of $sstr_2$ and $sstr_5$ in suppression of growth hormone secretion. The Endocrine Society Denver, 339 abstract.

Rocheville M., Lange D.C., Kumar U., Sasi R., Patel R.C. and Patel Y.C. (2000a). Subtypes of the somatostatin receptor assemble as functional homo- and heterodimers. J Biol Chem, 275, 7862-7869.

Rocheville M., Lange D.C., Kumar U., Patel S.C., Patel R.C. and Patel Y.C. (2000b). Receptors for dopamine and somatostatin: formation of hetero-oligomers with enhanced functional activity [see comments]. Science, 288, 154-157.

Ruszniewski P., Ducreux M., Chayvialle J.A., Blumberg J., Cloarec D., Michel H., Raymond J.M., Dupas J.L., Gouerou H., Jian R., Genestin E., Bernades P. and Rougier P. (1996). Treatment of the carcinoid syndrome with the longacting somatostatin analogue lanreotide: a prospective study in 39 patients. Gut, 39, 279–283.

Saveanu A., Gunz G., Dufour H., Caron P., Fina F., Ouafik L., Culler M.D., Moreau J.P., Enjalbert A. and Jaquet P. (2001). Bim-23244, a somatostatin receptor subtype 2- and 5-selective analog with enhanced efficacy in suppressing growth hormone (GH) from octreotide-resistant human GH-secreting adenomas. Journal of Clinical Endocrinology & Metabolism, 86, 140-145.

Scarpignato C. and Pelosini I. (2001). Somatostatin analogs for cancer treatment and diagnosis: an overview. Chemotherapy, 47 (Suppl 2), 1–29.

Sharma, K., Patel Y.C. and Srikat C.B. (1996). Subtype-selective induction of wild-type p53 and apoptosis, but not cell cycle arrest, by human somatostatin receptor 3. Mol Endocrinol, 10, 1688-1696.

Smith M.C., Liu J., Chen T., Schran H., Yeh C.M., Jamar F., Valkema R., Bakker W., Kvols L., Krenning E. and Pauwels S. (2000). OctreoTher: ongoing early clinical development of a somatostatin-receptor-targeted radionuclide antineoplastic therapy. Digestion, 62 (Suppl 1). 69–72.

Tiensuu Janson E.T., Westlin J.E., Eriksson B., Ahlstrom H., Nilsson S and Oberg K. (1994). [^{111}In-DTPA-D-Phe^{1}] octreotide scintigraphy in patients with carcinoid tumours: the predictive value for somatostatin analogue treatment. Eur J Endocrinol, 131, 577–581.
Trendle M.C., Moertel C.G. and Kvols L.K. (1997). Incidence and morbidity of cholelithiasis in patients receiving chronic octreotide for metastatic carcinoid and malignant islet cell tumors. Cancer, 79, 830–834.
van Eijck, C.H. Krenning E.P., Bootsma A.H., Oei H.Y., van Pel R.. Lindemans J., Jeekel J.J., Reubi J.C. and Lamberts S.W. (1994). Somatostatin-receptor scintigraphy in primary breast cancer [see comments]. Lancet, 343, 640-643.
Verhelst J.A., Pedroncelli A.M., Abs R., Montini M., Vandeweghe M.V., Albani G., Maiter D., Pagani M.D., Legros J.J., Gianola D., Bex M., Poppe K., Mockel J. and Pagani G.(2000). Slow-release lanreotide in the treatment of acromegaly: a study in 66 patients. Eur J Endocrinol, 143, 577–584.
Virgolini I., Traub T., Leimer M., Novotny C., Pangerl T., Ofluoglu S., Halvadjieva E., Smith-Jones P., Flores J., Li S.R., Angelberger P., Havlik E., Andreae F., Raderer M., Kurtaran A., Niederle B. and Dudczak R.(2000). New radiopharmaceuticals for receptor scintigraphy and radionuclide therapy. Q Journal of Nuclear Medicine, 44, 50–58.
Warnet A., Harris A.G., Renard E., Martin D., James-Deidier A. and Chaumet-Riffaud P. (1997). A prospective multicenter trial of octreotide in 24 patients with visual defects caused by nonfunctioning and gonadotropin-secreting pituitary adenomas. French Multicenter Octreotide Study Group. Neurosurgery, 41, 786–795.
Wymenga A.N., Eriksson B., Salmela P.I., Jacobsen M.B., Van Cutsem E.J., Fiasse R.H., Valimaki M.J., Renstrup J., de Vries E.G. and Oberg K.E. (1999). Efficacy and safety of prolonged-release lanreotide in patients with gastrointestinal neuroendocrine tumors and hormone-related symptoms. J Clin Oncol, 17, 1111.
Zatelli M.C., Tagliati F., Taylor J.E., Rossi R., Culler M.D. and Uberti E.C. (2001). Somatostatin receptor subtypes 2 and 5 differentially affect proliferation in vitro of the human medullary thyroid carcinoma cell line tt. Journal of Clinical Endocrinology & Metabolism, 86, 2161-2169.

Chapter 9

Antagonists of Growth Hormone-releasing Hormone in Oncology

A.V. Schally

Growth Hormone-releasing Hormone (GHRH)

Growth hormone-releasing hormone (GHRH) is secreted by the hypothalamus and, upon binding to specific GHRH receptors in the pituitary, stimulates the synthesis and the release of GH. GHRH is also present in several extrahypothalamic tissues, including placenta, ovary, testis, gastrointestinal tract and tumors of neuroendocrine origin (Bagnato et al., 1992). Thus, the presence of GHRH ligand was demonstrated in human prostatic, ovarian, endometrial, mammary and lung cancers, suggesting that GHRH could be a growth factor for these tumors. The identification of growth hormone-releasing hormone (GHRH) was facilitated by the demonstration of ectopic production of GHRH by carcinoid and pancreatic cell tumors (Frohman and Szabo, 1981).

The 44- and 40-amino acid forms of GHRH were first isolated from human pancreatic tumors and only subsequently identified in human hypothalamus (Guillemin et al., 1982; Rivier et al., 1982). GHRH is structurally related to vasoactive intestinal peptide (VIP) and secretin. The full intrinsic biological activity is retained by the NH_2-terminal 29 amino acid sequence [GHRH(1-29)NH_2].

Agonistic and Antagonistic Analogs of GHRH

Many agonistic analogs of GHRH(1-29)NH_2 were synthesized for clinical and veterinary applications (reviewed in Schally and Comaru-Schally, 1998a). D-Amino acid substitutions in positions 1, 2 or 3 resulted in analogs with increased GH-releasing activity. To avoid oxidative inactivation of the analogs, Met^{27} was replaced by norleucine in some peptides. We synthesized superactive agonists of GHRH(1-29) with increased metabolic stability, containing ornithine instead of lysine in positions 12 and 21, agmatine at the C terminus and other modifications (Izdebski et al., 1995). Extensive experimental investigations, but only a few veterinary or clinical studies, were performed with GHRH agonists (reviewed in Schally and Comaru-Schally, 1998a).

In the meantime it became apparent that antagonistic analogs of GHRH would be even more useful clinically. The GHRH antagonists could be tried in conditions such as acromegaly, diabetic retinopathy or diabetic nephropathy (glomerulosclerosis). However, the main applications of GHRH antagonists would be in the field of cancer. The clinical need for GHRH antagonists was first advocated by Pollak et al. (1989) on the grounds that somatostatin analogs do not adequately suppress GH and insulin-like growth factor (IGF)-1 levels in patients with tumors potentially dependent on IGF-1. In the course of synthesis of various agonists of hGHRH(1-29)NH_2, it was found that replacement of Ala^2 by D-Arg^2 within the NH_2-terminal 29 amino acid segment of GHRH leads to antagonists (Robberecht et al., 1985). An early GHRH antagonist, [Ac-Tyr^1,D-Arg^2]hGHRH(1-29)NH_2, inhibited the GHRH-stimulated adenylate cyclase activity in rat pituitary cells and suppressed GH release in rats. However, there was relatively little activity in this field until our group started systematic work on the development of more potent GHRH antagonists. Work in our laboratory yielded the potent GHRH antagonists MZ-4-71 and MZ-5-156 (Zarandi et al., 1994, 1997). The syntheses of our previous series of GHRH antagonists containing C-terminal agmatine were summarized previously (Schally et al., 1998b). Positively charged amino acids were then incorporated into GHRH antagonists to produce analogs such as JV-1-36 and JV-1-38, with further increased bioactivity (Varga et al., 1999; Schally and Varga 1999). These compounds show a high binding affinity to pituitary and tumoral GHRH receptors, and strongly inhibit pituitary GH secretion, in vitro and in vivo (Schally and Varga 1999; Schally et al., 2001).

After the synthesis and purification, our GHRH antagonists are characterized on the basis of in vitro and in vivo endocrine assays on rat pituitaries and oncological tests. Because endocrine tests are carried out using rat pituitaries and GHRH antagonists are being developed for clinical applications, it was essential to demonstrate the efficacy of these antagonists on the human pituitary receptor, since the rat pituitary GHRH-R shows an 18% difference in the amino acid sequence as compared to its human counterpart. We expressed human GHRH receptors in GH3 rat pituitary tumor cells using recombinant adenoviral vectors and studied the effects of GHRH antagonists (Kovacs et al., 2002). Cell culture and superfusion experiments showed that GHRH antagonists effectively inhibited the actions of GHRH on the GH3 cells transfected with hGHRH receptors and exhibited a similar spectrum of activity on the human and the rat GHRH-receptors. These results support the view that this class of compounds would be active clinically in human beings. This is of critical importance, because the tumor inhibition induced by GHRH antagonists is exerted in part through the suppression of GH release from the pituitary and the reduction in hepatic production of IGF-1 (Schally et al., 2001).

The antiproliferative activity of GHRH antagonists was evaluated in many tumor models in vivo and also in vitro. The purpose of this article is to review extensive oncological investigations with the previous series of analogs and new more potent antagonists of GHRH. Potential clinical applications of GHRH antagonists for the treatment of various cancers will be discussed in the light of the increasing evidence for the involvement of not only IGF-1 and IGF-2, but also tissue (local) GHRH in the process of tumorigenesis.

GHRH and GHRH Receptors in Human Cancers

GHRH and its receptors are expressed in many extrahypothalamic and extrapituitary tissues, suggesting a broad biological role for this peptide (Schally et al., 2001). Since the discovery of ectopic GHRH production (Frohman and Szabo, 1981), much evidence has accumulated on the involvement of GHRH and its receptors in the pathophysiology of cancer.

GHRH in Human Tumors

The expression of mRNA for GHRH and the presence of biologically or immunologically active GHRH was demonstrated in various human malignant tumors, including cancers of the breast, endometrium and ovary, prostate and the lung (Kahan et al., 1999, 2000; Kiaris et al., 1999). GHRH may function as an autocrine growth factor in the case of small cell lung cancer (SCLC) (Kiaris et al., 1999). Thus, H-69 and H-510A SCLC lines cultured in vitro express mRNA for GHRH, which is apparently translated into peptide GHRH and then secreted by the cells, as shown by the detection of GHRH-like immunoreactivity in media from the cells cultured in vitro. GHRH(1-29) stimulates the proliferation of H-69 and H-510A SCLCs in vitro and GHRH antagonists inhibit it (Kiaris et al., 1999). We also demonstrated a high incidence (86%) of mRNA for hGHRH in human prostate cancer specimens (Halmos et al., 2002). The expression of hGHRH was similarly found in LNCaP and PC-3 human prostate cancers (Plonowski et al., 2002a). Chopin and Herington (2001) also showed recently that the human prostate cancer lines ALVA-41, DU-145, LNCaP and PC-3 express mRNA for GHRH and produce immunoreactive GHRH peptide. The presence of biologically and immunologically active GHRH and mRNA for GHRH in human breast, endometrial and ovarian cancers supports the hypothesis that locally-produced GHRH may play a role in the proliferation of these tumors (Kahan et al., 1999). mRNA for GHRH was also present in human breast cancer cell lines MCF-7, MCF-7MIII, MDA-MB-231, MDA-MB-435, MDA-MB-468 and T47D (Garcia-Fernandez et al., 2002). The growth of T47D breast cancer line was stimulated by GHRH and inhibited by GHRH antagonists. GHRH is similarly present in human gastroenteropancreatic cancers (Busto et al., 2002b). We detected mRNA for GHRH in pancreatic (SW1990, PANC-1, MIA PaCa-2, Capan-1, Capan-2 and CFPAC1), gastric (NCI-N87, HS746T and AGS) and colonic (COLO 320DM and HT-29) cancer lines. In studies in vitro with pancreatic, colonic and gastric cancer lines, exogenously added GHRH(1-29)NH_2 increased the rate of cell proliferation. RT-PCR analyses show the presence of mRNA for GHRH in MNNG/HOS human osteosarcoma and SK-ES-1 Ewing's sarcoma (Busto et al., 2002a). Radioimmunoassays for GHRH on media from tissue cultures of both these sarcomas indicate that the mRNA for GHRH can be translated into an immunoreactive peptide product and released into the extracellular medium (Busto et al., 2002a).

Receptors for GHRH on Tumors

Oncological tests carried out in human cancer lines xenografted into nude mice or in vitro revealed that most of the effects of the GHRH antagonists may be exerted directly on tumors. Various attempts failed to detect the pituitary form of GHRH receptors in human cancer models (Schally and Varga, 1999), but peptide receptors on tumors that might mediate the effects of GHRH and its antagonists were identified recently (Rekasi et al., 2000; Halmos et al., 2000). Using ^{125}I-labeled GHRH antagonist JV-1-42 as a ligand, we were able to demonstrate the presence of specific high-affinity binding sites for GHRH and its antagonists on CAKI-1 renal, MiaPaCa-2 pancreatic, LNCaP and PC-3 prostatic and OV-1063 ovarian cancers (Rekasi et al., 2000; Halmos et al., 2000; Chatzistamou et al., 2001a). The isolation and sequencing of cDNAs encoding tumoral GHRH receptors revealed that they are splice variants (SV) of the pituitary GHRH receptors (Rekasi et al., 2000). RT-PCR analyses initially revealed the expression of receptor SVs in several cancers, including LNCaP prostatic, MiaPaCa-2 pancreatic, CAKI-1 renal, H-69 SCLC, MDA-MB-468 breast, and OV-1063 ovarian cancers. Tumoral SV_1, SV_2 and SV_4, have a retained intronic sequence at their 5' ends and lack the first three exons. The major part of the cDNA sequence of SV_1 is identical with the corresponding sequence of pituitary GHRH receptor cDNA, but the first 334 nucleotides of SV_1 and SV_2 are completely different from those in the pituitary GHRH receptor. The deduced protein sequence of SV_1 and SV_2 differs from that of the pituitary GHRH receptor only in the 25 amino acid sequence at the N-terminal extracellular domain (Rekasi et al., 2000). SV_2 may encode a GHRH receptor isoform truncated after the second transmembrane domain. Additional studies are needed to confirm that mRNAs for tumoral SV receptors are translated into the GHRH binding sites found by radioligand assay. SV_1 appears to be the major isoform of GHRH receptors expressed in neoplastic tissues, which may mediate the antiproliferative effect of GHRH antagonists (Rekasi et al., 2000; Halmos et al., 2000). Recently we found mRNA for the SV_1 isoform of GHRH receptors in human osteosarcoma line MNNG/HOS and SK-ES-1 Ewing's sarcoma line (Busto et al., 2002a) and in MCF-7MIII, MDA-MB-468 and T47D breast cancer cell lines and SV_2 isoform in MCF-7MIII and T47D cell lines (Garcia-Fernandez et al., 2002). mRNA for SV_1 isoform of GHRH receptors is also expressed in tumors of pancreatic (SW1990, PANC-1, MIA PaCa-2, Capan-1, Capan-2 and CFPAC1), colorectal (COLO 320DM and HT-29) and gastric (NCI-N87, HS746T and AGS) cancer cell lines; mRNA for SV_2 was also present in Capan-1, Capan-2, CFPAC1, HT-29 and NCI-N87 tumors (Busto et al., 2002b). We were also able to demonstrate the expression of SV of GHRH receptors in primary specimens of human cancers. SV_1 was present in 65% of the human prostate cancers and the presence of SV_2 was shown in 12 of the 20 (60%) specimens, but the expression of SV_4 was found in only three samples (15%) (Halmos et al., 2002). RT-PCR analyses of mRNA from LNCaP, MDA-PCa-2b and PC-3 prostate cancers similarly revealed the presence of SV_1 and SV_2 isoforms of GHRH receptors (Plonowski et al., 2002a). Chopin and Herington (2001) also found SV_1 of GHRH receptors in ALVA-41, LNCaP, DU-145 and PC-3 models of prostate cancer.

We also showed the activation of cell proliferation responses to GHRH analogs in 3T3 fibroblasts transfected with the SV_1 isoform of GHRH receptor (Kiaris et al., 2002), supporting the hypothesis that SV_1 mediates direct effects of GHRH and its analogs on tumors. Our findings suggest that in some tumors, GHRH and its tumoral receptor could form an autocrine/paracrine mitogenic loop, which might be involved in the control of the malignant growth. The inhibitory effect of GHRH antagonists on cancers could be based in part on the interference with the local stimulatory GHRH system.

Effects of GHRH Antagonists on Growth of Experimental Cancers

Our initial investigations of oncological activities of the GHRH antagonists were based only on the assumption that the blockade of the pituitary GH/hepatic IGF-1 axis might inhibit the growth of IGF-1 dependent cancers (Pinski et al., 1995). However, subsequently we discovered that GHRH antagonists can also suppress the proliferation of diverse tumors that are influenced by autocrine and/or paracrine production of IGF-1 and IGF-2. In addition, GHRH antagonists can inhibit the growth of some cancers, such as SCLC or prostate and breast cancers by blocking the action of autocrine/paracrine GHRH and GH itself. Hence, a wide range of cancers can be inhibited by GHRH antagonists.

Prostate Cancer

Both IGF-1 and IGF-2 appear to be involved in the malignant transformation and the progression of many tumors, including prostate cancer (Schally et al., 2000). Androgen-independent PC-3 and DU-145 prostate cancer cell lines produce and secrete IGF-1 or IGF-2 and possess IGF-1 receptors. In an attempt to develop a new approach to the treatment of androgen-independent prostate cancer, we evaluated the effects of GHRH antagonist MZ-4-71 in nude mice bearing DU-145 and PC-3 prostate cancer cell lines. Therapy with MZ-4-71 significantly decreased tumor growth, serum levels of GH and IGF-1 and liver IGF-1 levels (Jungwirth et al., 1997b). The concentration of IGF-1 and IGF-2 in PC-3 tumor tissue was reduced to non-detectable values after treatment with MZ-4-71. To investigate the mechanisms involved, we treated male nude mice bearing xenografts of DU-145 prostate cancer with GHRH antagonist MZ-5-156 and again found significant reductions in the volume of DU-145 tumors, serum IGF-1 and tumor IGF-2 levels (Lamharzi et al., 1998). RT-PCR analysis revealed that the expression of IGF-2 mRNA in DU-145 tumors was greatly decreased. Thus, GHRH antagonists may inhibit the growth of DU-145 prostate cancers also by reducing the production of IGF-2 in the tumor tissue. Direct effects of GHRH antagonists were demonstrated in vitro. Antagonists MZ-4-71 and MZ-5-156 significantly inhibited the rate of proliferation of prostatic (PC-3 and DU-145) cancer cell lines in vitro (Csernus et al., 1999), as shown by colorimetric and [^{3}H]-thymidine incorporation tests, reduced the expression of IGF-2 mRNA in the cells and the concentration of IGF-2 secreted into the culture medium. A new class of GHRH antagonists, such as JV-1-38 (Varga et al., 1999), has a higher and more protracted biological activity than the previously used antagonists MZ-4-71 or MZ-5-156. Recently we showed that antagonist JV-1-38 is more potent than MZ-5-156 in inhibiting growth of PC-3 tumors in nude mice (Plonowski et al., 2000). Although both antagonists had similar effects on serum IGF-1, JV-

1-38 caused greater reduction of the expression of mRNA for IGF-2 in the tumor tissue (Plonowski et al., 2000). We also demonstrated an increased inhibition of growth of PC-3 human androgen-independent prostate cancer in vivo by using a combination of GHRH antagonist JV-1-38 and bombesin/GRP antagonist RC-3940-II. However, the antiproliferative effect of GHRH antagonists in PC-3 prostate cancers is not always correlated with the suppression of serum IGF-1 or the expression of IGF-2 in tumors (Plonowski et al., 2002b). The antiproliferative effects of GHRH antagonists on prostate cancer could be also exerted by a direct interference with tumoral GHRH system. It is well known that the duration of clinical response to androgen deprivation is limited, as cancer cells acquire the ability to grow in the absence of androgens. One of the proposed mechanisms of relapse is the activation of proliferation pathways by intracellular cascades evoked by growth factors. Thus the inhibition of IGF-dependent or GHRH-dependent mitogenic loops by GHRH antagonists could delay or prevent the activation of these proliferation pathways. Studies in nude mice implanted orthotopically with LNCaP human androgen-sensitive prostate cancer show that castration alone does not cause a lasting suppression of serum PSA or inhibition of tumor growth (Rekasi et al., 2001). After an initial arrest of about 1 week, serum PSA levels start to rise, indicating that a relapse has occurred. GHRH antagonist JV-1-38 alone similarly does not affect serum PSA or tumor growth in intact mice. However, treatment with JV-1-38 combined with castration can powerfully decrease PSA serum concentration and reduce the weight of orthotopic LNCaP tumors (Rekasi et al., 2001).

These and other results show that GHRH antagonists greatly potentiate the tumor growth inhibition induced by androgen deprivation. GHRH antagonists may interfere with mechanisms involved in progression of prostate cancer toward androgen independence, and could be used clinically as agents preventing relapse in prostate cancer patients receiving androgen deprivation therapies. The antiproliferative effects of GHRH antagonists on prostate cancer could be exerted in part by a direct interference with this tumoral GHRH system.

GHRH antagonists might provide new approaches to therapy of patients with prostatic carcinoma who have relapsed following conventional androgen deprivation.

Breast Cancer

IGF-1 and IGF-2 might influence the growth of human breast cancers by endocrine, autocrine or paracrine mechanisms (Kahan et al., 2000; Schally et al., 2001). The presence of biologically and immunologically active GHRH and messenger ribonucleic acid for GHRH in human breast cancers supports the hypothesis that locally produced GHRH may also play a role in the proliferation of these tumors (Kahan et al., 1999). Antagonists of GHRH may offer a new approach to treatment of breast cancer. GHRH antagonists MZ-5-156 and JV-1-36 induced regression of estrogen-independent MDA-MB-468 human breast cancers xenografted into nude mice (Kahan et al., 2000) and in vitro inhibited the rate of proliferation of the MDA-MB-468 cell line. The expression of mRNA for human GHRH was found in some tumors. Since IGF-1 receptor signaling is defective in this line, these results suggest that GHRH antagonists also inhibit MDA-MB-468 breast cancers, through mechanisms involving interference with locally produced GHRH. GHRH antagonist JV-1-36 also inhibited growth and metastases of orthotopically implanted MDA-MB-435 human estrogen-independent breast cancers (Chatzistamou et al., 2001b). mRNA for IGF-1 or IGF-2 was not detected in MDA-MB-435 cells, indicating that the suppression of autocrine IGFs may not be involved in the antiproliferative mechanism. However, the expression of mRNA for GHRH receptor SV_1 I was found in MDA-MB-435 tumors. These results suggest that the antitumorigenic action of GHRH antagonists on MDA-MB-435 breast cancer could be mediated by tumoral GHRH receptors (Chatzistamou et al., 2001b).

Various GHRH antagonists also inhibit growth of MXT estrogen-independent mouse mammary cancers (Szepeshazi et al., 2001). This growth inhibition was associated with a decrease in cell proliferation and an increase in apoptosis in MXT cancers. The concentrations of GH and IGF-1 and the levels of mRNA for GH and IGF-1 in tumors were reduced by the therapy with GHRH antagonists. In vitro, the proliferation of MXT cancer cells was strongly stimulated by GH and less effectively by IGF-1, indicating that both GH and IGF-1 may act as growth factors for this mammary carcinoma. GHRH antagonist JV-1-38 inhibited the autonomous growth of MXT cells and the proliferation induced by IGF-1 or GH, and diminished ^{3}H-thymidine-incorporation stimulated by IGF-1 and GH. These findings and a sustained increase in cyclin B2 concentrations in the cells shown by immunoblotting indicate that JV-1-38 causes a block at the end of the G_2 phase of the cell cycle. These investigations indicate that GHRH antagonists could be potentially useful for the treatment of breast cancer.

Ovarian Cancer

IGF-1 and IGF-2 stimulate proliferation of human epithelial ovarian cancer cell lines (Chatzistamou et al., 2001a). We investigated the effects of antagonists of GHRH on the growth of human epithelial ovarian cancer cell lines xenografted into nude mice. Treatment with GHRH antagonists JV-1-36 or MZ-5-156 decreased growth of OV-1063 cancers and reduced the levels of mRNA for IGF-2 in tumors. JV-1-36 also inhibited cell proliferation in vitro. OV-1063 cancers express mRNA for tumoral SV_1 of GHRH receptors. Antagonist JV-1-36 also inhibited the growth of UCI-107 human ovarian cell carcinomas. These results indicate that antagonistic analogs of GHRH can inhibit the growth of epithelial ovarian cancers.

Renal Cell Carcinoma (RCC)

Since GH and IGF-1 may play a role in the development of renal cancers, we investigated the effects of GHRH antagonist MZ-4-71 on Caki-1 human RCC (Jungwirth et al., 1997a). Treatment with MZ-4-71 significantly inhibited growth of CAKI-1 tumors in nude mice and decreased serum levels of GH and

IGF-1, liver concentrations of IGF-1 and tumor levels of IGF-1 and IGF-2. GHRH antagonist JV-1-38 also inhibited the growth of orthotopic CAKI-1 RCC in nude mice and inhibited the development of metastases to lung and lymph nodes (Halmos et al., 2000). RT-PCR revealed the expression of SVs of hGH-RH receptor in CAKI-1 tumors (Halmos et al., 2000). These distinct receptors can mediate the inhibitory effect of GHRH antagonists in RCC. Further investigations are needed to evaluate the use of GHRH antagonists for the therapy of advanced RCC.

Brain Tumors

Gliomas contain IGF-1 and IGF-2 and express mRNA for IGF-1 receptors and a potential therapy for gliomas could be based on the inhibition of IGF system. The effects of GHRH antagonists MZ-5-156 and JV-1-36 were investigated in nude mice bearing xenografts of U-87MG human glioblastomas (Kiaris et al., 2000a). Therapy with GHRH antagonists inhibited the growth of U-87MG glioblastomas and decreased the levels of mRNA for IGF-2 in tumors (Kiaris et al., 2000a). Treatment with MZ-5-156 also decreased telomerase activity in U-87MG glioblastomas (Kiaris and Schally, 1999). mRNA for GHRH was detected in U-87MG tumors, suggesting that GHRH might play a role in the pathogenesis of this tumor. Antagonistic analogs of GHRH should be further developed for treatment of malignant glioblastoma.

Lung Cancer

Human SCLC and non-SCLC cell lines secrete and respond to IGF-1 and IGF-2, express IGF-1 and IGF-2 genes and IGF-1 receptors. SCLC lines, cultured in vitro, express mRNA for GHRH and secrete immunoreactive GHRH. GHRH can function as an autocrine growth factor in SCLCs. We were able to demonstrate that GHRH antagonists MZ-4-71 and MZ-5-156 significantly inhibited growth of SCLC H69 and non-SCLC H157 tumors in nude mice (Pinski et al., 1996) and decreased the levels of IGF-1 in serum and liver tissue. New GHRH antagonist JV-1-36 also powerfully inhibited growth of H-69 SCLC in vivo, but did not change serum IGF-1 or tumor IGF-2 levels and mRNA for IGF-2 (Kiaris et al., 1999, 2000b). H-69 and H-510A SCLC lines cultured in vitro express mRNA for GHRH, which apparently is translated into peptide GHRH and then secreted by the cells, as shown by the detection of GHRH-like immunoreactivity in conditioned media from the cells cultured in vitro. In addition, the levels of GH-RH-like immunoreactivity in serum from nude mice bearing H-69 xenografts were higher than in tumor free mice. GHRH(1-29)NH_2 stimulated the proliferation of H-69 and H-510A SCLCs in vitro, and GH-RH antagonist JV-1-36 inhibited it (Kiaris et al., 1999). Treatment with GHRH antagonist JV-1-38 also significantly inhibited tumor growth of H838 non-SCLC xenografted s.c. into nude mice (Szereday et al., 2002). These results suggest that GHRH can function as an autocrine growth factor in SCLC and non-SCLC. Treatment with antagonistic analogs of GHRH may offer a new approach to the treatment of SCLC and other cancers.

Pancreatic Cancer

IGF-1 and IGF-2 are implicated in the pathogenesis of pancreatic carcinoma. GHRH antagonists MZ-4-71 and MZ-5-156 inhibited the growth of nitrosamine-induced pancreatic cancers in hamsters and SW-1990 human pancreatic cancers xenografted into nude mice and reduced IGF-2 concentration in tumors (Szepeshazi et al., 2000b). In vitro, MZ-5-156 decreased SW-1990 cell proliferation and IGF-2 synthesis and secretion in the cells. Thus, the inhibitory effects of GHRH antagonists on the growth of pancreatic cancers may result from a reduction in the production of IGF-2 in the tumors, but the expression of GHRH and SV_1 isoform of GHRH receptors also indicates the involvement of autocrine GHRH.

Colorectal Cancer

Various findings support the involvement of IGF-1 and IGF-2 in the growth of colorectal cancers. The incidence of colon cancer is increased in acromegalics, suggesting that excessive secretion of GH or IGF-1 may be a factor. When we treated nude mice with xenografts of HT-29 human colon cancer with GHRH antagonists there was a major decrease in the growth of HT-29 cancer (Szepeshazi et al., 2000a) and reduction in IGF-2 concentrations and IGF-2 mRNA expression in tumors. IGF-1 and IGF-2 stimulated in vitro growth of HT-29 cancers. MZ-5-156 diminished IGF-2 production and the proliferation of HT-29 cells in vitro. These studies demonstrate that GHRH antagonists inhibit the growth of human colon cancers through a reduction in the production of IGF-2 by cancer cells, but the expression of GHRH and SV_1 isoform of GHRH receptors also indicate the involvement of autocrine GHRH.

Osteogenic Sarcomas

Osteosarcoma is the most common primary bone tumor in children and young adults and present therapeutic methods are inadequate. The growth of osteosarcomas is stimulated by IGF-1, IGF-2 and GH (Schally et al., 2001). Consequently, in our first oncological study we evaluated the effect of GHRH antagonist MZ-4-71 on human osteosarcoma cell line SK-ES-1 and Ewings sarcoma MNNG/HOS (Pinski et al., 1995). MZ-4-71 inhibited growth of SK-ES-1 and MNNG/HOS bone tumors in nude mice and decreased IGF-1 levels in serum and tumor tissue (Pinski et al., 1995). The growth rate of the two cell lines in vitro was also suppressed by MZ-4-71. In the next study (Braczkowski et al., 2002), we investigated the effects of GHRH antagonist JV-1-38. GHRH antagonist significantly inhibited the tumor volume and tumor weight of MNNG/HOS bone tumors and SK-ES-1 tumors by more than 50% after 4 weeks and increased tumor doubling time. JV-1-38 lowered serum IGF-1 level, decreased the expression of mRNA for IGF-1 in the liver and significantly reduced the concentration of IGF-2 and mRNA levels for IGF-2 in both sarcomas. The concentration of IGF-1 was lowered only in SK-ES-I tumors. In vitro, the proliferation of SK-ES-1 and MNNG/HOS cells was inhibited by JV-1-38. Thus, the inhibition of MNNG/HOS osteosarcoma and SK-ES-1 Ewing's sarcoma by GHRH antagonists is linked to a suppression of IGF-2 production in tumors, but in SK-ES-1 tumors effects on IGF-1 may also be involved. Other studies reveal (Busto et al., 2002a) that MNNG/HOS and SK-ES-1 bone sarcomas also express SV_1 of GH-RH receptors and produce GHRH peptide. Thus, an autocrine loop based on GHRH and SV_1 GHRH receptors might be involved in the pathophysiology of sarcomas. All these findings suggest that GHRH antagonists could be considered for the treatment of human malignant bone tumors.

Mechanism of Action of GHRH Antagonists

GHRH antagonists can inhibit tumor growth indirectly through suppression of the endocrine GH-IGF-1 axis, and also by direct action on the tumor cells (Schally and Varga, 1999; Schally et al., 2001) (Figs. 1-3). The indirect mechanism is important for those cancers that depend on IGF-1 as a growth factor. A strong positive association was reported between plasma IGF-1 levels and the risk of prostate, breast and colorectal cancers (Reviewed in Schally and Varga, 1999). GHRH antagonists decrease the levels of IGF-1 in serum by inhibiting the release of GH from the pituitary, which results in a suppression of hepatic IGF-1 production (Fig. 1). In some studies in nude mice bear-

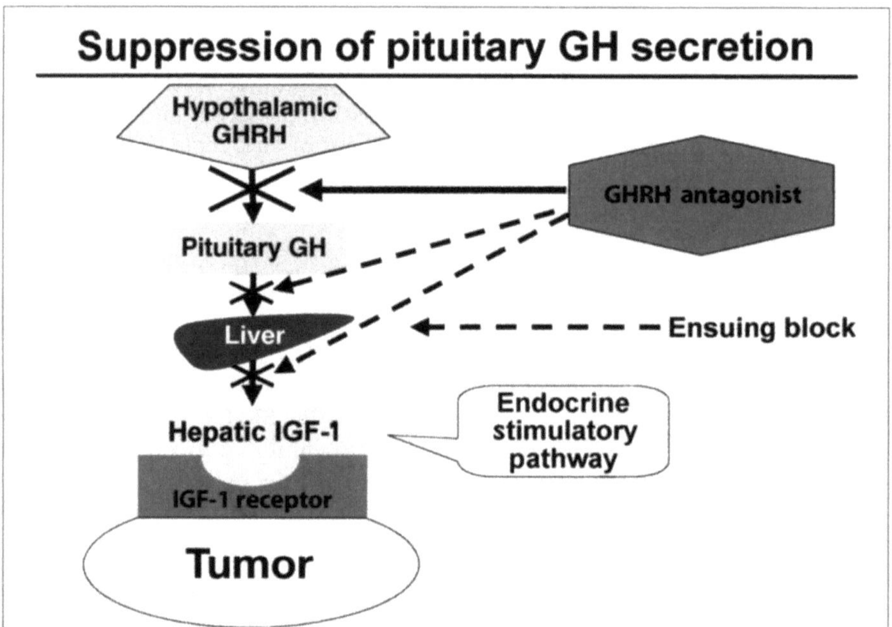

Fig. 1. Indirect action mediated through the suppression of the pituitary GH-hepatic IGF-1 axis. GHRH antagonists block the secretion of GH from the pituitary by inhibiting the binding of hypothalamic GHRH to pituitary GHRH receptors. This results in a decrease of the levels of circulating IGF-1 and lowering of the levels of circulating IGF-1, ultimately leading to inhibition of tumor growth

ing various cancers, tumor inhibition was accompanied by a decrease in levels of serum IGF-1. In such cases the antiproliferative effect of GHRH antagonists could be ascribed in part to the suppression of the GH-IGF-1 endocrine axis (Fig. 1). However, this indirect mechanism cannot account for tumor inhibition observed in other cancer models in which GHRH antagonists did not cause significant inhibition of serum IGF-1 levels. Moreover, GHRH antagonists inhibit the proliferation of various cancer cell lines in vitro, where the involvement of the GH-IGF-1 axis is clearly excluded. These direct inhibitory effects appear to be mediated by the tumoral SVs of GHRH receptors, by mechanisms dependent or independent of IGF-1 and IGF-2. GHRH and SVs of GHRH receptors are present in a variety of human cancers and may form an autocrine/paracrine stimulatory loop. Thus, in the case of H-69 SCLC and other cancers, the tumor inhibition is not associated with a suppression of production of IGF-1 and IGF-2, but appears to be due to the blockade of the stimulatory action of tumoral autocrine GHRH by GHRH antagonists (Fig. 2). Still, in many human cancer lines in vitro and in vivo, including prostatic, renal, pancreatic and colorectal cancers, glioblastomas, ovarian cancers and non-SCLCs, GHRH antagonists inhibit the production of IGF-1 and IGF-2 and the expression of IGF-2 mRNA by an action apparently

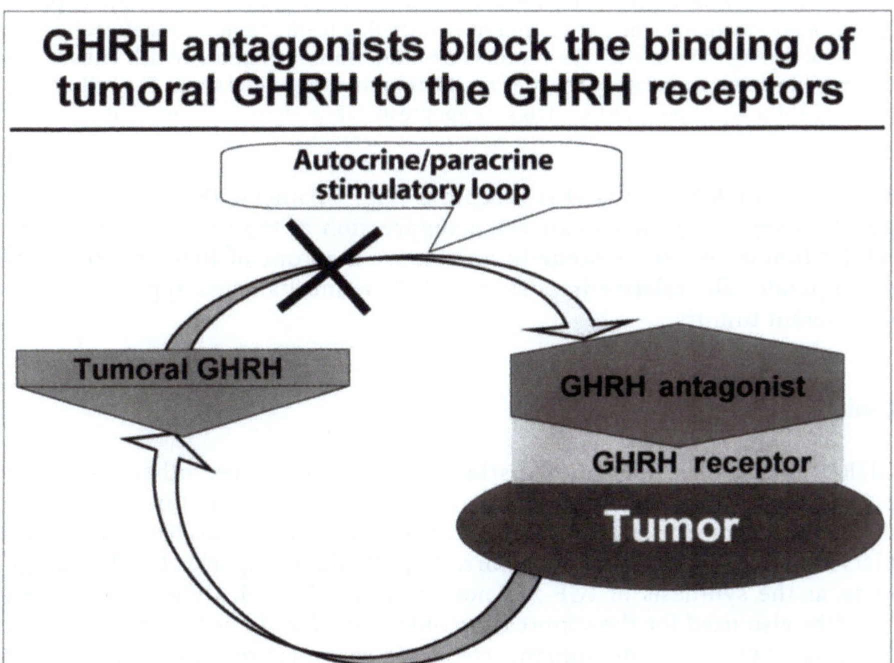

Fig. 2. Direct action. GHRH antagonists competitively inhibit the binding of tumoral autocrine/paracrine GHRH to splice variants (SVs) of GHRH receptor on tumors. This blocks the stimulatory effect of locally produced GHRH on tumor growth without the involvement of the IGF system

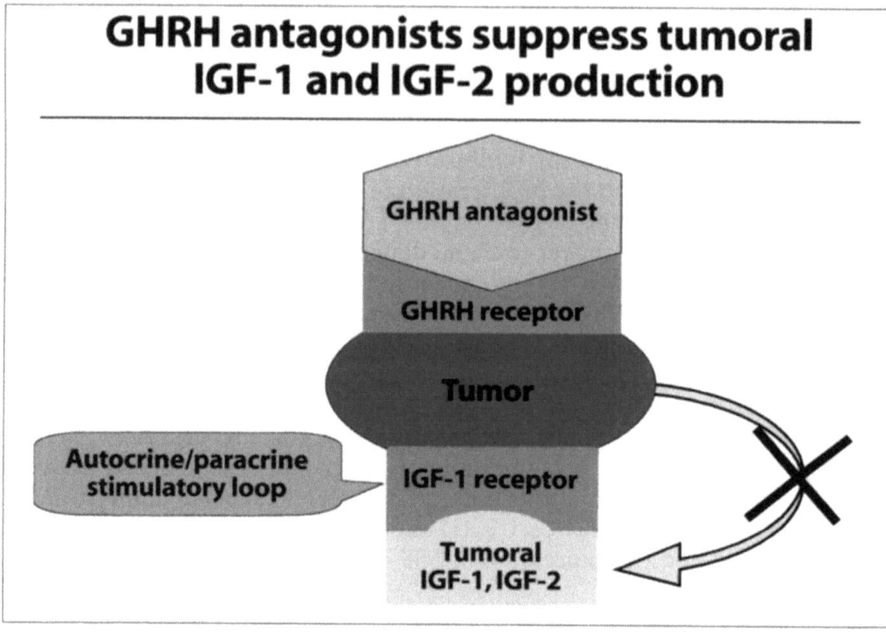

Fig. 3. Direct action. GHRH antagonists can inhibit tumor growth directly by suppressing the autocrine/paracrine production of IGF-1/IGF-2 by the tumor. This effect is likely mediated through SVs of GHRH receptors on tumors. In some tumors GHRH antagonists can also block the stimulatory effect of local GH on tumor proliferation. The cell cycle is arrested at the G_2-M point, which triggers apoptosis (Szepeshazi et al., 2001; not shown)

exerted through SVs of GHRH receptors (Fig. 3). Since IGF-1 and IGF-2 are potent mitogens for many cancers, a suppression of their production would inhibit tumor growth. In some tumors, more than one of these mechanisms may operate. The relative importance of these mechanisms appears to vary in different tumors.

Clinical Notes

GHRH antagonists may offer distinctive advantages over other classes of prospective antitumor agents. Therapy with GHRH antagonists should be devoid of severe side effects typical of chemotherapy. Because GHRH antagonists inhibit IGF-2-dependent tumors, they should be superior to GH antagonists, as the synthesis of IGF-2 is not controlled by GH. GHRH antagonists could be also used for the suppression of tumors that do not express somatostatin receptors, such as human osteogenic sarcomas or those that contain only low levels of SST receptors.

No clinical trials have been carried out so far with our GHRH antagonists. The administration of an early GHRH antagonist was reported to reduce GH hypersecretion in a patient with metastatic GHRH secreting carcinoid tumor, but the effect of large bolus doses lasted only 3-4 h (Jaffe et al., 1997). New generations of GHRH antagonists might prove to be of benefit in patients with acromegaly due to metastatic GHRH secreting tumors, but the principal applications of GHRH antagonists should be for cancer therapy.

References

Bagnato A., Moretti C., Ohnishi J., Frajese G. and Catt K.J. (1992). Expression of the growth hormone-releasing hormone gene and its peptide product in the rat ovary. Endocrinology, 130, 1097-1102.

Braczkowski R., Schally A.V., Plonowski A., Varga J.L., Groot K., Krupa M. and Armatis P. (2002). Inhibition of proliferation of human MNNG/HOS osteosarcoma and SK-ES-1 Ewing's sarcoma cell lines in vitro and in vivo by antagonists of growth hormone-releasing hormone: Effects on IGF-2. Cancer, 95, 1735-1745.

Busto R., Schally A.V., Braczkowski R., Plonowski A., Krupa M., Groot K., Armatis P. and Varga J.L. (2002a). Expression of mRNA for growth hormone-releasing hormone (GHRH), and splice variants of GHRH receptors in human osteosarcomas. Regul Peptides, 108, 47-53.

Busto R., Schally A.V., Varga J.L., Garcia-Fernandez M.O., Groot K., Armatis P. and Szepeshazi K. (2002b). The expression of growth hormone-releasing hormone (GHRH) and splice variants of its receptor in human gastroenteropancreatic carcinomas. Proc Natl Acad Sci USA, 99, 11866-11871.

Chatzistamou I., Schally A.V., Varga J.L., Groot K. and Armatis P. (2001a). Antagonists of growth hormone-releasing hormone and somatostatin analog RC-160 inhibit growth of OV-1063 human epithelial ovarian CA cell line xenografted into nude mice. J Clin Endocrinol Metab, 86, 2144-2152.

Chatzistamou I., Schally A.V., Varga J.L., Groot K., Busto R., Armatis P. and Halmos G. (2001b). Inhibition of growth and metastases of MDA-MB-435 human estrogen-independent breast cancers by an antagonist of growth hormone-releasing hormone. Anti-cancer Drugs, 12, 761-768.

Chopin L.K. and Herington A.C. (2001). A potential autocrine pathway for growth hormone releasing hormone (GHRH) and its receptor in human prostate cancer cell lines. Prostate, 49, 116-121.

Csernus V.J., Schally A.V., Kiaris H. and Armatis P. (1999) Inhibition of growth, production of insulin-like growth factor-2 (IGF-2) and expression of IGF-2 mRNA of human cancer cell lines by antagonistic analogs of growth hormone-releasing hormone in vitro. Proc Natl Acad Sci USA, 96, 3098-3103.

Frohman L.A. and Szabo M. (1981). Ectopic production of growth hormone-releasing factor by carcinoid and pancreatic islet tumors associated with acromegaly. Prog Clin Biol Res, 74, 259-271.

Garcia-Fernandez M.O., Schally A.V., Varga J.L., Groot K. and Busto R. (2003). The expression of growth hormone-releasing hormone (GHRH) and its receptor splice variants in human breast cancer lines; the evaluation of signaling mechanisms in the stimulation of cell proliferation. Breast Cancer Res Treat, 77, 15-26.

Guillemin R., Brazeau P., Bohlen P., Esch F., Ling N. and Wehrenberg W.B. (1982). Growth hormone-releasing factor from a human pancreatic tumor that caused acromegaly. Science, 218, 585-587.

Halmos G., Schally A.V., Varga J.L., Plonowski A., Rekasi Z. and Czompoly T. (2000). Human renal cell carcinoma expresses distinct binding sites for growth hormone-releasing hormone. Proc Natl Acad Sci USA, 97, 10555-10560.

Halmos G., Schally A.V., Comaru-Schally A.M., Nagy A. and Irimpen A. (2003). Targeted analogs of somatostatin carrying cytotoxic radicals or radionuclides do not bind to growth hormone secretagogue receptors on human myocardium. Life Sci, 72, 2669-2674.

Izdebski J., Pinski J., Horvath J.E., Halmos G., Groot K. and Schally A.V. (1995). Synthesis and biological evaluation of superactive agonists of growth hormone-releasing hormone. Proc Natl Acad Sci, USA, 92, 4872-4876.

Jaffe C.A., DeMott-Friberg R., Frohman L.A. and Barkan A.L. (1997). Suppression of growth hormone (GH) hypersecretion due to ectopic GH-releasing hormone (GHRH) by a selective GHRH antagonist. J Clin Endocrinol Metab, 82, 634-637.

Jungwirth A., Schally A.V., Pinski J., Groot K., Armatis A. and Halmos G. (1997a). Growth hormone-releasing hormone (GHRH) antagonist MZ-4-71 inhibits in vivo proliferation of Caki-I renal adenocarcinoma. Proc Natl Acad Sci USA, 94, 5810-5813.

Jungwirth A., Schally A.V., Pinski J., Halmos G., Groot K., Armatis P. and Vadillo-Buenfil M. (1997b). Inhibition of in vivo proliferation of androgen-independent prostate cancers by an antagonist of growth hormone-releasing hormone. Br J Cancer, 75, 1585-1592.

Kahan Z., Arencibia J., Csernus V., Groot K., Kineman R., Robinson W.R. and Schally A.V. (1999). Expression of growth hormone-releasing hormone (GHRH) messenger ribonucleic acid and the presence of biologically active GHRH in human breast, endometrial, and ovarian cancers. J Clin Endocrinol Metab, 84, 582-589.

Kahan Z., Varga J.L., Schally A.V., Rekasi Z., Armatis P., Chatzistamou I., Czompoly T. and Halmos G. (2000). Antagonists of growth hormone releasing hormone arrest the growth of MDA-MB-468 estrogen-independent human breast cancers in nude mice. Breast Cancer Res Treat, 60, 71-79.

Kiaris H. and Schally A.V. (1999). Decrease in telomerase activity in U-87MG human glioblastomas after treatment with an antagonist of growth hormone-releasing hormone. Proc Natl Acad Sci USA, 96, 226-231.

Kiaris H., Schally A.V., Busto R., Halmos G., Artavanis-Tsakonas S. and Varga J.L. (2002). Expression of a splice variant of the receptor for GHRH in 3T3 fibroblasts activates cell proliferation responses to GHRH analogs. Proc Natl Acad Sci USA, 99, 196-200

Kiaris H., Schally A.V. and Varga J.L. (2000a). Antagonists of growth hormone-releasing hormone inhibit the growth of U-87MG human glioblastomas in nude mice. Neoplasia, 2, 242-250.

Kiaris H., Schally A.V. and Varga J. (2000b). Suppression of tumor growth by growth hormone-releasing hormone antagonist JV-1-36 does not involve the inhibition of autocrine production of insulin like growth factor 2 in H-69 small cell lung carcinoma. Cancer Lett, 161, 149-155.

Kiaris H., Schally A.V., Varga J.L., Groot K. and Armatis P. (1999). Growth hormone-releasing hormone: an autocrine growth factor for small cell lung carcinoma. Proc Natl Acad Sci USA, 96, 14894-14898.

Kovacs M., Schally A.V., Lee E-J., Busto R., Armatis P., Groot K. and Varga J.L. (2002). Inhibitory effects of antagonistic analogs of growth hormone-releasing hormone (GHRH) on GH3 pituitary cells expressing the human GHRH receptor. J Endocrinol, 175, 425-434.

Lamharzi N., Schally A.V., Koppan M. and Groot K. (1998). Growth hormone-releasing hormone antagonist MZ-5-156 inhibits growth of DU-145 human androgen-independent prostate carcinoma in nude mice and suppresses the levels and mRNA expression of insulin like growth factor 2 in tumors. Proc Natl Acad Sci USA, 95, 8864-8868.

Pinski J., Schally A.V., Groot K., Halmos G., Szepeshazi K., Zarandi M. and Armatis P. (1995). Inhibition of growth of human osteosarcomas by antagonists of growth hormone-releasing hormone. J Nat Cancer Inst, 87, 1787-1794.

Pinski J., Schally A.V., Jungwirth A., Groot K., Halmos G., Armatis P., Zarandi M. and Vadillo-Buenfil M. (1996) Inhibition of growth of human small-cell and non-small-cell lung carcinomas by antagonists of growth hormone-releasing hormone (GHRH). Int J Oncol, 9, 1099-1105.

Plonowski A., Schally A.V., Busto R., Krupa M., Varga J.L. and Halmos G. (2002a). Expression of growth hormone-releasing hormone (GHRH) and splice variants of GHRH receptors in human experimental prostate cancers. Peptides, 23, 1127-1133.

Plonowski A., Schally A.V., Krupa A., Hebert F., Groot K. and Varga J.L. (2002b). The inhibition of proliferation of PC-3 human prostate cancer by antagonists of growth hormone-releasing hormone is not correlated with the suppression of serum IGF-1 or tumoral IGF-2 and vascular endothelial growth factor. Prostate, 52, 173-182.

Plonowski A., Schally A.V., Varga J.L., Rekasi Z., Hebert F., Halmos G. and Groot K. (2000). Potentiation of the inhibitory effect of growth hormone-releasing hormone antagonists on PC-3 human prostate cancer by bombesin antagonists indicative of interference with both IGF and EGF pathways. Prostate, 44, 172-180.

Pollak M.N., Polychronakos C. and Guyda H. (1989). Somatostatin analogue SMS 201-995 reduces serum IGF-1 levels in patients with neoplasm potentially dependent on IGF-1. Anticancer Res, 9, 889-891.

Rekasi Z., Czompoly T., Schally A.V. and Halmos G. (2000). Isolation and sequencing of cDNAs for splice variants of growth hormone-releasing hormone receptors from human cancers. Proc Natl Acad Sci USA, 97, 10561-10566.

Rekasi Z., Schally A.V., Plonowski A., Czompoly T., Csernus B. and Varga J.L. (2001). Regulation of prostate-specific antigen (PSA) gene expression and release in LNCaP prostate cancer by antagonists of growth hormone-releasing hormone and vasoactive intestinal peptide. Prostate, 48, 188-199.

Rivier J., Spiess J., Thorner M. and Vale W. (1982). Characterization of a growth hormone-releasing factor from a human pancreatic islet tumor. Nature, 300, 276-278.

Robberecht P., Coy D., Waelbroeck M., Heiman M., deNeef P., Camus J-C. and Christophe J. (1985). Structural requirements for the activation of rat anterior pituitary adenylate cyclase by growth hormone-releasing factor (GRF): discovery of (N-Ac-Tyr^1, D-Arg^2)-GRF(1-29)-NH_2 as a GRF antagonist on membranes. Endocrinology, 117, 1759-1764.

Schally A.V. and Comaru-Schally A.M. (1998a). Agonistic analogs of growth hormone-releasing hormone (GHRH): endocrine and growth studies. In Growth Hormone Secretagogues in Clinical Practice, eds Bercu B.B. and Walker R.F., pp. 131-144. New York, Marcel Dekker.

Schally A.V., Comaru-Schally A.M., Nagy A., Kovacs M., Szepeshazi K., Plonowski A., Varga J.L. and Halmos G. (2001). Hypothalamic hormones and cancer. Frontiers Neuroendocrinol, 22, 248-291.

Schally A.V., Comaru-Schally A.M., Plonowski A., Nagy A., Halmos G. and Rekasi Z. (2000). Peptide analogs in the therapy of prostate cancer. Prostate, 45, 158-166.

Schally A.V., Kovacs M., Toth K. and Comaru-Schally A.M. (1998b). Antagonistic actions of growth hormone-releasing hormone: endocrine and oncological studies. In Growth Hormone Secretagogues in clinical practice, eds Bercu B.B. and Walker R.F., pp. 145-162. New York, Marcel Dekker.

Schally A.V. and Varga J.L. (1999). Antagonistic analogs of growth hormone-releasing hormone: new potential antitumor agents. Trends Endocrinol Metab, 10, 383-391.

Szepeshazi K., Schally A.V., Groot K., Armatis P., Halmos G., Hebert F., Szende B., Varga J.L. and Zarandi M. (2000a). Antagonists of growth hormone-releasing hormone (GHRH) decrease IGF-2 Production of HT-29 human colon cancer cells and inhibit tumour growth. Br J Cancer, 82, 1724-1731.

Szepeshazi K., Schally A.V., Groot K., Armatis P., Hebert F. and Halmos G. (2000b). Antagonists of growth hormone-releasing hormone (GHRH) inhibit in vivo proliferation of experimental pancreatic cancers and decrease IGF-2 levels in tumors. Eur J Cancer, 36, 128-136.

Szepeshazi K., Schally A.V., Armatis P., Groot K., Hebert F., Feil A., Varga J.L. and Halmos G. (2001). Antagonists of GHRH decrease production of GH and IGF-1 in MXT mouse mammary cancers and inhibit tumor growth. Endocrinology, 142, 4371-4378.

Szereday Z., Schally A.V., Varga J.L., Hebert F., Armatis P., Groot K., Szepeshazi K., Halmos G. and Busto R. (2002). Antagonists of growth hormone-releasing hormone inhibit the proliferation of experimental non-small cell lung carcinoma. Cancer Res (in press).

Varga J.L., Schally A.V., Csernus V.J., Zarandi M., Halmos G. and Rekasi Z. (1999). Synthesis and biological evaluation of antagonists of growth hormone-releasing hormone with high and protracted in vivo activities. Proc Natl Acad Sci USA, 96, 692-697.

Zarandi M., Horvath J.E., Halmos G., Pinski J., Nagy A., Groot K., Rekasi Z. and Schally A.V. (1994). Synthesis and biological activities of highly potent antagonists of growth hormone-releasing hormone. Proc Natl Acad Sci USA, 91, 12298-12301.

Zarandi M., Kovacs M., Horvath J., Toth K., Halmos G., Groot K., Nagy A., Kele Z. and Schally A.V. (1997). Synthesis and in vitro evaluation of new potent antagonists of growth hormone- releasing hormone (GHRH). Peptides, 18, 423-430.

CHAPTER 10

GH Receptor Antagonists: Basic Knowledge and Clinical Perspectives

A.J. VAN DER LELY

GHR Antagonists: the Past

GH is a protein that contains 191 amino acids with two disulfide bonds and four α helices (Abdel-Meguid et al., 1987; de Vos et al., 1992). Its molecular mass is approximately 22 kDa. GH is secreted by the anterior pituitary gland (Theill and Karin, 1993; Ohlsson et al., 1998). GH signal transduction begins with GH binding to a transmembrane GH receptor (Lesniak et al., 1973). GH has two distinct binding domains that bind to two identical GHRs at the cell surface. The initial (high-affinity) binding of the GH binding site I at the GHR is followed by binding at the GH site II, which produces functional receptor dimerization of the two GHRs (de Vos et al., 1992; Carter-Su et al., 2000).

Transgenic mice that express a GH analogue with a so-called perfect amphiphilic helix 3 (bGH-M8) possess decreased circulating IGF-1 concentrations and exhibit a dwarf phenotype (Chen et al., 1990, 1991a). The observed small phenotype and the fact that bGH-M8 inhibited binding of radioactive iodinated GH to membranes resulted in the first report of a GHR antagonist (Chen et al., 1990; Chen et al., 1991a). Subsequently, it was found that GH analogs with a single amino acid substitution of glycine 120 in the third helix, with any amino acid other than alanine, converted GH from an agonist to an antagonist (Chen et al., 1991b; Fuh et al., 1992).

Kopchick and co-workers proposed that the antagonistic properties of this GH antagonist were due to inability to interact with the second GHR, suggesting that the mechanism by which the GH antagonist acts is by preventing functional GHR dimerization (Chen et al., 1991a, 1991b, 1994; Okada et al., 1992).

This GH antagonist has a relatively small size of 22 kDa. GH is normally cleared via the kidneys and/or GHR internalization and has a half-life of approximately 15 min (Veldhuis et al., 2000). When the resulting GHR antagonist molecule – with the original substitution of glycine 120 as well as eight mutations in site I – was combined with PEG-5000, the final molecule, known as PEG-hGH G120K (B2036 peg), was shown to maintain its GHR binding and antagonistic properties (Thorner et al., 1999), with a half-life of more than 100 h (Rodvold and van der Lely, 1999). PEG-hGH G120K is currently in the final stages of clinical trials for subcutaneous injection in the treatment of acromegaly. The generic name is pegvisomant and its trade name will be Somavert®, which is administered by daily subcutaneous (s.c.) injection.

GHR Antagonists: the Present and Future

Should Acromegaly be Treated with GHR Antagonists?

Acromegaly is virtually always caused by a benign GH-secreting pituitary adenoma and is associated with a proven increased mortality rate (Melmed, 1990, 2001; Orme et al., 1998). Available medical treatment modalities are dopamine agonists and somatostatin analogs. Both these classes of drugs still leave at least one-third of patients eligible for a more effective medical therapy. In 2000, six patients with acromegaly resistant to maximal doses of octreotide therapy were described, who normalized their IGF-1 levels while receiving short-term therapy with pegvisomant (Herman-Bonert et al., 2000).

Two important studies have tried to establish the efficacy of long-term pegvisomant therapy in the treatment of acromegaly (Trainer et al., 2000; van der Lely et al., 2001a). The first was a double-blind placebo-controlled study in 112 patients with active acromegaly, who were treated with either placebo or one of three s.c. dosages (10, 15 or 20 mg) of pegvisomant for 12 weeks (Trainer et al., 2000). In the pegvisomant-treated patients, a dose-related improvement in symptoms and signs was observed. Serum IGF-1 concentrations decreased significantly in all treatment groups, and 82% of patients treated with the highest dose achieved normal serum IGF-1 concentrations at the end of the study.

More aspects of long-term efficacy and safety became available after the publication of the results of a database, containing the data of 152 patients with acromegaly who were treated with pegvisomant for up to 18 months. Of patients treated for 12 months, pegvisomant normalized IGF-1 levels in 90% (Fig. 1) (van der Lely et al., 2001a). During long-term pegvisomant therapy, GH levels increase substantially. However, these patients did show a significant increase in their mean tumor volume (Utiger, 2000; Ho, 2001; van der Lely et al., 2001a). On the other hand, two patients who were not pretreated with radiotherapy, demonstrated a clinically significant increase in tumor size (van der Lely et al., 2001a, 2001b). Another two patients developed a significant but reversible increase in serum liver enzyme concentrations (van der Lely et al., 2001a).

Pegvisomant is the most effective medical treatment for acromegaly to date. Therefore, we might conclude that active acromegaly should indeed be treated with pegvisomant, although a tight control of tumor size and liver enzyme profiles is warranted. In the near future, especially those patients with active acromegaly despite maximal medical treatment with long-acting somatostatin analogs are the most likely candidates for this promising compound.

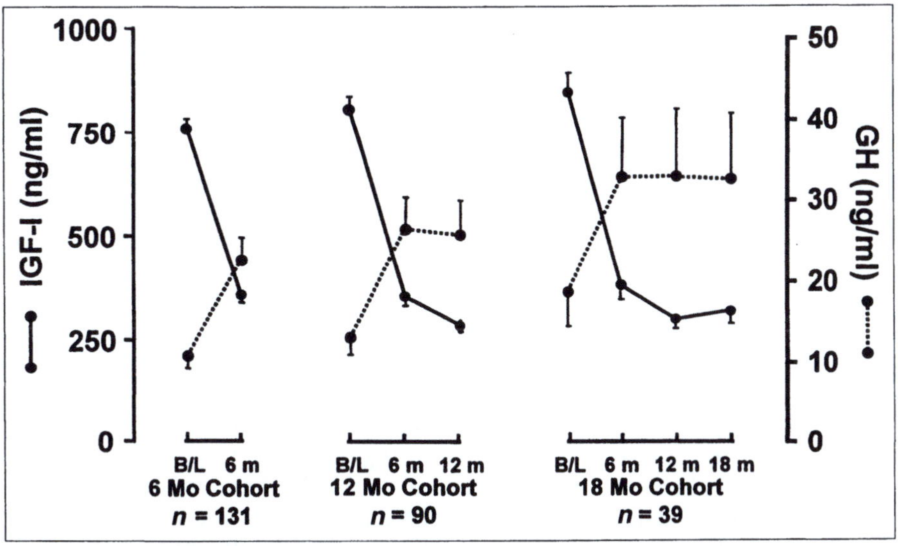

Fig. 1. Serum concentrations of insulin-like growth factor-I (•—•) and growth hormone (•---•) in patients who completed at least 6 months (n = 131), 12 months (n = 90) or 18 months (n = 39) of daily pegvisomant treatment. The cohorts are sequentially constructed, such that all the patients in the 18 month treatment cohort were also included in the 6 and 12 month cohorts, and the patients in the 12 month cohort were also included in the 6 month cohort. For all cohorts, the baseline visit was considered the visit immediately prior to beginning pegvisomant therapy in the initial study protocol. Baseline values were calculated using only data from patients in each cohort. All changes from baseline for both insulin-like growth factor I and growth hormone were statistically significant ($p < 0.05$) for all cohorts. Reproduced by permission from van der Lely et al., 2001a.

Should We Use GHR Antagonists in the Treatment of Cancer?

Cancer is a very complex issue that, with respect to the potential beneficial role of GHR antagonists, should be divided into two possible indications: modification of the induction of cancer and modification of the growth of tumors. The potential use of GHR antagonists is of particular interest, as some recent epidemiological studies have linked IGF-1 with the risk of developing prostate, breast or colon cancer (Hankinson et al., 1998; Chan et al., 1998; Ma et al., 1999).

One preclinical study has tried to address the impact of the presence of a GHR antagonist in transgenic mice expressing a GH antagonist, and in nontransgenic littermates following carcinogenic exposure. As expected, the transgenic animals had significantly lower IGF-1 concentrations and had a dwarf phenotype. Interestingly, the transgenic animals had a decreased tumor incidence (68.2% tumor-free at 39 weeks vs. 31.6% in controls; Pollak et al., 2001).

With respect to modulating tumor growth, IGF-1 is regarded as potent growth factor (Osborne et al., 1990; O'Dell and Day, 1998; Khandwala et al., 2000). Most of the work on the ability of GH receptor antagonists to modify tumor growth has been performed using xenograft or syngenic models in mice. Several experiments have been performed with pegvisomant using a variety of colon cancer models. In one study of a xenografted human colorectal cancer, pegvisomant reduced the volume and weight by 39% and 44%, respectively (Duan et al., 1999). Pegvisomant was also found to be an effective therapy in an animal model with hepatic metastases of colon cancer. Moreover, the combination of pegvisomant and irinotecan (a topoisomerase 1 inhibitor) was superior to either therapy alone (Friend, 2000). In other studies, using tissue and animal models for breast cancer and meningiomas, pegvisomant again showed remarkable beneficial effects on growth and/or tumor size (Friend et al., 1999, 2000; McCutcheon et al., 2001).

The answer to the question at the beginning of this section, "Should we use GHR antagonists in the treatment of cancer?", should therefore be that experimental *preclinical* data suggest that GHR antagonists have very promising beneficial effects in oncology. However, clinical studies must provide the final answer on whether pegvisomant can keep its promises in patient care.

Should We Use GHR Antagonists for the Treatment of Diabetic Complications?

Decades ago it was suggested that GH might play an important role in the development of diabetic microvascular complications (Yde, 1969; Hansen and Johansen, 1970; Lundbaek et al., 1970). Therefore, one might expect some benefits of a blockade of the effects of the increased GH levels in especially poorly controlled diabetes in order to minimize the development of long-term diabetic complications. Naturally, GHR antagonists are interesting candidates for this purpose, and, indeed, some results have already been obtained, that support some potential beneficial effects of pegvisomant. Studies in diabetic mice, transgenic for a GHR antagonist, show that these animals are protected against the development of diabetic renal changes (Chen et al., 1995, 1996; Bellush et al., 2000). Moreover, these beneficial effects were observed without an alteration in glycaemic control. Also, administration of pegvisomant to diabetic mice prevented renal enlargement and glomerular hypertrophy, as well as reduced urinary albumin excretion (Flyvbjerg et al., 1999; Segev et al., 1999).

Another microvascular complication of diabetes is diabetic retinopathy. Nondiabetic, ischemia-associated neovascularization of the retina was inhibited in GHR antagonist-expressing animals (Smith et al., 1997). However, in a recent small pilot study, in 25 type 1 and type 2 diabetes patients with proliferative retinopathy treated with pegvisomant for 12 weeks, a 55% reduction in serum IGF-1 was observed, without regression of retinopathy. Moreover, while 16 patients had an unchanged degree of retinopathy, nine patients even showed progression (Growth Hormone Antagonist for Proliferative Diabetic Retinopathy Study Group, 2001). These results do not support a beneficial effect of pegvisomant on diabetic retinopathy. It would, however, be of interest in future studies to study patients with less severe diabetic eye disease.

The answer to the question at the beginning of this section, "Should we use GHR antagonists for the treatment of diabetic complications?", should therefore be that experimental data suggest that GHR antagonists may present a new concept in the treatment of diabetic renal complications. With respect to diabetic retinopathy, future studies are warranted.

References

Abdel-Meguid S.S., Shieh H.S., Smith W.W., Dayringer H.E., Violand B.N. and Bentle L.A. (1987). Three-dimensional structure of a genetically engineered variant of porcine growth hormone. Proc Natl Acad Sci USA 84, 6434-6437.

Bellush L.L., Doublier S., Holland A.N., Striker L.J., Striker G.E. and Kopchick J.J. (2000). Protection against diabetes-induced nephropathy in growth hormone receptor/binding protein gene-disrupted mice. Endocrinology, 141, 163-168.

Carter-Su C., Rui L. and Herrington J. (2000). Role of the tyrosine kinase JAK2 in signal transduction by growth hormone. Pediatr Nephrol, 14, 550-557.

Chan J.M., Stampfer M.J., Giovannucci E., Gann P.H., Ma J., Wilkinson P., Hennekens C.H. and Pollak M. (1998). Plasma insulin-like growth factor-I and prostate cancer risk: a prospective study. Science, 279, 563-566.

Chen N.Y., Chen W.Y., Bellush L., Yang C.W., Striker L.J., Striker G.E. and Kopchick J.J. (1995). Effects of streptozotocin treatment in growth hormone (GH) and GH antagonist transgenic mice. Endocrinology, 136, 660-667.

Chen N.Y., Chen W.Y. and Kopchick J.J. (1996). A growth hormone antagonist protects mice against streptozotocin induced glomerulosclerosis even in the presence of elevated levels of glucose and glycated hemoglobin. Endocrinology, 137, 5163-5165.

Chen W.Y., Chen N., Yun J., Wagner T.E. and Kopchick J.J. (1994). In vitro and in vivo studies of the antagonistic effects of human growth hormone analogs. J Biol Chem, 269, 20806.

Chen W.Y., White M.E., Wagner T.E. and Kopchick J.J. (1991a). Functional antagonism between endogenous mouse growth hormone (GH) and a GH analog results in dwarf transgenic mice. Endocrinology, 129, 1402-1408.

Chen W.Y., Wight D.C., Mehta B.V., Wagner T.E. and Kopchick J.J. (1991b). Glycine 119 of bovine growth hormone is critical for growth-promoting activity. Mol Endocrinol, 5, 1845-1852.

Chen W.Y., Wight D.C., Wagner T.E. and Kopchick J.J. (1990). Expression of a mutated bovine growth hormone gene suppresses growth of transgenic mice. Proc Nat Acad Sci USA, 87, 5061-5065.

de Vos A.M., Ultsch M. and Kossiakoff A.A. (1992). Human growth hormone and extracellular domain of its receptor: crystal structure of the complex. Science, 255, 306-312.

Duan H., Dagnaes-Hansen F., Rasmussen L., Friend K.E., Orskov H., Bennet W.F. and Flyvbjerg A. (1999). GH receptor antagonist treatment inhibits growth of human colorectal carcinoma, COLO205 in nude mice. Program of the 5th International Symposium on Insulin-like Growth Factors, Brighton, 1999 (Abstract P13).

Flyvbjerg A., Bennett W.F., Rasch R., Kopchick J.J. and Scarlett J.A. (1999). Inhibitory effect of a growth hormone receptor antagonist (G120K-PEG) on renal enlargement, glomerular hypertrophy, and urinary albumin excretion in experimental diabetes in mice. Diabetes, 48, 377-382.

Friend K.E. (2000). Targeting the growth hormone axis as a therapeutic strategy in oncology. Growth Horm IGF Res, 10 (suppl A), S45-S46.

Friend K.E., Flyvbjerg A., Bennet W.F. and McCutcheon I.E. (2000). The growth hormone receptor antagonist pegvisomant exhibits antitumor activity in multiple preclinical tumor models. Proceedings of the 11th NCI-EORTC-AACR Symposium, Amsterdam, The Netherlands (Abstract 420) .

Friend K.E., Radinsky R. and McCutcheon I.E. (1999). Growth hormone receptor expression and function in meningiomas: effect of a specific receptor antagonist. J Neurosurg, 91, 93-99.

Fuh G., Cunningham B.C., Fukunaga R., Nagata S., Goeddel D.V. and Wells J.A. (1992). Rational design of potent antagonists to the human growth hormone receptor. Science, 256, 1677-1680.

Growth Hormone Antagonist for Proliferative Diabetic Retinopathy Study Group (2001). The effect of a growth hormone receptor antagonist drug on proliferative diabetic retinopathy. Ophthalmology, 108, 2266-2272.

Hankinson S.E., Willett W.C., Colditz G.A., Hunter D.J., Michaud D.S., Deroo B., Rosner B., Speizer F.E. and Pollak M. (1998). Circulating concentrations of insulin-like growth factor-I and risk of breast cancer. Lancet, 351, 1393-1396.

Hansen A.P. and Johansen K. (1970). Diurnal patterns of blood glucose, serum free fatty acids, insulin, glucagon and growth hormone in normals and juvenile diabetics. Diabetologia, 6, 27-33.

Herman-Bonert V.S., Zib K., Scarlett J.A. and Melmed S. (2000). Growth hormone receptor antagonist therapy in acromegalic patients resistant to somatostatin analogs. J Clin Endocrinol Metab, 85, 2958-2961.

Ho K.K. (2001). Place of pegvisomant in acromegaly. Lancet, 358, 1743-1744.

Khandwala H.M., McCutcheon I.E., Flyvbjerg A. and Friend K.E. (2000). The effects of insulin-like growth factors on tumorigenesis and neoplastic growth. Endocr Rev, 21, 215-244.

Lesniak M.A., Roth J., Gorden P. and Gavin J.R. III (1973). Human growth hormone radioreceptor assay using cultured human lymphocytes. Nature New Biol, 241, 20-22.

Lundbaek K., Jensen V.A., Olsen T.S., Orskov H., Christensen N.J., Johansen K., Hansen A.P. and Osterby R. (1970). Growth hormone and diabetic angiopathy. Lancet, 2, 472.

Ma J., Pollak M.N., Giovannucci E., Chan J.M., Tao Y., Hennekens C.H. and Stampfer M.J. (1999). Prospective study of colorectal cancer risk in men and plasma levels of insulin-like growth factor (IGF)-I and IGF-binding protein-3. J Natl Cancer Inst, 91, 620-625.

McCutcheon I.E., Flyvbjerg A., Hill H., Li J., Bennett W.F., Scarlett J.A. and Friend K.E. (2001). Antitumor activity of the growth hormone receptor antagonist pegvisomant against human meningiomas in nude mice. J Neurosurg, 94, 487-492.

Melmed S. (1990). Acromegaly. N Engl J Med, 322, 966-977.

Melmed S. (2001). Acromegaly and cancer: not a problem? J Clin Endocrinol Metab, 86, 2929-2934.

O'Dell S.D. and Day I.N. (1998). Insulin-like growth factor II (IGF-II). Int J Biochem Cell Biol, 30, 767-771.

Ohlsson C., Bengtsson B.A., Isaksson O.G., Andreassen T.T. and Slootweg M.C. (1998). Growth hormone and bone. Endocr Rev, 19, 55-79.

Orme S.M., McNally R.J., Cartwright R.A. and Belchetz P.E. (1998). Mortality and cancer incidence in acromegaly: a retrospective cohort study. United Kingdom Acromegaly Study Group. J Clin Endocrinol Metab, 83, 2730-2734.

Osborne C.K., Clemmons D.R. and Arteaga C.L. (1990). Regulation of breast cancer growth by insulin-like growth factors. J Steroid Biochem Mol Biol, 37, 805-809.

Pollak M., Blouin M.J., Zhang J.C. and Kopchick J.J. (2001). Reduced mammary gland carcinogenesis in transgenic mice expressing a growth hormone antagonist. Br J Cancer, 85, 428-430.

Rodvold K. A. and van der Lely A. J. (1999). Pharmacokinetics and pharmacodynamics of B2036PEG, a novel growth hormone receptor antagonist, in acromegalic subjects. The Endocrine Society 81st Annual Meeting. June 12-15 1999, San Diego, CA, Abstract P1-049.

Segev Y., Landau D., Rasch R., Flyvbjerg A. and Phillip M. (1999). Growth hormone receptor antagonism prevents early renal changes in nonobese diabetic mice. J Am Soc Nephrol, 10, 2374-2381.
Smith L.E., Kopchick J.J., Chen W., Knapp J., Kinose F., Daley D., Foley E., Smith R.G. and Schaeffer J.M. (1997). Essential role of growth hormone in ischemia-induced retinal neovascularization. Science, 276, 1706-1709.
Theill L.E. and Karin M. (1993). Transcriptional control of GH expression and anterior pituitary development. Endocr Rev, 14, 670-689.
Thorner M.O., Strasburger C.J., Wu Z., Straume M., Bidlingmaier M., Pezzoli S.S., Zib K., Scarlett J.C. and Bennett W.F. (1999). Growth hormone (GH) receptor blockade with a PEG-modified GH (B2036- PEG) lowers serum insulin-like growth factor-I but does not acutely stimulate serum GH. J Clin Endocrinol Metab, 84, 2098-2103.
Trainer P.J., Drake W.M., Katznelson L., Freda P.U., Herman-Bonert V., van der Lely A.J., Dimaraki E.V., Stewart P.M., Friend K.E., Vance M.L., Besser G.M., Scarlett J.A., Thorner M.O., Parkinson C., Klibanski A., Powell J.S., Barkan A.L., Sheppard M.C., Malsonado M., Rose D.R., Clemmons D.R., Johannsson G., Bengtsson B.A., Stavrou S., Kleinberg D.L., Cook D.M., Phillips L.S., Bidlingmaier M., Strasburger C.J., Hackett S., Zib K., Bennett W.F. and Davis R.J. (2000). Treatment of acromegaly with the growth hormone-receptor antagonist pegvisomant. N Engl J Med, 342, 1171-1177.
Utiger R.D. (2000). Treatment of acromegaly. N Engl J Med, 342, 1210-1211.
van der Lely A.J., Hutson R.K., Trainer P.J., Besser G.M., Barkan A.L., Katznelson L., Klibanski A., Herman-Bonert V., Melmed S., Vance M.L., Freda P.U., Stewart P.M., Friend K.E., Clemmons D.R., Johannsson G., Stavrou S., Cook D.M., Phillips L.S., Strasburger C.J., Hackett S., Zib K.A., Davis R.J., Scarlett J.A. and Thorner M.O. (2001a). Long-term treatment of acromegaly with pegvisomant, a growth hormone receptor antagonist. Lancet, 358, 1754-1759.
van der Lely A.J., Muller A., Janssen J.A., Davis R.J., Zib K.A., Scarlett J.A. and Lamberts S.W. (2001b). Control of tumor size and disease activity during cotreatment with octreotide and the growth hormone receptor antagonist pegvisomant in an acromegalic patient. J Clin Endocrinol Metab, 86, 478-481.
Veldhuis J.D., Bidlingmaier M., Wu Z. and Strasburger C.J. (2000). A selective recombinant human (rh) GH-receptor antagonist fails to impede metabolic removal of endogenous or exogenous GH in healthy adults: evidence that the GH receptor does not participate primarily in the in vivo GH elimination process. 11th International Congress of Endocrinology 2000, Sydney, Australia, p. 405.
Yde H. (1969). Abnormal growth hormone response to ingestion of glucose in juvenile diabetics. Acta Med Scand, 186, 499-504.

GHRELIN AND GHRELIN MIMETICS/GHS

CHAPTER 11

Hypothalamic Circuits Responsive to Ghrelin: Regulation by Leptin and Insulin

S.L. DICKSON, L.Y.C. TUNG AND A.K. HEWSON

Ghrelin

Circulating Ghrelin

Since its discovery in 1999 (Kojima et al., 1999), ghrelin has emerged as a potentially important circulating hunger-inducing peptide (Wren et al., 2001a; Cummings et al., 2001). It was isolated from the oxyntic glands of the rat stomach (Kojima et al., 1999) and this appears to be the major source of circulating ghrelin as levels are reduced by 80% following gastrectomy (Dordonville de la Cour et al., 2001). Ghrelin mRNA has also been detected in a number of other organs, including the pituitary (Korbonits et al., 2001), hypothalamus (Kojima et al., 1999), kidney (Mori et al., 2000), bowel (Date et al., 2000) and placenta (Gualillo et al., 2001).

Actions of Ghrelin and Ghrelin Mimetics

Central or peripheral injection of ghrelin stimulates food intake in satiated rats (Wren et al., 2000, 2001; Nakazato et al., 2001) and, following chronic subcutaneous administration, induces fat accumulation in rodents (Tschöp et al., 2000). These effects are mediated, at least in part, via activation of the cloned growth hormone secretagogue receptor (GHS-R) (Howard et al., 1996), for which synthetic ligands (the growth hormone secretagogues; GHS) have been available for around 20 years. These compounds are so-called based on their potent growth hormone-releasing effects (Bowers et al., 1984) and are now recognized as ghrelin mimetics. The effects of chronic exposure to GHS and ghrelin on appetite and fat accumulation are, however, GH-independent, as they were observed in GH-deficient *lit/lit* mice (Lall et al., 2001; Tschöp et al., 2000).

Ghrelin Release

Ghrelin release appears to be under physiological control. Plasma ghrelin concentrations are lower in states of positive energy balance, both in chronic states, such as obesity (Tschöp et al., 2001), and in acute states, such as following food intake (Cummings et al., 2001). Conversely, ghrelin levels are higher in states of negative energy balance, such as fasting (Cummings et al., 2001) and anorexia nervosa (Otto et al., 2001). It has been suggested that ghrelin has a physiological role in meal initiation, as there appears to be a marked preprandial rise in plasma ghrelin levels in humans (Cummings et al., 2001).

Central Actions of Ghrelin

Circuits Mediating Effects on Appetite and Growth Hormone Secretion

The past decade of GHS research has provided a wealth of information regarding the likely circuits through which ghrelin acts. In 1993, we provided the first evidence that GHS are centrally active, as systemic injection of GHS resulted in an increase in the activity of a subpopulation of arcuate nucleus neurones, shown in both electrophysiological studies and studies mapping expression of the immediate early gene, C-*fos* (Dickson et al., 1993, 1995). Neurochemical identification of the cells expressing *fos* protein following GHS administration revealed that around 50% of the cells activated are neuropeptide Y (NPY)-containing, while 23% contain the endogenous growth hormone-releasing hormone (GHRH; Dickson and Luckman, 1997). Consistent with this, GHS-receptors have been identified on subpopulations of both NPY (Willesen et al., 1999) and GHRH-containing neurones (Tannenbaum and Bowers, 2001).

Evidence for a Role for NPY/AGRP in Ghrelin-induced Feeding

It seems likely that the stimulatory action of ghrelin/GHS on food intake is mediated via these orexigenic neuropeptide Y (NPY) neurones, although there is some debate as to whether it is NPY itself that mediates this response or perhaps agouti-related peptide (AGRP), which is colocalized within the same neurones (Hahn et al., 1998). Indeed, NPY knockout mice show normal fat accumulation following chronic GHS exposure (Tschöp et al., 2002), raising the possibility that it may not be NPY itself that mediates ghrelin/GHS-induced adiposity. AGRP is an endogenous antagonist of the anorectic peptide α-melanocyte stimulating hormone (MSH) (Lu et al., 1994). Thus, AGRP could also mediate ghrelin/GHS effects on food intake. Ghrelin administration has been shown to increase both NPY mRNA and AGRP mRNA in the arcuate nucleus (Kamegai et al., 2001). Moreover, antiserum or antagonists to either NPY or AGRP have been shown to abolish ghrelin–induced feeding (Nakazato et al., 2001; Shintani et al., 2001).

Ghrelin and Other Circulating Regulators of Energy Balance

NPY/AGRP neurones integrate information from circulating satiety and hunger factors.

Arcuate nucleus NPY/AGRP neurones appear to respond to states of positive and negative energy balance. Expression of arcuate nucleus NPY and AGRP mRNAs are greatly enhanced in conditions of hypoinsulinaemia/hypoleptinaemia (e.g. fasting, insulin-deficient diabetes, *ob/ob* mice) and can

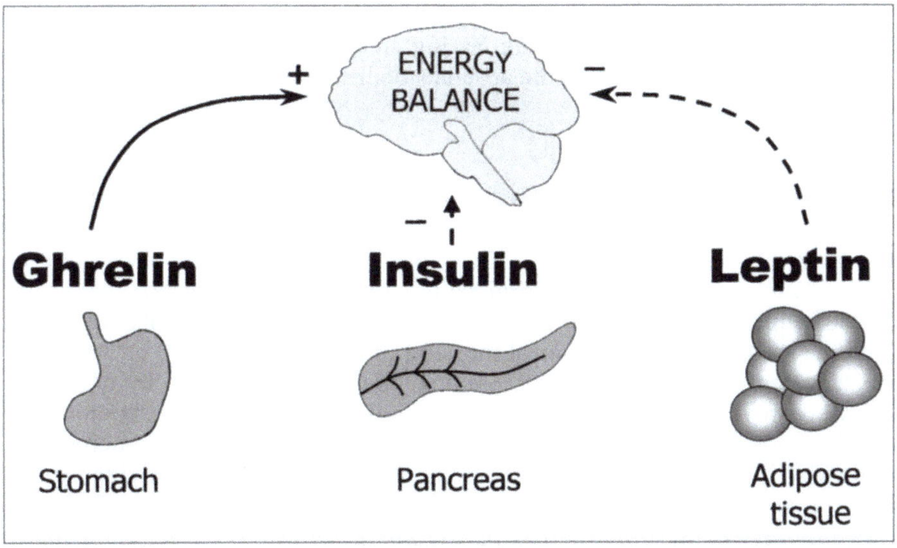

Fig. 1. The hypothalamus receives and integrates information from satiety signals, such as leptin and insulin, and also from the recently discovered gastric peptide ghrelin

be reversed by appropriate replacement of insulin or leptin but not in insulin/leptin-resistant states (e.g. obese *fa/fa* Zucker rats, *db/db* mice; Schwartz et al., 1991, 1992; Marks et al., 1993; Stephens et al., 1995; Cusin et al., 1996). This suggests an inhibitory action of insulin and leptin on arcuate neurone NPY/AGRP gene expression and this is believed to mediate the central inhibitory effect of these hormones on food intake (Friedman, 2000; Baskin et al., 1999). As mentioned above, this is in contrast to the known actions of ghrelin to increase NPY and AGRP gene expression (Kamegai et al., 2001) and stimulate food intake (Tschöp et al., 2000). Thus, arcuate nucleus NPY/AGRP neurones appear to receive and integrate a variety of information (e.g. about nutritional state) from a number of circulating factors (e.g. ghrelin, leptin, insulin; fig. 1). It will be interesting to discover also whether the newly discovered gut peptide $PYY_{3\text{-}36}$ (Batterham *et al.*, 2002) signals information to suppress food intake via this route.

Enhanced Response to Ghrelin/GHS in Fasting

Previously, we showed that there is a 2-3-fold increase in the number of cells expressing Fos protein in response to GHS/ghrelin in the arcuate nucleus of 48 h fasted rats, when compared to normally fed rats (Luckman et al., 1999; Hewson and Dickson, 2000). This suggests that the hypothalamus may be more responsive to GHS/ghrelin in the fasting state or, conversely, that the fed state is associated with a suppressed responsiveness. Thus, either new subpopulations of arcuate nucleus cells are recruited to become activated following GHS/ghrelin in fasting rats, or the activity of a subpopulation of

GHS/ghrelin-responsive cells is suppressed by food intake. One possible explanation for this is that in the fasting state, GHS/ghrelin's hypothalamic actions are left unopposed, in the absence of circulating satiety signals such as leptin and insulin.

Effects of Central Infusion of Leptin and Insulin on Central Responsiveness to GHS

Recently, we examined the possibility that the increased responsiveness of arcuate nucleus neurones to GHS/ghrelin administration in fasted rats may be due to reduced insulin/leptin levels. Thus, in separate experiments, we examined the effects of chronic central infusion of leptin (1.2 μg/day) or insulin (2 mU/day) on GHS-induced Fos protein in the arcuate nucleus. By using the intracerebroventricular route, we can be confident that any effects observed are due to a direct central action of leptin or insulin rather than being secondary to a peripheral action of these hormones, e. g., on blood glucose. We found that chronic central infusion of either insulin or leptin to 48 h fasted rats suppressed the potentiation of the Fos response to GHRP-6 normally seen in the fasted state (Hewson et al., 2002) (Fig. 2).

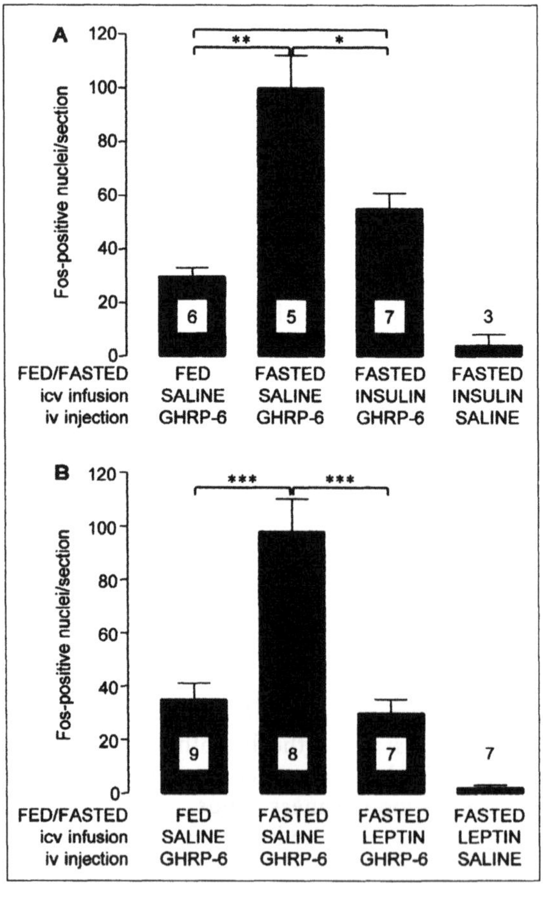

Fig. 2. Mean (± SEM) number of Fos-positive cells in the arcuate nucleus of male rats injected intravenously with GHRP-6 following central infusion of saline and (A) insulin (2 mU/day) or (B) leptin (1.2 μg/day) for 6 days and allowed free access to food throughout (FED) or fasted for the last 48 h of the infusion period (FASTED). * $p = 0.01$, ** $p = 0.004$ and *** $p = 0.001$, Mann-Whitney U-test. Numbers within or above columns indicate the number of animals in each group

Central Actions of GHS in Leptin- and Insulin-resistant Zucker Rats

Further evidence that a subpopulation of ghrelin/GHS-responsive cells in the arcuate nucleus are subject to inhibition by the satiety hormones insulin and leptin is suggested by experiments in obese (*fa/fa*) Zucker rats. The *fa* mutation causes a defect in the leptin receptor (leptin resistance) and subsequently the development of insulin resistance. We found that these rats display a two-fold greater Fos response to GHRP-6 injection compared to lean controls (Fig. 3), despite the manifest hyperleptinemia and hyperinsulinemia (Hewson *et al.*, 2002). The most likely explanation is the inability of leptin and insulin to exert an inhibitory effect on arcuate neurones due to leptin and insulin resistance. This is further supported by the fact that the obese Zucker rats appear to be resistant to changes in central responsiveness to GHS associated with the fasting state; thus, fasting did not potentiate the Fos response to GHS in these rats. Fed obese Zucker rats display a Fos response to GHRP-6 similar to that seen in Wistar and lean Zucker rats following a 48 h fast. Since, in obese Zucker rats, leptin and insulin cannot signal information to the hypothalamus about the size of the energy store, it is perceived to be in a fasted state (even when fed) and the hypothalamus displays increased sensitivity to GHS administration. Perhaps not surprisingly, the Fos response to GHRP-6 in obese Zucker rats was not further increased following a 48 fast, in direct contrast to the marked increase seen in lean Zucker rats, which was associated with clear falls in plasma insulin and lepin levels.

Effects of leptin and insulin on ghrelin-responsive neurones

Using an in vitro electrophysiological approach to record the activity of arcuate nucleus cells in a hypothalamic slice preparation in which synaptic trans-

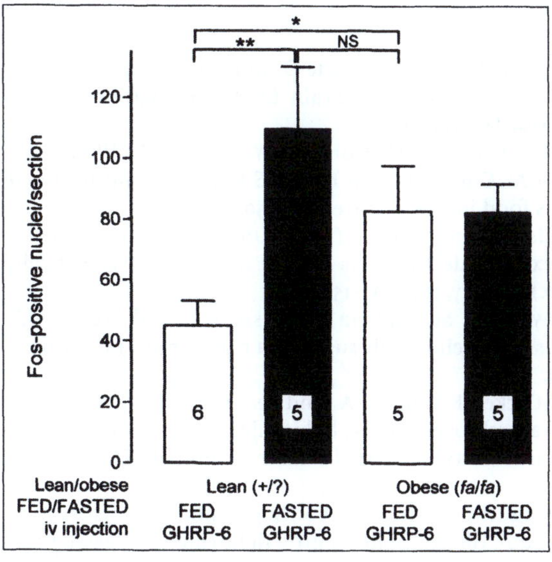

Fig. 3. Mean (± SEM) number of Fos-positive cells in the arcuate nucleus following intravenous administration of GHRP-6 or saline to male rats fed *ad libitum*, fasted for 48 h or fasted for 48 h and refed for 2 h. * $p = 0.003$, ** $p = 0.02$; ns, not significant, Mann-Whitney U-test. Numbers within columns indicate the number of animals in each group

mission is blocked, we have been able to determine whether GHS-responsive neurones also respond to either leptin or insulin. In separate studies we found that arcuate cells activated by GHS tended to be directly inhibited by leptin (Tung et al., 2001) and by insulin (unpublished observation). This suggests that both leptin and insulin can directly suppress the activity of GHS-responsive cells. Whilst this extracellular approach does not allow for neurochemical identification of the cell being recorded from, a cell excited by GHS and inhibited by leptin would certainly fit the expected profile of an NPY neurone, based on the evidence above. It should be noted, however, that the electrical responses of arcuate nucleus neurones to both GHS and leptin are heterogeneous and that other neuronal populations (e.g. GHRH and POMC) might be expected to respond to both GHS and leptin, albeit with different profiles to NPY neurones.

Conclusions

Studies employing both immediate early gene mapping and electrophysiology have shown that the central circuits through which ghrelin operates are subject to inhibitory control by the circulating satiety hormones leptin and insulin. This lends further support to the hypothesis that ghrelin may play a physiological role in the regulation of food intake, as well as an adaptive role in the response to negative energy balance.

Acknowledgments. The authors wish to thank Professor Claes Ohlsson and Maud Petersson at the Department of Clinical Pharmacology, Sahlgrenska University Hospital, Gothenburg, Sweden, for performing the insulin, leptin and glucose assays. This research was supported by the EC Fifth Framework (QLRT-1999-02038) and by the Medical Research Council (MRC), UK.

References

Baskin D.G., Lattemann D.F., Seeley R.J., Woods S.C., Porte D. and Schwartz M.W. (1999). Insulin and leptin: dual adiposity signals to the brain for the regulation of food intake and body weight. Brain Res, 848, 114-123.

Batterham R.L., Cowley M.A., Small C.J., Herzog H., Cohen M.A., Dakin C.L., Wren A.M., Brynes A.E., Low M.J., Ghatei M.A., Cone R.D. and Bloom S.R. (2002). Gut hormone PYY3-36 physiologically inhibits food intake. Nature, 418, 650-654.

Bowers C.Y., Momany F.A., Reynolds G.A. and Hong A. (1984). On the in vitro and in vivo activity of a new synthetic hexapeptide that acts on the pituitary to specifically release growth-hormone. Endocrinology, 114, 1537-1545.

Cummings D.E., Purnell J.Q., Frayo R.S., Schmidova K., Wisse B.E. and Weigle D.S. (2001). A preprandial rise in plasma ghrelin levels suggests a role in meal initiation in humans. Diabetes, 50, 1714-1719.

Cusin I., Rohner Jeanrenaud F., Stricker Krongrad A. and Jeanrenaud B. (1996). The weight-reducing effect of an intracerebroventricular bolus injection of leptin in genetically Obese fa/fa rats-reduced sensitivity compared with lean animals. Diabetes, 45, 1446-1451.

Date Y., Kojima M., Hosoda H., Sawaguchi A., Mondal M.S., Suganuma T., Matsukura S., Kangawa K. and Nakazato M. (2000). Ghrelin, a novel growth hormone-releasing acy-

lated peptide, is synthesized in a distinct endocrine cell type in the gastrointestinal tracts of rats and humans. Endocrinology, 141, 4255-4261.
Dickson S.L., Leng G., Dyball R.E.J. and Smith R.G. (1995). Central actions of peptide and nonpeptide growth-hormone secretagogues in the rat. Neuroendocrinology, 61, 36-43.
Dickson S.L., Leng G. and Robinson I.C.A.F. (1993). Growth-hormone release evoked by electrical-stimulation of the arcuate nucleus in anesthetized male-rats. Brain Res, 623, 95-100.
Dickson S.L. and Luckman S.M. (1997). Induction of c-fos messenger ribonucleic acid in neuropeptide Y and growth hormone (GH)-releasing factor neurons in the rat arcuate nucleus following systemic injection of the GH secretagogue, GH-releasing peptide 6. Endocrinology, 138, 771-777.
Dordonville De la Cour C.D., Bjorkqvist M., Sandvik A.K., Bakke I., Zhao C.M., Chen D. and Hakanson R. (2001). A-like cells in the rat stomach contain ghrelin and do not operate under gastrin control. Reg Peptides, 99, 141-150.
Friedman J.M. (2000). Obesity in the new millennium. Nature, 404, 632-634.
Gualillo O., Caminos J.E., Blanco M., Garcia-Caballero T., Kojima M., Kangawa K., Dieguez C. and Casanueva F.F. (2001). Ghrelin, a novel placental-derived hormone. Endocrinology, 142, 788-794.
Hahn T.M., Breininger J.F., Baskin D.G. and Schwartz M.W. (1998). Coexpression of Agrp and NPY in fasting-activated hypothalamic neurons. Nature Neurosci, 1, 271-272.
Hewson A.K. and Dickson S.L. (2000). Systemic administration of ghrelin induces Fos and Egr-1 proteins in the hypothalamic arcuate nucleus of fasted and fed rats. J Neuroendocrinol, 12, 1047-1049.
Hewson A.K., Tung L.Y.C., Connell D.W., Tookman L. and Dickson S.L. (2002). The rat arcuate nucleus integrates peripheral signals provided by leptin, insulin and a ghrelin mimetic. Diabetes, 51, 3412-3419.
Howard A.D., Feighner S.D., Cully D.F., Arena J.P., Liberator P.A., Rosenblum C.I., Hamelin M., Hreniuk D.L., Palyha O.C., Anderson J., Paress P.S., Diaz C., Chou M., Liu K.K., Mckee K.K., Pong S.S., Chaung L.Y., Elbrecht A., Dashkevicz M., Heavens R., Rigby M., Sirinathsinghji D.J.S., Dean D.C., Melillo D.G., Patchett A.A., Nargund R., Griffin P.R., DeMartino J.A., Gupta S.K., Schaeffer J.M., Smith R.G. and Van der Ploeg L.H.T. (1996). A receptor in pituitary and hypothalamus that functions in growth hormone release. Science, 273, 974-977.
Kamegai J., Tamura H., Shimizu T., Ishii S., Sugihara H. and Wakabayashi I. (2001). Chronic central infusion of ghrelin increases hypothalamic neuropeptide Y and agouti-related protein mRNA levels and body weight in rats. Diabetes, 50, 2438-2443.
Kojima M., Hosoda H., Date Y., Nakazato M., Matsuo H. and Kangawa K. (1999). Ghrelin is a growth-hormone-releasing acylated peptide from stomach. Nature, 402, 656-660.
Korbonits M., Kojima M., Kangawa K. and Grossman A.B. (2001). Presence of ghrelin in normal and adenomatous human pituitary. Endocrine, 14, 101-104.
Lall S., Tung L.Y.C., Ohlsson C., Jansson J.O. and Dickson S.L. (2001). Growth hormone (GH)-independent stimulation of adiposity by GH secretagogues. Biochem Biophys Res Commun, 280, 132-138.
Lu D.S., Willard D., Patel I.R., Kadwell S., Overton L., Kost T., Luther M., Chen W.B., Woychik R.P., Wilkison W.O. and Cone R.D. (1994). Agouti protein is an antagonist of the melanocyte-stimulating-hormone receptor. Nature, 371, 799-802.
Luckman S.M., Rosenzweig I. and Dickson S.L. (1999). Activation of arcuate nucleus neurons by systemic administration of leptin and growth hormone-releasing peptide-6 in normal and fasted rats. Neuroendocrinology, 70, 93-100.
Marks J.L., Waite K. and Li M. (1993). Effects of streptozotocin-induced diabetes-mellitus and insulin-treatment on neuropeptide- Y messenger RNA in the rat hypothalamus. Diabetologia, 36, 497-502.

Mori K., Yoshimoto A., Takaya K., Hosoda K., Ariyasu H., Yahata K., Mukoyama M., Sugawara A., Hosoda H., Kojima M., Kangawa K. and Nakao K. (2000). Kidney produces a novel acylated peptide, ghrelin. Febs Lett, 486, 213-216.
Nakazato M., Murakami N., Date Y., Kojima M., Matsuo H., Kangawa K. and Matsukura S. (2001). A role for ghrelin in the central regulation of feeding. Nature, 409, 194-198.
Otto B., Cuntz U., Fruehauf E., Wawarta R., Folwaczny C., Riepl R.L., Heiman M.L., Lehnert P., Fichter M. and Tschop M. (2001). Weight gain decreases elevated plasma ghrelin concentrations of patients with anorexia nervosa. Eur J Endocrinol, 145, R5-R9.
Schwartz M.W., Marks J.L., Sipols A.J., Baskin D.G., Woods S.C., Kahn S.E. and Porte D. (1991). Central insulin administration reduces neuropeptide- Y messenger RNA expression in the arcuate nucleus of food-deprived lean (fa/fa) but not obese (fa/fa) zucker rats. Endocrinology, 128, 2645-2647.
Schwartz M.W., Sipols A.J., Marks J.L., Sanacora G., White J.D., Scheurink A., Kahn S.E., Baskin D.G., Woods S.C., Figlewicz D.P. and Porte D. (1992). Inhibition of hypothalamic neuropeptide- Y gene-expression by insulin. Endocrinology, 130, 3608-3616.
Shintani M., Ogawa Y., Ebihara K., Aizawa-Abe M., Miyanaga F., Takaya K., Hosoda K., Hayashi T., Inoue G., Kojima M., Kangawa K. and Nakao K. (2001). Ghrelin is a novel orexigenic peptide that antagonizes leptin action through the activation of hypothalamic NeuropeptideY/Y1 pathway. Diabetes, 50, A15.
Stephens T.W., Basinski M., Bristow P.K., Buevalleskey J.M., Burgett S.G., Craft L., Hale J., Hoffmann J., Hsiung H.M., Kriauciunas A., Mackellar W., Rosteck P.R., Schoner B., Smith D., Tinsley F.C., Zhang X.Y. and Heiman M. (1995). The role of neuropeptide-Y in the antiobesity action of the obese gene-product. Nature, 377, 530-532.
Tannenbaum G.S. and Bowers C.Y. (2001). Interactions of growth hormone secretagogues and growth hormone-releasing hormone/somatostatin. Endocrine 14, 21-27.
Tschöp M., Smiley D.L. and Heiman M.L. (2000). Ghrelin induces adiposity in rodents. Nature, 407, 908-913.
Tschöp M., Statnick M.A., Suter T.M. and Heiman M.L. (2002). GH-releasing peptide-2 increases fat mass in mice lacking NPY: Indication for a crucial mediating role of hypothalamic agouti- related protein. Endocrinology, 143, 558-568.
Tschöp M., Weyer C., Tataranni P.A., Devanarayan V., Ravussin E. and Heiman M.L. (2001). Circulating Ghrelin levels are decreased in human obesity. Diabetes, 50, 707-709.
Tung Y.C.L., Hewson A.K. and Dickson S.L. (2001). Actions of leptin on growth hormone secretagogue-responsive neurones in the rat hypothalamic arcuate nucleus recorded in vitro. J Neuroendocrinol, 13, 209-215.
Willesen M.G., Kristensen P. and Romer J. (1999). Co-localization of growth hormone secretagogue receptor and NPY mRNA in the arcuate nucleus of the rat. Neuroendocrinology, 70, 306-316.
Wren A.M., Seal L.J., Cohen M.A., Brynes A.E., Frost G.S., Murphy K.G., Dhillo W.S., Ghatei M.A. and Bloom S.R. (2001a). Ghrelin enhances appetite and increases food intake in humans. J Clin Endocrinol Metab, 86, 5992-5995.
Wren A.M., Small C.J., Abbott C.R., Dhillo W.S., Seal L.J., Cohen M.A., Batterham R.L., Taheri S., Stanley S.A., Ghatei M.A. and Bloom S.R. (2001b). Ghrelin causes hyperphagia and obesity in rats. Diabetes, 50, 2540-2547.
Wren A.M., Small C.J., Ward H.L., Murphy K.G., Dakin C.L., Taheri S., Kennedy A.R., Roberts G.H., Morgan D.G.A., Ghatei M.A. and Bloom S.R. (2000). The novel hypothalamic peptide ghrelin stimulates food intake and growth hormone secretion. Endocrinology, 141, 4325-4328.

Chapter 12

Physiological Function of Growth Hormone Secretagogue Receptors in the Cardiovascular System

H. Ong, D. Lamontagne, A. Demers and S. Marleau

Introduction

Growth hormone secretagogues (GHS) consist of a series of small enkephalin derived peptides identified as growth hormone-releasing peptides (GHRPs) (Bowers, 1993) and non-peptidyl derivatives modeled from GHRPs (Smith et al., 1997). To this class of compounds is recently added a new member, ghrelin, an endogenous 28 amino acid polypeptide isolated from the stomach (Kojima et al., 1999). GHS share a common activity in stimulating the release of growth hormone (GH) from the pituitary in several animal species and in man (Ghigo et al., 2001). The GH release is mediated through the binding of GHS to a G protein-coupled receptor identified by expression cloning as GHS-R1a or ghrelin receptor, for which mRNA expression as well as protein receptor localization are mainly confined to the hypothalamus and the pituitary (Howard et al., 1996).

GHS Receptor Distribution

Peripheral GHS Receptor Distribution

Beyond their somatotroph activity, GHS feature numerous central and peripheral effects on appetite (Wren et al., 2001), energy metabolism and adiposity (Tschöp et al., 2000), insulin secretion (Date et al., 2002), immune function (Hattori et al., 2001) and cardiovascular function (De Gennaro Colonna et al., 1997; Bisi et al., 1999; Bodart et al., 2002; Weekers et al., 2000; MacAndrew et al., 2001). The question about the nature of the receptors mediating the multiple effects of GHS and the distribution of their specific receptors in the target tissues has been addressed by different groups, using both RT-PCR and equilibrium-binding techniques. RT-PCR assay has been used based on the two types of cDNAs isolated from mammalian pituitary: type 1a, encoding seven transmembrane passages functional protein of 41 kDa identified in the hypothalamus and pituitary; and type 1b, encoding a putative protein containing the transmembrane passages 1-5, with no functional activity so far identified. GHS-R1a transcripts were found to be predominantly expressed in the pituitary but also to a much lesser extent in other tissues, such as the adrenals, thyroid, pancreas, spleen, and myocardium (Fig. 1) (Gnanapavan et al., 2002). No GHS-R1a transcript was detected in the gas-

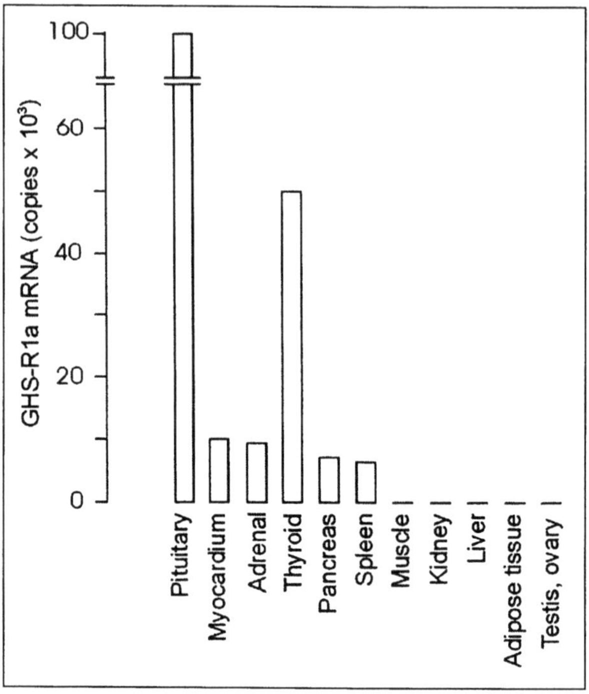

Fig. 1. GHS-R1a mRNA expression in human tissues. RT-PCR results of GHS-R1a receptor expression in human pituitary and peripheral tissues. Adapted from Gnanapavan et al. (2002)

trointestinal tract, kidney, liver, sketelal muscle or reproductive tissues. By contrast, GHS-R1b distribution is ubiquitous, GHS-R1b mRNA being detected in all the peripheral tissues tested (Gnanapavan et al., 2002). Binding studies, using GHRP derivatives or ghrelin as radioligands, have shown that GHS binding sites are widely expressed in a large number of endocrine and non-endocrine human tissues (Papotti et al., 2000). As shown in Table 1, using

Table 1. Binding affinity and maximum density receptors for radiolabeled hexarelin derivative ([125I]-Tyr-Ala- Hexarelin) to GHS receptors in various tissues

Competitive ligand Tissue	Hexarelin	IC_{50} (x 10^{-8} M) Ghrelin	MK 0677	B_{max} (fmol/mg protein)
Pituitary	3.7 ± 1.1	19.3 ± 3.3	18 ± 1.7	1194
Myocardium	3.7 ± 0.8	> 200	> 200	4144
Adrenal	3.4 ± 0.6	17 ± 2.5	18.3 ± 1.4	2819
Thyroid	4.6 ± 0.8	16.3 ± 2.6	17.3 ± 2	957
Pancreas	N/A	N/A	N/A	< 10
Spleen	N/A	N/A	N/A	< 10
Skeletal muscle	5.1 ± 2	> 200	> 200	1500
Kidney	3.8 ± 0.9	> 200	> 200	1391
Liver	4.5 ± 1.6	> 200	> 200	1550
Adipose tissue	3.8 ± 1.0	> 200	> 200	405

Adapted from Papotti et al., J Clin Endocrinol Metab, 2000, 851, 3803.

[^{125}I]Tyr-Ala-hexarelin as the radioligand, the highest density of GHS binding sites was found in the myocardium, followed by the adrenal gland, liver, skeletal muscle, kidney, and the pituitary gland. Although significant binding sites were detected in the thyroid, very low binding signal was found in the spleen, pancreas and stomach. It is interesting to note that the GHS binding data reported for various human tissues did not correlate with GHS-R1a mRNA levels detected in the same tissues. A similar observation has been made for human breast carcinomas, in which significant maximum binding sites (B_{max} value within the range of 2000 fmol/mg protein) were detected using [^{125}I]Tyr-Ala-hexarelin, showing a dissociation constant (K_d) value of 1.7-2 nM, although, no cDNA corresponding to GHS-R1a could be found in these carcinoma cells (Cassoni et al., 2001). These results suggest that the radiolabeled hexarelin derivative binds not only to GHS-R1a but also to other specific receptors expressed in peripheral tissues.

As reported previously, the covalent binding of the photoactivatable hexarelin derivative revealed the existence of GHS receptor subtype of 57 kD in pituitary membranes, which was also detected in the adrenals (Ong et al., 1998a, 1998b; Fig. 2). Whether this receptor subtype is present in different peripheral tissues has yet to be determined.

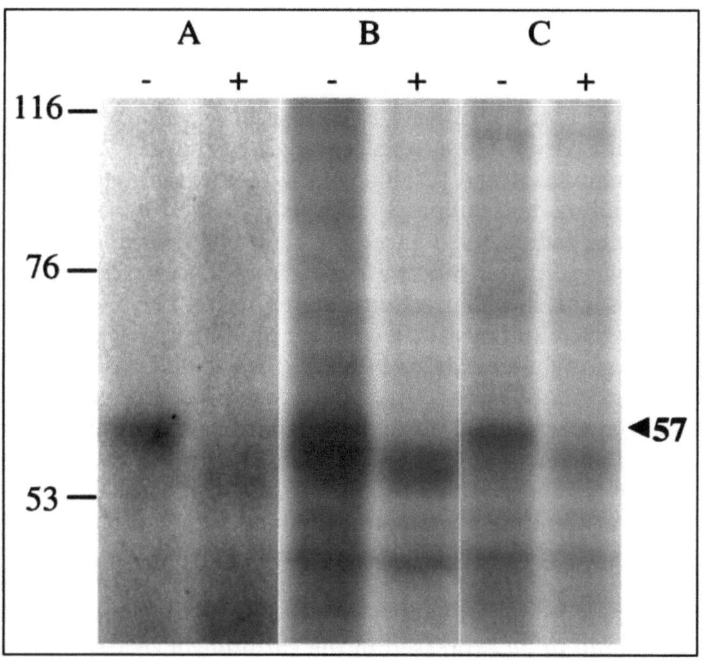

Fig. 2. GHS receptor subtype in human and bovine pituitary and in bovine adrenals. Covalent photolabeling of the GHS receptor subtype with [^{125}I]Tyr-Bpa-Ala-hexarelin in membranes obtained from bovine, human pituitary and bovine adrenals, as previously described (Ong et al., 1998b). Autoradiograms of the SDS-PAGE of the photolabeled membranes from bovine pituitary (A), human pituitary (B) and bovine adrenals (C) in the absence (–) or presence (+) of 10 μM hexarelin featured a specific band at 57 kDa

GHS Receptors in the Cardiovascular System

Among the peripheral tissues, the cardiovascular system appears as one of the major target of GHS, as demonstrated by in vivo and in vitro studies (De Gennaro Colonna et al., 1997; Bisi et al., 1999; Bedendi et al., 2001; Filigheddu et al., 2001). GHS-R1a transcripts in the myocardium revealed the presence of specific binding sites mediating the cardiovascular activities of GHRPs, although transcript numbers were 100-fold lower than those found in the pituitary (Gnanapavan et al., 2002). This finding is consistent with the distribution of GHS-R1a in both left and right atria documented by binding studies using [^{125}I]His^{9}-ghrelin as radioligand in human cardiac membranes (Katugampola et al., 2001). These binding sites showed a B_{max} value of 7.8-9.7 fmol/mg protein and a K_d of 0.43-0.48 nM. The binding sites are also detected in the coronary artery and are characterized by a B_{max} value of 6.2 fmol/mg protein and a K_d of 0.22 nM. Using [^{125}I]Tyr-Ala-hexarelin as radioligand in human cardiac membranes, Papotti et al. (2000) obtained binding sites with a B_{max} value of 4.1 nmol/mg of protein and an IC_{50} of 37 nM, using hexarelin as the competitor agent. In cardiac tissue, the highest level of binding sites was found in the ventricular myocardium followed by atria, coronaries and endocardium (Muccioli et al., 2000). As shown in Table 1, the IC_{50} values differed strikingly according to the ligant used in competition binding assays, with ghrelin and MK-0677 having IC_{50} values more than 50-fold higher than hexarelin (> 2000 nM). By contrast, ghrelin and MK-0677 competes with [^{125}I]Tyr-Ala-hexarelin for binding sites in human pituitary membranes with IC_{50} values of 193 and 180 nM, respectively, as compared to an IC_{50} value of 37 nM for hexarelin in that tissue. These results suggested distinct GHS binding sites within the human heart and pituitary. In agreement, the apparent inconsistency in the binding data obtained when using either the radiolabeled hexarelin derivative or radiolabeled ghrelin as radioligands could be explained by the presence of additional binding sites, distinct from GHS-R1a, for which hexarelin binds with a higher affinity than ghrelin. In order to characterize these novel cardiac binding sites, a covalent binding approach using the photoactivatable benzoylphenylalanine (Bpa) radiolabeled derivative of hexarelin, [^{125}I]Tyr-Bpa-Ala-hexarelin, was used as radioligand (Bodart et al., 1999). The covalent binding studies, performed in cardiac membranes from various animal species and in man, led to the identification of the specific cardiac binding sites of hexarelin with a M_r of 84 kDa. The saturation binding curves gave a B_{max} of 91 fmol/mg protein and the binding affinity, assessed by competition curves using hexarelin as competitor, gave an IC_{50} value of 2.3 μM (Bodart et al., 1999). Further characterization of this binding site revealed a structure identical to that of CD36 (Bodart et al., 2002), a multiligand receptor that was found to be expressed in the cardiomyocytes and the microvascular endothelium (Febbraio et al., 2001). Using hexarelin and ghrelin as competitors for the binding of the radioiodinated photoactivatable derivative of hexarelin in rat heart membrane preparations, we show that hexarelin appears to bind with higher affinity to these binding sites, identified as CD36, than does ghrelin (Fig. 3). Taken together, these results suggest the existence of at least two classes of binding sites for GHS within the heart: (a) GHS-R1a

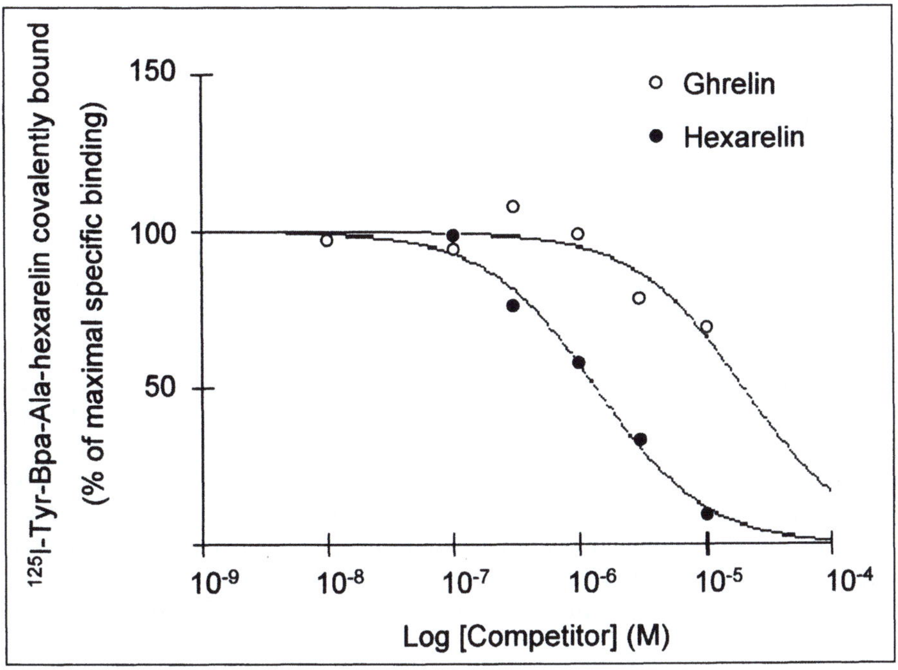

Fig. 3. Competition curves of hexarelin and ghrelin for the binding of [^{125}I] Tyr-Bpa-Ala-hexarelin in rat cardiac membranes. A fixed concentration of [^{125}I] Tyr-Bpa-Tyr-Ala-hexarelin (0.33 nM) was incubated with rat cardiac membranes in presence of increasing concentrations of hexarelin or ghrelin as competitors. (●) Hexarelin, (○) ghrelin

receptor, as the high-affinity and low-density binding site; and (b) the multi-ligand receptor CD36, as the binding site of low affinity and high density. Hexarelin derivatives bind to both GHS-R1a and CD36. By contrast, ghrelin binds specifically to GHS-R1a.

Physiological Functions of GHS in the Cardiovascular System

Cardioprotective Effect of GHS

The first evidence of the cardiovascular activity of GHS was the cardioprotective effect of GHS against ischemia-reperfusion (I/R) injury, known as "myocardial stunning", which consists of impaired systolic and diastolic function, as evidenced by reduced contractility and relaxation of the heart. Long-term pretreatment of rats with GHS, including the pyrazolinone-piperidine peptidomimetic derivative CP 424,391 and the GHRPs hexarelin and GHRP-2, for a period of 1-3 weeks, afforded protection against post-ischemic ventricular dysfunction induced by I/R in Langendorff perfused hearts from GH-deficient rats (De Gennaro Colonna et al., 1997), aged rats (Rossoni et al., 1998) and rabbits (Weekers et al., 2000; MacAndrew et al.,

2001). In addition, we report here the cardioprotective role of hexarelin in preserving the integrity of the endothelial function against ischemic injury, as assessed by the dilator response to serotonin in Langendorff-perfused rat hearts (Fig 4). Sprague-Dawley rat hearts were submitted to I/R protocols as previously described (Bouchard and Lamontagne, 1996). Hearts subjected to a severe 30 min low-flow ischemia showed an altered vasodilatation response to serotonin, which was abolished by 10 μM hexarelin added to the perfusate. The protective effect exerted by hexarelin on serotonin-induced endothelial vasodilator response was of the same magnitude than the one obtained by ischemic preconditioning. Full recovery of the left ventricle end-diastolic pressure (LVEDP) upon reperfusion of the hearts from GHS pretreated animals comparable to that observed following ischemic preconditioning. Interestingly, the signaling pathways involved, and more specifically the upregulation of protein kinase C (PKC) activity, is a common feature of GHS-R1a stimulation and ischemic preconditioning. In agreement, the cardioprotection afforded by both conditions was abolished by chelerythrine (Fig. 4). It has also been reported that an increase in PKC activity is associated with a selective improvement of diastolic stiffness in I/R (Musters et al., 1999). Furthermore, GHS action in somatotrophs is associated with an increase of

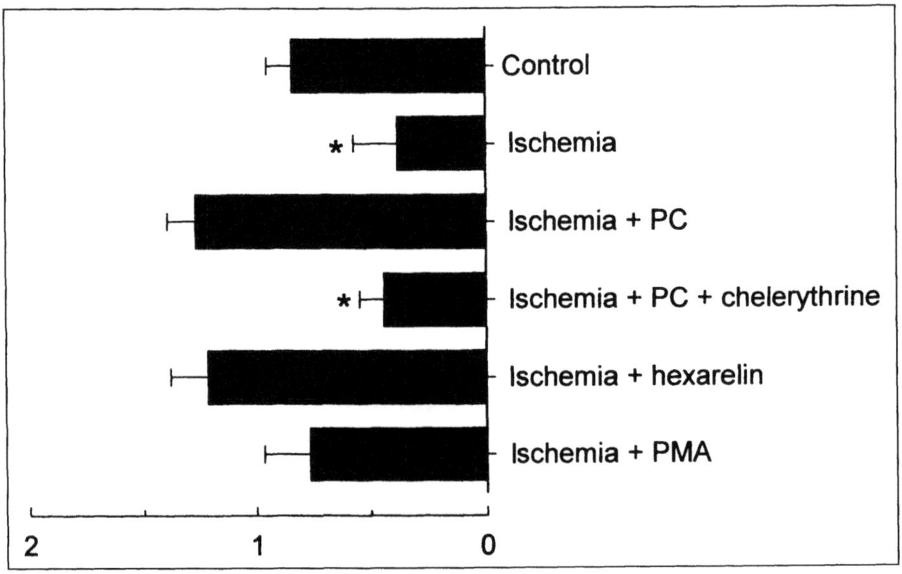

Fig. 4. Cardioprotective effect of hexarelin in preserving the integrity of the endothelial function against ischemic injury. The ratio of the dilator response to the endothelium-dependent dilator, serotonin (5-HT; 10 μM), on that of the endothelium-independent dilator, sodium nitroprussiate (SNP; 3 μM), in Langendorff-perfused rat hearts in time-matched controls, and in hearts exposed to a 30 min low-flow ischemia (1 ml/min), without or with a 5 min zero-flow ischemic preconditioning (PC), in either the absence or presence of the PKC inhibitor, chelerythrine (1 μM) was presented. Additional experiments were performed in ischemic hearts perfused with either hexarelin (10 μM) or the PKC activator, PMA (10 nM). * $p < 0.05$ compared with control hearts

inositol (1,4,5)-trisphosphate ($InsP_3$) and diacylglycerol following the activation of phospholipase Cβ, leading to an increase in PKC activity (Wu et al., 1997). It is therefore conceivable that this signaling pathway is also involved upon activation of cardiac GHS-R1a receptors by GHS. Hexarelin also induced a vasoconstrictive response in isolated, perfused rat hearts, and a role for PKC as an intracellular signal transduction pathway is supported by both chelerythrine and bisindoylmaleimide inhibition of hexarelin-induced vasoconstriction (Bodart et al., 1999). As the increase in intracellular $InsP_3$, induced by the binding of GHS to GHS-R1a, is linked to intracellular calcium (Ca) release and Ca influx, it may be that long-term GHS treatment is associated with an adaptative activation of Ca reuptake pathways, thereby preventing cytosolic Ca overload in myocardial cells. Interestingly, the creatine kinase release profile of GHS-treated hearts subjected to I/R conditions displays a significantly lower amount of creatine release than hearts from controls, indicating preservation of the myocardial cell membranes, integrity with hexarelin pretreatment (Berti et al., 1999). This cardioprotective effect induced by GHS appears to be GH/IGF-1-independent, as hexarelin is still capable to induce the recovery of LVEDP at reperfusion, in hearts from obese Zucker rats featuring an impaired secretion of GH (De Gennaro Colonna et al., 2000) as well as in hypophysectomized rats (Locatelli et al., 1999). Recently, the cardioprotective effect of hexarelin against cytotoxic agents such as doxorubicin and TNFα on H9C2 cells (fetal cardiomyocyte-derived cells), have been reported (Filigheddu et al., 2001). Hexarelin exerts its effect through inhibition of apoptosis, which involves activation of the AkT kinase signaling pathway. This inhibitory effect of hexarelin on cardiomyocyte apoptosis was suggested as the mechanism of cardioprotection against ischemia observed in vivo.

Taken together, the data show that GHS bind to two classes of binding sites so far identified in the myocardium: GHS-R1a receptor and/or CD36. The signaling pathways triggered by the binding of GHS to the two receptors involves PKC activation, which plays a key role in the cardioprotective effect of these compounds. The direct effect of GHS in myocardial cells is similar to that of ischemic preconditioning, thus preventing injury associated with Ca overload in these cells.

Cardiotropic Effect of GHS

The beneficial effect of hexarelin pretreatment on LVDP during the reperfusion period in the I/R study (Rossoni et al., 1998) and on the stroke volume index, as determined by transthoracic echocardiography in rats 4 weeks after myocardial infarction (Tivesten et al., 2000), suggests a direct inotropic effect of hexarelin on the myocardium. In support, acute administration of hexarelin in humans induces an increase of left ventricular ejection fraction (LVEF) in hypopituitary patients with severe GH deficiency, as well as in normal volunteers, suggesting that this effect is unlikely to be IGF-1-dependent but rather results from a direct effect of the peptide on the myocardium. Although the subtype of GHS receptors mediating the inotropic effect of hexarelin remains speculative, studies on isolated papillary muscle showed that hexarelin induced a transient increase of the contractile force which was abolished by propranolol. This suggests that hexarelin exerts an indirect effect on papillary muscle contractility by inducing the transient release of endogenous catecholamines from nerve endings within cardiac tissue (Bedendi et al., 2001). Furthermore, the absence of any direct effect of hexarelin on calcium transients in isolated ventricular cells suggests that hexarelin may not feature any contractile activity involving L-type calcium current (Bedendi et al., 2001).

Vasoactive Properties of GHS

The vasoactive properties of GHS were first demonstrated by the negative modulatory effect of these compounds on the hyperreactivity of the coronary vasculature (De Gennaro Colonna et al., 1997) and aortic rings (Rossoni et al., 1998) to vasoconstrictors such as angiotensin II and endothelin-1. Long-term pretreatment of rats with hexarelin normalized the vasopressor response to angiotensin II and endothelin-1, and this was associated with a parallel increase of PGI_2 and nitric oxide (NO) production. Interestingly, ghrelin, the endogenous ligand, displayed a vasodilatory effect as shown by an increase of forearm blood flow, through a NO-independent mechanism following its intra-arterial infusion (Okumura et al., 2002). This finding is consistent with the hemodynamic response to i.v. infusion of ghrelin in normal subjects. Ghrelin significantly decreased mean arterial pressure with an increase in the cardiac index and stroke volume index (Nagaya et al., 2001). The vasodilatory activity of ghrelin has been recently evidenced in human endothelium-denuded internal mammary artery precontracted with endothelin-1 (Wiley and Davenport, 2002). Whether the regulation of the vascular tone by GHS following their chronic or acute administration is mediated by GHS-R1a receptor remains to be ascertained, inasmuch as gene expression of this G protein-coupled receptor has been detected in the aorta and the heart (Nagaya et al., 2001). By contrast, the acute administration of hexarelin in micromolar concentrations induced a potent and transient coronary vasoconstriction in perfused rat heart (Bodart et al., 1999). This vasoconstrictive effect of hexarelin is mediated through the binding of hexarelin to CD36, a multiligand receptor expressed in the microvascular endothelium (Bodart et al., 2002).

Conclusions

Beyond somatotroph activity, GHS feature interesting pharmacological properties which may lead to potential clinical applications. The cardioprotective activity of GHS may find its application in preventing I/R injury from low-flow bypass surgery. The interaction of GHS with the multiligand receptor CD36 opens new perspectives for the use of these compounds in the regulation of atherosclerosis development and the negative modulation of angiogenesis, as CD36 is reported to play a key role in lipid metabolism in the macrophages and in the proliferation of the microvasculature.

References

Bedendi I., Gallo M.P., Malan D., Levi R.C. and Alloatti G. (2001). Role of endothelial cells in modulation of contractility induced by hexarelin in rat ventricle. Life Sci, 69, 2189-2201.

Berti F., Rossoni G., and De Gennaro Colonna V. (1999). Hexarelin, a synthetic growth hormone secretagogue, exhibits protectant activity in experimental myocardial ischemia and reperfusion. In Growth hormone secretagogues, eds E. Ghigo, M. Boghen, F.F. Casanueva and C. Dieguez, pp. 301-314. New York, Elsevier Science.

Bisi G., Podio V., Valetto M.R., Broglio F., Bertuccio G., Del Rio G., Arvat E., Boghen M.F., Deghenghi R., Muccioli G., Ong H. and Ghigo E. (1999). Acute cardiovascular and hormonal effects of GH and hexarelin, a synthetic GH-releasing peptide, in humans. J Endocrinol Invest, 22, 266-272.

Bodart V., Bouchard J.F., McNicoll N., Escher E., Carriere P., Ghigo E., Sejlitz T., Sirois M.G., Lamontagne D. and Ong, H. (1999). Identification and characterization of a new growth hormone-releasing peptide receptor in the heart. Circ Res, 85, 796-802.

Bodart V., Febbraio M., Demers A., McNicoll N., Pohankova P., Perreault A., Sejlitz T., Escher E., Silverstein R.L., Lamontagne D. and Ong, H. (2002). CD36 mediates the cardiovascular action of growth hormone-releasing peptides in the heart. Circ Res, 90, 844-849.

Bouchard J.F. and Lamontagne D. (1996). Mechanisms of protection afforded by preconditioning to endothelial function against ischemic injury. Am J Physiol, 271, H1801-H186.

Bowers C.Y. (1993). GH-releasing peptides-structure and kinetics. J Pediatr Endocrinol, 6, 21-31.

Cassoni P., Papotti M., Ghè C., Catapano F., Sapino A., Graziani A., Deghenghi R., Reissmann T., Ghigo E. and Muccioli G. (2001). Identification, characterization, and biological activity of specific receptors for natural (ghrelin) and synthetic growth hormone secretagogues and analogs in human breast carcinomas and cell lines. J Clin Endocrinol Metab, 86, 1738-1745.

Date Y., Nakazato M., Hashiguchi S., Dezaki K., Mondal M.S., Hosoda H., Kojima M., Kangawa K., Arima T., Matsuo H., Yada T. and Matsukura S. (2002). Ghrelin is present in pancreatic α-cells of humans and rats and stimulates insulin secretion. Diabetes, 51, 124-129.

De Gennaro Colonna V., Rossoni G., Bernareggi M., Muller E.E. and Berti F. (1997). Cardiac ischemia and impairment of vascular endothelium function in hearts from growth hormone-deficient rats: protection by hexarelin. Eur J Pharmacol, 334, 201-207.

De Gennaro Colonna V., Rossoni G., Cocchi D., Rigamonti A.E., Berti F. and Muller E.E. (2000). Endocrine, metabolic and cardioprotective effects of hexarelin in obese Zucker rats. J Endocrinol, 166, 529-536.

Febbraio M., Hajjar D.P., and Silverstein R.L. (2001). CD36: a class B scavenger receptor involved in angiogenesis, atherosclerosis, inflammation, and lipid metabolism. J Clin Invest, 108, 785-791.

Filigheddu N., Fubini A., Baldanzi G., Cutrupi S., Ghè C., Catapano F., Broglio F., Bosia A., Papotti M., Muccioli G., Ghigo E., Deghenghi R. and Graziani A. (2001). Hexarelin protects H9c2 cardiomyocytes from doxorubicin-induced cell death. Endocrine, 14, 113-119.

Ghigo E., Arvat E., Giordano R., Broglio F., Gianotti L., Maccario M., Bisi G., Graziani A., Papotti M., Muccioli G., Deghenghi R. and Camanni F. (2001). Biologic activities of growth hormone secretagogues in humans. Endocrine, 14, 87-93.

Gnanapavan S., Kola B., Bustin S.A., Morris D.G., McGee P., Fairclough P., Bhattacharya S., Carpenter R., Grossman A.B., and Korbonits M. (2002). The tissue distribution of the mRNA of ghrelin and subtypes of its receptor, GHS-R, in humans. J Clin Endocrinol Metab, 87, 2988.

Hattori N., Saito T., Yagyu T., Jiang B.-H., Kitagawa K., and Inagaki C. (2001). GH, GH receptor, GH secretagogue receptor, and ghrelin expression in human T cells, B cells, and neutrophils. J Clin Endocrinol Metab, 86, 4284-4291.

Howard A.D., Feighner S., Cully D.F., Arena J.P., Liberator P.A., Resenblum C.I., Hamelin M., Hreniuk D.L., Palyha O.C., Anderson J., Paress P.S., Diaz C., Chou M., Liu K.K., McKee K.K., Pong S.S., Chaung L.Y., Elbrecht A., Dashkevicz M., Heavens R., Rigby M., Sirinathsinghji D.J., Dean D.C., Mellilo D.G. and Van der Ploeg L.H. (1996). A receptor in pituitary and hypothalamus that functions in growth hormone release. Science, 273, 974-977.

Katugampola S.D., Pallikaros Z. and Davenport M. (2001). ^{125}I-His(9)-ghrelin, a novel radiologand for localizing GHS orphan receptors in human and rat tissue: up-regulation of receptors with atherosclerosis. Br J Pharmacol, 134, 143-149.

Kojima M., Hosoda H., Date Y., Nakazato M., Matsuo H. and Kangawa K. (1999). Ghrelin is a growth-hormone-releasing acylated peptide from stomach. Nature, 402, 656-660.

Locatelli V., Rossoni G., Schweiger F., Torsello A., De Gennaro C.V., Bernareggi M., Deghenghi R., Muller E.E. and Berti F. (1999). Growth hormone-independent cardioprotective effects of hexarelin in the rat. Endocrinology, 140, 4024-4031.

MacAndrew J.T., Ellery S.S., Parry M.A., Pan L.C. and Black S.C. (2001). Efficacy of a growth hormone-releasing peptide mimetic in cardiac ischemia/reperfusion injury. Eur J Pharmacol, 432, 195-202.

Muccioli G., Broglio F., Valetto M.R., Ghè C., Catapano F., Graziani A., Papotti M., Bisi G., Deghenghi R. and Ghigo E. (2000). Growth hormone-releasing peptides and the cardiovascular system. Ann Endocrinol, 61, 27-31.

Musters R.J., van der Meulen E.T., Zuidwijk M., Muller A., Simonides W.S., Banerjee A. and van Hardeveld C. (1999). PKC-dependent preconditionning with norepinephrine protects sarcoplasmic reticulum function in rat trabeculae following metabolic inhibition. J Mol Cell Cardiol, 31, 1083-1094.

Nagaya N., Kojima M., Uematsu M., Yamagishi M., Hosoda H., Oya H., Hayashi Y. and Kangawa K. (2001). Hemodynamic and hormonal effects of human ghrelin in healthy volunteers. Am J Physiol Regulatory Integrative Comp Physiol, 280, R1483-R1487.

Okumura H., Nagaya N., Enomoto M., Nakagawa E., Oya H. and Kangawa K. (2002). Vasodilatory effect of ghrelin and endogenous peptides from the stomach. J Cardiovasc Pharmacol, 39, 779-783.

Ong H., Bodart V., McNicoll N., Lamontagne D. and Bouchard J.F. (1998a). Binding sites for growth hormone-releasing peptide. Growth Horm IGF Res, 8 (Suppl B), 137-140.

Ong H., McNicoll N., Escher E., Collu R., Deghenghi R., Locatelli V., Ghigo E., Muccioli G., Boghen M. and Nilsson A. (1998b). Identification of a pituitary growth hormone-releasing peptide (GHRP) receptor subtype by photoaffinity labeling. Endocrinology, 139, 432-435.

Papotti M., Ghè C., Cassoni P., Catapano F., Deghenghi R., Ghigo E. and Muccioli G. (2000). Growth hormone secretagogue binding sites in peripheral human tissues. J Clin Endocrinol Metab, 85, 3803-3807.

Rossoni G., De Gennaro Colonna V., Bernareggi M., Polvani G.L., Muller E.E. and Berti F. (1998). Protectant activity of hexarelin or growth hormone against postischemic ventricular dysfunction in hearts from aged rats. J Cardiovasc Phamacol, 32, 260-265.

Smith R.G., Van der Ploeg L.H.T., Howard A.D., Feighner S.D., Cheng K., Hickey G.J., Wyvratt M.J. Jr, Fisher M.H., Nargund R.P. and Patchett A.A. (1997). Peptidomimetic regulation of growth hormone secretion. Endoc Rev, 18, 621-645.

Tivesten Å., Bollano E., Caidahl K., Kujacic V., Sun X.Y., Hedner T., Hjalmarson Å., Bengtsson B.-Å. and Isgaard J. (2000). The growth hormone secretagogue hexarelin improves cardiac function in rats after experimental myocardial infarction. Endocrinology, 141, 60-66.

Tschöp M., Smiley D.L. and Heiman M.L. (2000). Ghrelin induces adiposity in rodents. Nature, 407, 908-913.

Weekers F., Van Herck E., Isgaard J. and Van den Berghe G. (2000). Pretreatment with growth hormone-releasing peptide-2 directly protects against the diastolic dysfunction of myocardial stunning in an isolated, blood-perfused rabbit heart model. Endocrinology, 141, 3993-3999.
Wiley K.E. and Davenport A.P. (2002). Comparison of vasodilators in human mammary arteries: ghrelin is a potent physiological antagonist of endothelin. Br J Pharmacol, 136, 1146-1152.
Wren A.A., Small C.J., Abbott C.R., Dhillo W.S., Seal L.J., Cohen M.A., Batterham R.L., Taheri S., Stanley S.A., Ghatei M.A. and Bloom S.R. (2001). Ghrelin causes hyperphagia and obesity in rats. Diabetes, 50, 2540-2547.
Wu D., Clarke I.J. and Chen C. (1997). The role of protein kinase C (PKC) in growth hormone (GH) secretion induced by GH-releasing factor (GRF) and GH-releasing peptides (GHRP) in cultured ovine somatotrophs. J Endocrinol, 154, 219-230.

CHAPTER 13

Endocrine and Extraendocrine Activity of Ghrelin and the GHS: Basic Research

E. BRESCIANI, A. TORSELLO, R. AVALLONE, I. BULGARELLI, C. NETTI, V. SIBILIA, G. RINDI, E.E. MÜLLER AND V. LOCATELLI

Introduction

Until few years ago it was generally accepted that the secretion of growth hormone (GH) was mainly regulated by stimulatory and inhibitory influences of two hypothalamic hypophysiotropic hormones, the growth hormone releasing hormone (GHRH) and somatostatin (SS), respectively. GHRH and SS were considered the final common pathway by which neurotransmitters, peripheral hormone, and environmental, metabolic and immune stimuli could influence the secretion of GH (Locatelli and Torsello, 1997; Müller et al., 1999). However, at the end of 1970s, the observation that several synthetic peptidyl and non-peptidyl molecules, derived from the pentapeptide met-enkephalin and named "growth hormone secretagogues" (GHS), were able to potently stimulate GH secretion from cultured pituitary cells (Bowers et al., 1980), experimental animals (Bowers et al., 1984), and humans (Ilson et al., 1989; Bowers et al., 1990) was suggestive of the existence of another endogenous factor physiologically involved in the regulation of GH release. In 1996, the identification of a specific GHS receptor (GHS-R) distinct from that of GHRH (Howard et al., 1996; Pong et al., 1996) further supported this hypothesis, and made possible the recent discovery of its endogenous agonist. The endogenous natural ligand of the GHS-R was isolated from a peripheral tissue, the stomach, and not, as generally expected, from the hypothalamus, and was named "ghrelin" (ghre is the Proto-Indo-European root of the word "grow") (Kojima et al., 1999).

Ghrelin

Structure

Ghrelin is a peptidic linear molecule of 28 amino acidic residues (molecular weight = 3314) with no significant homology with any of the GHS synthesized up to now. In the original study that led to its identification and structural characterization, Kojima and coworkers used a cell line stably transfected with the GHS-R in order to record the variations of intracellular calcium ($[Ca^{2+}]_{in}$) that follow receptor activation. This technique was used to screen homogenates obtained from different organs and tissues. The final result was the discovery that the maximal increase in intracellular calcium followed the cell exposure to a homogenate from the stomach. Sequential steps of purification allowed the identification of the N-terminal amino acid sequence of the molecule responsible for this action. This short sequence was used for the identification and sequencing of the mRNA encoding the full protein. However, the peptide synthesized using the sequence deduced from its cDNA, was ineffective in increasing $[Ca^{2+}]_{in}$ in cells transfected with the GHS-R. Moreover, the syntheic peptide had a lower molecular weight than the natural ghrelin purified from the stomach, suggesting that the endogenous ghrelin carried some kind of modifications that were essential for its biological activity. More detailed research revealed, in fact, the serine residue in position 3 (Ser^3) was esterified with n-octanoic acid, a peculiar post transductional modification capable of increasing the lipophilicity of the molecule and confering biological properties similar to those of the native ghrelin.

The analysis of a cDNA library from rat stomach demonstrated that the ghrelin gene encodes for a 117 amino acid peptide, named prepro-ghrelin, which shares an elevated sequence homology (82.9%) with the human form, indicating that the protein is highly conserved among different animal species (Kojima et al., 1999).

It is interesting that ghrelin mostly circulates as des-octanoyl ghrelin, i.e. without the esterification of Ser^3, a form of the protein that is devoid of endocrine properties and incapable of stimulating GHS-R (Kojima et al., 1999; Bednarek et al., 2000; Muccioli et al., 2001; Hosoda et al., 2000b).

Acylated ghrelin crosses the blood-brain barrier in both directions, from blood to brain and from brain to blood, using a saturable transport system that requires the presence of the unique octanoyl residue of the ghrelin molecule. In contrast, desacyl ghrelin crosses the blood-brain barrier by non-saturable passive mechanisms and is retained by the brain once within the central nervous system (Banks et al., 2002).

After the discovery of ghrelin, another form of the protein was isolated and named des-Gln^{14}-ghrelin. This is a 27 amino acid protein, with a peptidic sequence similar to that of ghrelin but lacking the Gln in position 14. Similarly to ghrelin, this molecule also requires the n-octanoylation of Ser^3 for its biological activity. Surprisingly, these two peptides, so similar in chemical structure and pharmacologic activity, result from the alternative splicing of a unique gene that produces two distinct mRNAs (Hosoda et al., 2000a).

Shortly after the publication of the original report describing the characterization of ghrelin and des-Gln^{14}-ghrelin, a paper from Tomasetto et al. (2000) reported the independent isolation from the gastrointestinal tract of the mouse of a protein that, due to its partial homology with motilin, was named motilin-related peptide. Comparisons of the protein sequences revealed that the motilin-related peptide and ghrelin were the same molecule (Fig. 1).

Rat ghrelin	GSS■LSP■H■KA■QR■■SK■PPAKLQPR
Human ghrelin	GSS■LSP■H■RV■QR■■SK■PPAKLQPR
Motilin	FVPI■TYG■L■RM■E-■■RN■GQ

Fig. 1. Sequence homology between human and rat ghrelin, and rat motilin. Identical amino acids are highlighted in grey. Amino acid residues in position 11 and 12 (underlined) are different in human and rat ghrelin

Structure-Activity Relationship

To develop new and more active synthetic agonists, recent studies aimed at investigating the minimal amino acidic sequence of ghrelin needed to activate the human GHS-R. By using a cell line stably transfected with the human GHS-R1a, it was shown that all the synthetic peptides encompassing the first four or five residues of ghrelin, and carrying the esterification of Ser^3, were capable of activating the human GHS-R1a as efficiently as the full-length ghrelin (Bednarek et al., 2000; Matsumoto et al., 2001). Based on these in vitro results, it was postulated that the active core required for the activation of the receptor was the tetrapeptide Gly-Ser-Ser(n-octanoil)-Phe. However, similar short ghrelin analogs did not stimulate GH release in vivo in the rat (Torsello et al., 2002), suggesting that the C-terminal portion of the molecule could play a key role in determining the bioactive conformation of ghrelin. On the other hand, the possibility cannot be ruled out that in transfected cells overexpression of human GHS-R1a, or a lack of other receptor populations physiologically expressed in normal pituitary cells, may be responsible for unphysiological stimulations of $[Ca^{2+}]_{in}$. Interestingly, other researchers have demonstrated that adenosine can increase $[Ca^{2+}]_{in}$ in cells transfected with human GHS-R1a; however, adenosine does not stimulate GH secretion, nor synergize with GHRH on primary rat pituitary cell culture in vitro (Tullin et al., 2000).

Ghrelin Expression and Distribution

Ghrelin is mainly expressed from the neck to the base of the oxyntic gland of the stomach, and its levels progressively decline along the gastrointestinal tract, with few cells present in the pyloric and intestinal mucosa (Kojima et al., 1999). Immunoelectron microscopy analysis (Rindi et al., 2002) demonstrated that, in the stomach, ghrelin-positive cells correspond to those endocrine cell types that in earlier ultrastructural classifications were labeled as X cells in the dog (Solcia et al., 1975), A-like or X cells in the rat (Capella et al., 1971; Forssmann et al., 1969) and P/D_1 in man (Capella et al., 1978; Solcia et al., 1979), and whose hormonal products and physiological functions have not previously been determined. They can now be reclassified under a single functional type, ultrastructurally and cytochemically different from others, known as endocrine cells of the oxyntic mucosa, such as the histamine-producing ECL cell, the somatostatin D cell or the serotonin EC cell (Rindi et al., 2002). In man, ghrelin cells are characterized by the presence of round, solid or thin-haloed secretory granules with a mean diameter of 147 ± 30 nm in standard aldehyde-osmium preparations, abundant cytoplasm microfilaments and frequent lysosomal dense (lipofuscin) bodies (Rindi et al., 2002). Gastric ghrelin cells are of closed type, i.e. they have no continuity with the gastric lumen, although they are closely associated with the capillary network running through the lamina propria, suggesting a specific endocrine/paracrine role for ghrelin (Dornonville de la Cour et al., 2001; Date et al., 2000).

Ghrelin expression is not confined to the gastrointestinal system, but is variably present in different tissues, including adrenal gland, mammary gland, buccal mucosa, esophagus, Fallopian tube, fat tissue, gall bladder, lymphocytes, ileum, kidney, left and right colon, lung, lymph node, muscle, myocardium, ovary, pancreas, pituitary, placenta, prostate, skin, spleen, testis, thyroid and vein (Gnanapavan et al., 2002). Recent experimental evidence suggests that ghrelin expression in the stomach would be related to a precise role in the control of gastric acid secretion (Masuda et al., 2000; Date et al., 2001; Sibilia et al., 2002). However, given its almost ubiquitous expression, the physiological role of ghrelin remains largely unknown.

Similarly to ghrelin, the expression of the GHS-R1a is almost ubiquitous (Guan et al., 1997; Muccioli et al., 1998; Papotti et al., 2000). Two different receptors for ghrelin have been cloned and designated 1a and 1b; they are synthesized by alternative processing of an unspliced pre-mRNA. The cDNA of the 1a encodes a 366 amino acid protein with seven transmembrane regions and a molecular weight of about 41 kDa. The cDNA for the isoform 1b encodes a shorter 289 amino acids protein with five transmembrane regions only, representing a truncated form of the GHS-R1a receptor.

Binding of ghrelin or synthetic GHS to the GHS-R1a activates the intracellular phospholipase C signaling pathway, leading to increased intracellular calcium and activation of the protein kinase C pathway, followed by the release of calcium ions from the intracellular stores (Smith et al., 1997; Kojima et al., 2001). Another concomitant mechanism is the inhibition of potassium channels, which in turn allows the entry of calcium through voltage-gated T and L channels (Chen et al., 1996). However, all the actions described are relative to the interaction with GHS-R1a only; in fact, apparently GHS-R1b neither binds GHS nor activates any intracellular signaling (Howard et al., 1996). Thus, the functional role of the GHS-R1b receptor remains to be defined. This issue is particularly relevant when considering that this isoform is more widely expressed than GHS-R1a. The lack of correspondence between the expression of ghrelin and its known functional receptor suggests that it can also activate additional receptor subtypes (Gnanapavan et al., 2002).

Ontogeny of Ghrelin

The study of ghrelin ontogeny in the rat reveals that ghrelin-immunoreactive cells are detectable in the fetal stomach from pregnancy day 18. The number of ghrelin-immunoreactive cells in the fetal stomach increases as the stomach grows (Hayashida et al., 2002), until a stable level is reached at puberty, without significant gender-related differences (Gualillo et al., 2001b; Sakata et al., 2002). Similarly, in the human fetal stomach, cells immunoreactive for ghrelin are detectable from the 10th week of gestation; furthermore, it has been observed that these cells develop long before histamine enterochromaffin-like cells (Rindi et al., 2002).

In the human and rat placenta, ghrelin expression shows a pregnancy-related time course of expression (Gualillo et al., 2001a; Torsello et al., 2003a). In the rat placenta, ghrelin expression increases during pregnancy and also remains elevated at term, whereas in the human placenta ghrelin expression is confined to the first half of pregnancy (Gualillo et al., 2001a). The precise role of fetal and placenta-derived ghrelin is still unclear at present, but its pattern of expression is certainly suggestive of an involvement in the regulation of fetal growth and differentiation, beginning from the early phases of development.

In the human pancreas, numerous ghrelin-immunoreactive cells (~10% of all endocrine pancreatic cells) are detectable from 10 weeks of gestation to early postnatal life (Rindi et al., 2002; Wierup et al., 2002). Interestingly, the onset of ghrelin expression in the pancreas precedes by far that in the stomach. Pancreatic ghrelin cells appear to be still present in the adult, but they are fewer and much less abundant than in the stomach (Wierup et al., 2002). Ghrelin cells are often located at the periphery of the islets, as single cells or small clusters of cells, but no co-localization could be detected at any stage, even though ghrelin-immunoreactive cells are often located in the immediate vicinity of glucagon- or somatostatin-positive cells (Wierup et al., 2002). It has to be mentioned, however, that we failed to detect ghrelin-immunoreactive cells in adult pancreas (Rindi et al., 2002).

In the human lung, ghrelin immunoreactive cells were observed in decreasing amounts from embryonic to late fetal periods (Rindi et al., 2002; Volante et al., 2002). Ghrelin-immunoreactive cells were demonstrated in newborns and children under 2 years but are extremely rare in adults (Rindi et al., 2002; Volante et al., 2002).

In the pituitary gland of the rat, the expression of ghrelin was high after birth but declined significantly with puberty, whereas in the hypothalamus it was barely detectable at birth and remained very low through ageing (Torsello et al., 2003a).

In summary, experimental evidence suggests that ghrelin could play a physiological role during fetal and postnatal life, but the significance of its role still remains obscure.

Regulation of Ghrelin Secretion

The stomach has been recognized as the major source of circulating ghrelin, as gastrectomy or the selective surgical removal of the fundus dramatically reduces the plasma circulating levels of the hormone, up to about 80% in the rat (Dornonville de la Cour et al., 2001; Date et al., 2000) and 65% in humans (Ariyasu et al., 2001). It has been suggested that the residual ghrelin secretion still present after gastrectomy in man could be due to the pancreas (Wierup et al., 2002). However, the regulation of the secretion of the peptide is still largely unknown. It has been observed that the expression of the ghrelin mRNA in the stomach and its plasma levels are chiefly related to variations of the energy balance. In the rat, circulating levels of ghrelin exhibited a diurnal pattern, with bimodal peaks occurring before dark and light periods. These two peaks were consistent with maximum and minimum volumes of gastric content, respectively (Murakami et al., 2002). In particular, plasma ghrelin peaks did not correlate with those of GH, but they were inversely related with those of leptin, a hormone endowed with anorexigenic properties, involved in the control of energy balance (Bagnasco et al., 2002). In man, plasma ghrelin levels increased during starvation, decreased after food ingestion and reached a peak in the night, showing a secretory profile similar to that of GH (Cummings et al., 2001; Shiiya et al., 2002). These results are consistent with a possible physiological role played by ghrelin in the control of feeding behavior and the secretion of GH. In the rat, the expression of ghrelin in the stomach is also controlled by other hormones involved in metabolic regulation, since the administration of insulin or leptin for 5 days was able to increase ghrelin mRNA levels (Toshinai et al., 2001). In the pituitary, ghrelin mRNA expression can be positively modified by the administration of GHRH (Kamegai et al., 2001a).

Ghrelin and the GHS: Endocrine Effects

Similarly to synthetic GHS, ghrelin dose-dependently stimulates GH release from primary pituitary cells in a dose-dependent manner (Kojima et al., 1999); however, its activity is much more evident in vivo, in both experimental animals and humans (Tolle et al., 2001; Seoane et al., 2000; Arvat et al., 2000; Takaya et al., 2000).

Intravenous ghrelin administration effectively stimulates the secretion of GH: a single intravenous bolus of the peptide elicits a rapid onset of plasma GH, which peaks within 5-15 min in the rat and 15-20 min in man (Kojima et al., 1999).

It is remarkable that the GH-releasing activity of ghrelin and the GHS is much more consistent than that of maximal doses of GHRH in man (Arvat et al., 2001). However, experiments performed in rats indicate that the GH-releasing activity of the hormone is also related to the route of administration, as it is more pronounced by the peripheral route (i.v.) than by the central one (Tamura et al., 2002). Although the predominant effect is the secretion of GH, the activity of these molecules is not fully specific for GH release. They can in fact elicit small but consistent increments of the plasma concentrations of PRL, ACTH and cortisol (Locatelli and Torsello, 1997; Kojima et al., 1999; Arvat et al., 2001).

Previous studies demonstrated that the GH-realeasing action of GHS was partially reduced by GHRH deficiency, indicating that the latter was essential for their full pharmacological activity (Locatelli and Torsello, 1997). Similarly, the endocrine activity of ghrelin in vivo depends, in addition to the route of administration, on the functional integrity of the GHRH system; in fact, in the adult rat, pretreatment with an antibody against GHRH, or a functional antagonist of GHRH (Bowers, 2001), or lesion of the arcuate nucleus are able to reduce their efficacy (Tamura et al., 2002).

At variance with the adult rat, we have reported that in 10 day-old rats the complete lack of GHRH and somatostatin, obtained by passive immunization against both factors, did not change the GH-releasing activity of GHRP-6 or hexarelin, indicating that GHRH activation may represent an intermediate, although not obligatory, step of GHS action (Locatelli et al., 1994).

It is noteworthy that, in vivo, coadministration of ghrelin and GHRH produces a synergistic effect on the release of GH, but not on the release of PRL, ACTH and cortisol (Hataya et al., 2001). However, the secretory response to ghrelin is not amplified by the combined administration of hexarelin, a synthetic GHS (Arvat et al., 2001). The synergistic effect of ghrelin and GHRH, as already reported for the GHS, probably derives from an interacion that takes place in the hypothalamus, as it is present in vitro in cultured pituitary cells (Yamazaki et al., 2002). Among the possible explanations of this phenomenon, we can consider both that GHS can act as a functional antagonist of somatostatin (Kojima et al., 2001), and that ghrelin and GHS would promote the release of an unknown hypothalamic factor, the "U" factor, that would be responsible for the aforementioned mechanism (Bowers, 1998).

Even if ghrelin is the most potent GH secretagogue so far discovered, being on molar basis even more potent than hexarelin and GHRP-2 (Arvat et al., 2001; Bowers, 2001), its plasma levels do not seem to be regulated by GH in a classic feedback mechanism fashion; in fact, in adult patients with isolated GH deficiency, ghrelin plasma levels are similar to those of control subjects and do not decrease after 1 year of GH replacement therapy (Janssen et al., 2001). On the other hand, it has been recently evidenced that in man the i.v. administration of somatostatin or cortistatin-14 (CRS-14), a natural analog of SS receptors, strongly inhibits the spontaneous release of ghrelin, indicating the existence of a tight functional relationship between the two systems. Although the mechanism responsible for such an inhibitory effect has not so far been defined, it is possible that the actions of SS and CRS-14 are mediated by interactions with the known somatostatinergic receptors, largely expressed in the gastric mucosa (Broglio et al., 2002).

It was not surprising that ghrelin, a gastrointestinal hormone, is endowed with endocrine effects on the pancreatic hormones. In particular, it was observed in the rat that ghrelin can stimulate insulin secretion, both in vitro on pancreatic tissue and in vivo (Date et al., 2002; Adeghate and Ponery, 2002; Lee et al., 2002). In contrast, in the isolated and perfused rat pancreas, ghrelin antagonizes glucose-stimulated insulin release (Egido et al., 2002).

Understanding of the effects of ghrelin on insulin secretion is further complicated by results obtained in humans. A recent clinical study has demonstrated that in humans acute ghrelin administration produces an increment of glucose blood levels and a reduction of those of insulin (Broglio et al., 2001), a result in keeping with the already reported effects in elderly subjects after long-term treatment with GHS (Svensson et al., 1998).

Further studies performed in different experimental and controlled conditions are warranted to explain such discrepancies.

Ghrelin and GHS: Extraendocrine Effects in Experimental Research

Orexigenic Effects

Before the discovery of ghrelin, some studies demonstrated that GHS administered peripherally or centrally is orexigenic in the rat (Locke et al., 1995; Torsello et al., 1998; Torsello et al., 2000) and that this effect is not strictly related to its GH-releasing properties and is probably mediated by different receptors (Torsello et al., 1998) (Table 1). The orexigenic effect is also inde-

Table 1 Endocrine and extraendocrine effects of GHS and ghrelin

	Hexarelin and some GHS	Ghrelin
Endocrine effects		
	GH releasing activity (rat) (Bowers et al., 1984) PPL, ACTH and corticosteron releasing activity (rat) (Thomas et al., 1997)	GH releasing activity (rat) (Kojima et al., 1984) PPL, ACTH and corticosteron releasing activity (rat) (Thomas et al., 1997) Insulin release (in vitro) (Date et al., 2002; Lee et al., 2002)
Extraendocrine effects		
	↑ Food intake (rat) (Torsello et al., 2000) ↑ Adiposit and body weight (Tschop et al., 2002)	↑ Food intake (rat) (Tschop et al., 2000) ↑ Adiposit and body weight (↓ lipidic oxidation) (Tschop et al., 2000; Inui, 2001)
	Cardioprotective effect in ischemic heart (also in hypophysectomized rats) (De Gennaro Colonna et al., 1997; Rossoni et al., 1998; Locatelli et al., 1999)	Improvement of left ventricular dysfunction and cardiac cachexy (rat) (Nagaya et al., 2001a)
	↓ Gastric acid secretion (conscious rat) (Sibilia et al., 2002)	↑ Gastric acid secretion and motility (anesthesized rat) (Masuda et al., 2000)
		↓ Gastric acid secretion (conscious rat) (Sibilia et al., 2002)
		Antagonism of ethanol-induced ulcers (rat) (Sibilia et al., 2002)
	↑ Bone mineral cotent and turnover (rat) (Sibilia et al., 2002)	
	↑ Penile erection (rat) (Melis et al., 2000)	↑ Penile erection (Melis et al., 2002)
		↓ REM sleep (rat) (Tolle et al., 2002), ↑ NREM sleep in mice (Obal et al., 2002)
	Antipoliferative effects in different cell lines (Ghè et al., 2002)	Antipoliferative effects in human mammary carcinoma cells (Cassoni et al., 2001)
	Antiapoptotic effects in cardiomyocytes in vitro (Filigheddu et al., 2001)	Antiapoptotic effects in cardiomyocytes in vitro (Filigheddu et al., 2001) Anxiogenic effect (mice) (Asakawa et al., 2001)

pendent from GHRH, but requires the integrity of the hypothalamic nuclei and the involvement of neuropeptide Y (NPY), a potent stimulator of the appetite of hypothamic origin (Torsello et al., 2000). Similarly to synthetic GHS, ghrelin also promotes feeding, with an efficacy similar to that of NPY (Tschop et al., 2000; Shintani et al., 2001; Wren et al., 2001); this result is further supported by the observation that the central administration of an anti-ghrelin antiserum twice daily for 5 days significantly decreased both daily food intake and body weight (Murakami et al., 2002). The mechanism of action of ghrelin is not completely defined; however, much experimental evidence supports the involvement of NPY and the agouti related protein (AGRP), another hypothalamic peptide with orexigenic properties. In the rat, in fact, both acute and chronic treatment with ghrelin cause an increase of the hypothalamic mRNA levels of NPY and AGRP (Kamegai et al., 2001b). Interestingly, ghrelin effects can be antagonized by coadministration with antagonists of AGRP or antagonists of the Y1 or Y5 receptor for NPY (Nakazato et al., 2001), as well as by destruction of the arcuate nucleus (Tamura et al., 2002).

The persistence of the orexigenic effect of ghrelin in NPY knock-out mice would indicate that AGRP system can substitute for the lack of NPY (Tschop et al., 2002).

The increase of appetite is associated to body weight increase. However, the latter does not depend on an increase of somatic or muscular development, which are typical effects of GH, but instead on increased adipogenesis and reduced lipid oxidation (Inui, 2001).

Effects on the Cardiovascular System

In 1997 it was reported for the first time that prolonged treatment with hexarelin could protect the heart of rats with experimental GH deficiency from ischemia-reperfusion damage (De Gennaro Colonna et al., 1997). A more recent report indicated that the protective effect does not depend on an increased GH secretion, since the effect is also present, and is even magnified, in hypophysectomized rats (Locatelli et al., 1999). However, similarly to the orexigenic activity, not all GHSs share the same efficacy in preventing ischemia-reperfusion damage, again indicating the possible involvement of different receptors in their mechanism of action (Locatelli et al., 1999). This hypothesis is further supported by our recent demonstration that in hypophysectomized rats ghrelin is much less effective than hexarelin in protecting the myocardium from ischemia-reperfusion damage (Torsello et al., 2003b). The different pharmacologic activity could depend on activation of different receptor species. In the heart, hexarelin binds primarily to the scavenger receptor B CD36, whereas ghrelin and the other less effective GHS-would activate mainly the GHS-R 1a (Bodart et al., 2002).

The cardiac activity of ghrelin is different, however, in different animal species. In humans, in fact, unlike in rats, the acute administration of the peptide was found effective in reducing the afterload and in increasing cardiac output, both in normal subjects and in patients with severe GH deficiency, without any change in heart rate (Nagaya et al., 2001b).

Effects on the Motility and Gastric Secretion

It is not surprising, based on its gastrointestinal origin, that ghrelin can influence stomach activity, particularly motility and acid secretion. In urethane-anesthetized rats, central administration of the peptide evokes an increase of gastric motility and acid secretion (Masuda et al., 2000; Date et al., 2001). However, in conscious rats ghrelin effectively inhibits gastric acid secretion after central and systemic administration, suggesting a possible physiological role of ghrelin in the control of gastric secretory function (Sibilia et al., 2002). The central long-lasting gastric inhibitory action of ghrelin seems appropriate from a teological point of view, considering that fasting increases ghrelin serum levels and that during fasting a decrease in acid secretion is relevant for the maintenance of gastric mucosal integrity. It has also been shown that the peripheral or central administration of ghrelin exerts a potent and dose-related gastroprotective action against ethanol-induced gastric ulcers; an effect mediated by endogenous nitric oxide release and that requires the integrity of sensory nerve fibers (Sibilia et al., 2003).

Antiproliferative Activity on Tumoral Cells

Recent studies have revealed that ghrelin and some synthetic GHSs also possess an antiproliferative activity on different tumoral cell lines (Cassoni et al., 2000; Ghè et al., 2002). It is of note that the expression of GHS-R subtypes has been found also in tumoral tissues from organs which do not express these receptors in physiological conditions, such as the breast (Cassoni et al., 2001). It has also been reported that des-acyl ghrelin, reportedly a biologically inactive peptide unable to bind GHS-R1a or to stimulate GH release in vivo and in vitro, caused inhibition of tumoral proliferation, indicating that it may activate a receptor distinct from GHS-R 1a (Cassoni et al., 2001).

Expression and Release of Ghrelin in Pathological Conditions

Since the secretion of ghrelin is regulated by energy balance, it is likely that the plasma levels of ghrelin should be lower in obese subjects (Tschop et al., 2001) and higher in anorexia nervosa patients (Otto et al., 2001) than in normal subjects. Generally, ghrelin circulating levels in man are inversely correlated to body mass index, adipose tissue mass, dimension of the adipocytes, and insulin and leptin plasma levels (Ravussin et al., 2001; Tschop et al., 2001). It is therefore possible that higher or lower secretion of ghrelin would compensate for metabolic dysregulations such as those of these pathologic situations.

Possible mutations of the ghrelin gene have also been proposed to explain the impaired regulation of body weight in obese mammals, as suggested by a study reporting an association between mutations in the preproghrelin/ghrelin gene and obesity (Ukkola et al., 2001).

Finally, ghrelin-immunoreactive cells have been detected in tumors of the diffuse endocrine system, and especially in well-differentiated endocrine tumors of the pituitary, the gastroenteropancreatic tract and the lung (Korbonits et al., 2001; Papotti et al., 2001; Rindi et al., 2002b). Tumor cells have also been shown by RT-PCR analysis to express GHS-R, suggesting a potential autocrine loop (Korbonits et al., 2001; Papotti et al., 2001). The potential secretory property of ghrelin-expressing tumor cells is not known.

Conclusions

Ghrelin, a peptide produced predominantly by the oxyntic gland of the stomach, is the most potent GH secretagogue discovered so far. Ghrelin, as well as GHS, can act directly on the pituitary; however, their principal site of action is in the hypothalamus, where they can can directly or indirectly synergize with GHRH. Administration of ghrelin and GHS also elicits modest but significant increases of plasma levels of ACTH, PRL and cortisol, by mechanisms different and independent from those involved in GH release.

In addition to their endocrine effects, ghrelin and the GHS are endowed with relevant extraendocrine effects. These pharmacologic properties may be relevant to define possible therapeutic uses of ghrelin and GHS in the care of endocrine and extraendocrine pathological conditions.

References

Adeghate E. and Ponery A.S. (2002). Ghrelin stimulates insulin secretion from the pancreas of normal and diabetic rats. J Neuroendocrinol, 14 (7), 555-560.

Ariyasu H., Takaya K., Tagami T., Ogawa Y., Hosoda K., Akamizu T., Suda M., Koh T., Natsui K., Toyooka S., Shirakami G., Usui T., Shimatsu A., Doi K., Hosoda H., Kojima M., Kangawa K. and Nakao K. (2001). Stomach is a major source of circulating ghrelin and feeding state determines plasma ghrelin-like immunoreactivity levels in humans. J Clin Endocrinol Metab, 86, 4573-4578.

Arvat E., Di Vito L., Broglio F., Papotti M., Muccioli G., Dieguez C., Casanueva F.F., Deghenghi R., Camanni F. and Ghigo E. (2000). Preliminary evidence that ghrelin, the natural GH secretagogue (GHS)-receptor ligand, strongly stimulates GH secretion in humans. J Endocrinol Invest, 23, 493-495.

Arvat E., Maccario M., Di Vito L., Broglio F., Benso A., Gottero C., Papotti M., Muccioli G., Dieguez C., Casanueva F.F., Deghenghi R., Camanni F. and Ghigo E. (2001). Endocrine activities of ghrelin, a natural growth hormone secretagogue (GHS), in humans: comparison and interactions with hexarelin, a nonnatural peptidyl GHS, and GH-releasing hormone. J Clin Endocrinol Metab, 86, 1169-1174.

Asakawa A., Inui A., Kaga T., Yuzuriha H., Nagata T., Fujimiya M., Katsuura G., Makino S., Fujino M. A. and Kasuga M. (2001). A role of ghrelin in neuroendocrine and behavioral responses to stress in mice. Neuroendocrinology, 74 (3), 143-147.

Bagnasco M., Kalra P.S. and Kalra S.P. (2002). Ghrelin and leptin pulse discharge in fed and fasted rats. Endocrinology, 143 (2), 726-729.

Banks W.A., Tschop M., Robinson S.M. and Heiman M.L. (2002). Extent and direction of ghrelin transport across the blood-brain barrier is determined by its unique primary structure. J Pharmacol Exp Ther, 302 (2), 822-827.

Bednarek M.A., Feighner S.D., Pong S.S., McKee K.K., Hreniuk D.L., Silva M.V., Warren V.A., Howard A.D., Van Der Ploeg L.H. and Heck J.V. (2000). Structure-function studies on the new growth hormone-releasing peptide, ghrelin: minimal sequence of ghrelin necessary for activation of growth hormone secretagogue receptor 1a. J Med Chem, 43, 4370-4376.

Bodart V., Febbraio M., Demers A., McNicoll N., Pohankova P., Perreault A., Sejlitz T., Escher E., Silverstein R.L., Lamontagne D. and Ong H. (2002). CD36 mediates the cardiovascular action of growth hormone-releasing peptides in the heart. Circ Res, 90 (8), 844-849.

Bowers C.Y., Momany F., Reynolds G.A., Chang D., Hong A. and Chang K. (1980). Structure-activity relationship of a synthetic pentapeptide that specifically releases growth hormone in vitro. Endocrinology, 106, 663-667.

Bowers C.Y., Momany F.A., Reynolds G.A. and Hong A. (1984). On the in vitro and in vivo activity of a new synthetic hexapeptide that acts on the pituitary to specifically release growth hormone. Endocrinology, 114, 1537-1545.

Bowers C.Y., Reynolds G.A., Durham D., Barrera C.M., Pezzoli S.S. and Thorner M.O. (1990). Growth hormone (GH)-releasing peptide stimulates GH release in normal men and acts synergistically with GH-releasing hormone. J Clin Endocrinol Metab, 70, 975-982.

Bowers C.Y. (1998). Growth hormone-releasing peptide (GHRP). Cell Mol Life Sci, 54, 1316-1319.

Bowers C.Y. (2001). Unnatural growth hormone-releasing peptide begets natural ghrelin. J Clin Endocrinol Metab, 86, 1464-1469.

Broglio F., Arvat E., Benso A., Gottero C., Muccioli G., Papotti M., van der Lely A.J., Deghenghi R. and Ghigo E. (2001). Ghrelin, a natural GH secretagogue produced by the stomach, induces hyperglycemia and reduces insulin secretion in humans. J Clin Endocrinol Metab, 86 (10), 5083-5086.

Broglio F., Koetsveld Pv. P., Benso A., Gottero C., Prodam F., Papotti M., Muccioli G., Gauna C., Hofland L., Deghenghi R., Arvat E., Van Der Lely A.J. and Ghigo E. (2002). Ghrelin secretion is inhibited by either somatostatin or cortistatin in humans. J Clin Endocrinol Metab, 87 (10), 4829-4832.

Capella C., Vassallo G. and Solcia E. (1971). Light and electron microscopic identification of the histamine-storing argyrophil (ECL) cell in murine stomach and of its equivalent in other mammals. Z Zellforsch Mikrosk Anat, 118, 68-84.

Capella C., Hage E., Solcia E. and Usellini L. (1978). Ultrastructural similarity of endocrine-like cells of the human lung and some related cells of the gut. Cell Tissue Res, 186, 25-37.

Cassoni P., Papotti M., Catapano F., Ghè C., Deghenghi R., Ghigo E. and Muccioli G. (2000). Specific binding sites for synthetic growth hormone secretagogues in non-tumoral and neoplasticc human thyroid tissue. J Endocrinol, 165, 139-146.

Cassoni P., Papotti M., Ghè C., Catapano F., Sapino A., Graziani A., Deghenghi R., Reissmann T., Ghigo E. and Muccioli G. (2001). Identification, characterization, and biological activity of specific receptors for natural (ghrelin) and synthetic growth hormone secretagogues and analogs in human breast carcinomas and cell lines. J Clin Endocrinol Metab, 86 (4), 1738-1745.

Chen C., Wu D. and Clarcke I.J. (1996). Signal transduction systems employed by synthetic GH-releasing peptides in somatotrophs. J Endocrinol, 148, 381-386.

Cummings D.E., Purnell J.Q., Frayo R.S., Schmidova K., Wisse B.E. and Weigle D.S. (2001). A preprandial rise in plasma ghrelin levels suggests a role in meal initiation in humans. Diabetes, 50 (8), 1714-1719.

Date Y., Kojima M., Hosoda H., Sawaguchi A., Mondal M.S., Suganuma T., Matsukura S., Kangawa K. and Nakazato M. (2000). Ghrelin, a novel growth hormone-releasing acylated peptide, is synthesized in a distinct endocrine cell type in the gastrointestinal tracts of rats and humans. Endocrinology, 141, 4255-4261.

Date Y., Nakazato M., Murakami N., Kojima M., Kangawa K. and Matsukura S. (2001). Ghrelin acts in the central nervous system to stimulate gastric acid secretion. Biochem Biophys Res Commun, 280, 904-907.

Date Y., Nakazato M., Hashiguchi S., Dezaki K., Mondal M.S., Hosoda H., Kojima M., Kangawa K., Arima T., Matsuo H., Yada T. and Matsukura S. (2002). Ghrelin is present in pancreatic α cells of humans and rats and stimulates insulin secretion. Diabetes, 51 (1), 124-129.

De Gennaro Colonna V., Rossoni G., Bernareggi M., Muller E.E. and Berti F. (1997). Hexarelin, a growth hormone-releasing peptide, discloses protectant activity against cardiovascular damage in rats with isolated growth hormone deficiency. Cardiologia, 42 (11), 1165-1172.

Dornonville de la Cour C., Bjorkqvist M., Sandvik A.K., Bakke I., Zhao C.M., Chen D. and Hakanson R. (2001). A-like cells in the rat stomach contain ghrelin and do not operate under gastrin control. Regul Pept, 99 (2-3), 141-150.

Egido E.M., Rodriguez-Gallardo J., Silvestre R.A. and Marco J. (2002). Inhibitory effect of ghrelin on insulin and pancreatic somatostatin secretion. Eur J Endocrinol, 146 (2), 241-244.

Filigheddu N., Fubini A., Baldanzi G., Cutrupi S., Ghe C., Catapano F., Broglio F., Bosia A., Papotti M., Muccioli G., Ghigo E., Deghenghi R. and Graziani A. (2001). Hexarelin protects H9c2 cardiomyocytes from doxorubicin-induced cell death. Endocrine, 14 (1), 113-119.

Forssmann W.G., Orci L., Pictet R., Renold A.E. and Rouiller C. (1969). The endocrine cells in the epithelium of the gastrointestinal mucosa of the rat. An electron microscope study. J Cell Biol 40, 692-715.

Ghè C., Cassoni P., Catapano F., Marrocco T., Deghenghi R., Ghigo E., Muccioli G. and Papotti M. (2002). The antiproliferative effect of synthetic peptidyl GH secretagogues in human CALU-1 lung carcinoma cells. Endocrinology, 143 (2), 484-491.

Gnanapavan S., Kola B., Bustin S.A., Morris D.G., McGee P., Fairclough P., Bhattacharya S., Carpenter R., Grossman A.B. and Korbonits M. (2002). The tissue distribution of the mRNA of ghrelin and subtypes of its receptor, GHS-R, in humans. J Clin Endocrinol Metab, 87, 2988-2991.

Gualillo O., Caminos J., Blanco M., Garcia-Caballero T., Kojima M., Kangawa K., Dieguez C. and Casanueva F. (2001a). Ghrelin, a novel placental-derived hormone. Endocrinology, 142 (2), 788-794.

Gualillo O., Caminos J.E., Kojima M., Kangawa K., Arvat E., Ghigo E., Casanueva F.F. and Dieguez C. (2001b). Gender and gonadal influences on ghrelin mRNA levels in rat stomach. Eur J Endocrinol, 144 (6), 687-690.

Guan X.M., Yu H., Palyha O.C., McKee K.K., Feighner S.D., Sirinathsinghji D.J. Smith R.G., Van Der Ploeg L.H.T. and Howard A.D. (1997). Distribution of mRNA encoding the growth hormone secretagogue receptor in brain and peripheral tissues. Brain Res Mol Brain Res, 48, 23-9.

Hataya Y., Akamizu T., Takaya K., Kanamoto N., Ariyasu H., Saijo M., Moriyama K., Shimatsu A., Kojima M., Kangawa K. and Nakao K. (2001). A low dose of ghrelin stimulates growth hormone (GH) release synergistically with GH-releasing hormone in humans. J Clin Endocrinol Metab, 86, 4552-4555.

Hayashida T., Nakahara K., Mondal M.S., Date Y., Nakazato M., Kojima M., Kangawa K. and Murakami N. (2002). Ghrelin in neonatal rats: distribution in stomach and its possible role. J Endocrinol, 173 (2), 239-245.

Hosoda H., Kojima M., Matsuo H. and Kangawa K. (2000a). Purification and characterization of rat des-Gln14-ghrelin, a second endogenous ligand for the growth hormone secretagogue receptor. J Biol Chem, 275, 21995-20000.

Hosoda H., Kojima M., Matsuo H. and Kangawa K. (2000b). Ghrelin and des-acyl ghrelin peptide in gastrointestinal tissue. Biochem Biophys Res Commun, 279, 910-913.

Howard A.D., Feighner S.D., Cully D.F., Arena J.P., Liberator P.A., Rosenblum C.I., Hamelin M., Hreniuk D.L., Palyha O.C., Anderson J., Paress P.S., Diaz C., Chou M., Liu K.K., McKee K.K., Pong S.S., Chaung L.Y., Elbrecht A., Dashkevicz M., Heavens R., Rigby M., Sirinathsinghji D.J., Dean D.C., Melillo D.G., Van der Ploeg L.H. et al. (1996). A receptor in pituitary and hypothalamus that functions in growth hormone release. Science, 273, 974-976.

Ilson B.E., Jorkasky D.K., Curnow R.T. and Stote R.M. (1989). Effect of a new synthetic hexapeptide to selectively stimulate growth hormone release in healthy human subjects. J Clin Endocrinol Metab, 69, 212-214.

Inui A. (2001). Ghrelin: an orexigenic and somatotrophic signal from the stomach. Nature Rev Neurosci, 2, 551-560.

Janssen J.A., Van der Toorn F.M., Hofland L.J., Van Koetsveld P., Broglio F., Ghigo E., Lamberts S.W. and Jan van der Lely A. (2001). Systemic ghrelin levels in subjects with growth hormone deficiency are not modified by one year of growth hormone replacement therapy. Eur J Endocrinol, 145, 711-716.

Kamegai J., Tamura H., Shimizu T., Ishii S., Sugihara H. and Oikawa S. (2001a). Regulation of the ghrelin gene: growth hormone-releasing hormone upregulates ghrelin mRNA in the pituitary. Endocrinology, 142 (9), 4154-4157.

Kamegai J., Tamura H., Shimizu T., Ishii S., Sugihara H. and Wakabayashi I. (2001b). Chronic central infusion of ghrelin increases hypothalamic neuropeptide Y and Agouti-related protein mRNA levels and body weight in rats. Diabetes, 50 (11), 2438-2443.

Kojima M., Hosoda H., Date Y., Nakazato M., Matsuo H. and Kangawa K. (1999). Ghrelin is a growth-hormone-releasing acylated peptide from stomach. Nature, 402, 656-660.

Kojima M., Hosoda H., Matsuo H. and Kangawa K. (2001). Ghrelin: discovery of the natural endogenous ligand for the growth hormone secretagogue receptor. Trends Endocrinol Metabol, 12, 118-122.

Korbonits M., Bustin S.A., Kjima M., Jordan S., Adams E.F., Lowe D.G., Kangawa K. and Grossman AB (2001). The expression of the growth hormone secretagogue receptor ligand in normal and abnormal human pituitary and other neuroendocrine tumors. J Clin Endocrinol Metab, 86, 881-887.

Lee H.M., Wang G., Englander E.W., Kojima M. and Greeley G.H. Jr. (2002). Ghrelin, a new gastrointestinal endocrine peptide that stimulates insulin secretion: enteric distribution, ontogeny, influence of endocrine and dietary manipulations. Endocrinology, 143 (1), 185-190.

Locatelli V., Grilli R., Torsello A., Cella S.G., Wehremberg W.B. and Müller E.E. (1994). Growth hormone-releasing hormone and somatostatin are not involved in the stimulation of growth hormone release by growth hormone-releasing hexapeptide in the infant rat. Pediat Res, 36 (2), 169-175.

Locatelli V. and Torsello A. (1997). Growth hormone secretagogues: focus on the growth hormone-releasing peptides. Pharmacol Res, 36, 415-423.

Locatelli V., Rossoni G., Schweiger F., Torsello A., De Gennaro Colonna V., Bernareggi M., Deghenghi R., Muller E. E. and Berti F. (1999). Growth hormone-independent cardioprotective effects of hexarelin in the rat. Endocrinology, 140, 4024-4031.

Locke W., Kirgis H.D., Bowers C.Y. and Abdoh A.A. (1995). Intracerebroventricular growth-hormone-releasing peptide 6 stimulates eating without affecting plasma growth hormone responses in rats. Life Sci, 56, 1347-1352.

Masuda Y., Tanaka T., Inomata N., Ohnuma N., Tanaka S., Itoh Z., Hosoda H., Kojima M. and Kangawa K. (2000). Ghrelin stimulates gastric acid secretion and motility in rats. Biochem Biophys Res Commun, 276, 905-908.

Matsumoto M., Hosoda H., Kitajima Y., Morozumi N., Minamitake Y., Tanaka S., Matsuo H., Kojima M., Hayashi Y. and Kangawa K. (2001). Structure-activity relationship of ghrelin: pharmacological study of ghrelin peptides. Biochem Biophys Res Commun, 287 (1), 42-146.

Melis M.R., Spano M.S., Succu S., Locatelli V., Torsello A., Muller E.E., Deghenghi R. and Argiolas A. (2000). EP 60761- and EP 50885-induced penile erection: structure-activity studies and comparison with ipomorphine, oxytocin and N-methyl-D-aspartic acid. Int J Impot Res, 12, 255-262.

Melis M.R., Mascia M.S., Succu S., Torsello A., Muller E.E., Deghenghi R. and Argiolas A. (2002). Ghrelin injected into the paraventricular nucleus of the hypothalamus of male rats induces feeding but not penile erection. Neurosci Lett, 329, 339-343.

Muccioli G., Ghè C., Ghigo M.C., Papotti M., Arvat E., Boghen M.F., Nilsson M.H., Deghenghi R., Ong H. and Ghigo E. (1998). Specific receptors for synthetic GH secretagogues in the human brain and pituitary gland. J Endocrinol, 157, 99-106.

Muccioli G., Papotti M., Locatelli V., Ghigo E. and Deghenghi R. (2001). Binding of ^{125}I-labeled ghrelin to membranes from human hypothalamus and pituitary gland. J Endocrinol Invest, 24, RC7-RC9.

Müller E.E., Locatelli V. and Cocchi D. (1999). Neuroendocrine control of growth hormone secretion. Physiol Rev, 79, 511-607.

Murakami N., Hayashida T., Kuroiwa T., Nakahara K., Ida T., Mondal M. S., Nakazato M., Kojima M. and Kangawa K. (2002). Role for central ghrelin in food intake and secretion profile of stomach ghrelin in rats. J Endocrinol, 174 (2), 283-288.

Nagaya N., Uematsu M., Kojima M., Ikeda Y., Yoshihara F., Shimizu W., Hosoda H., Hirota Y., Ishida H., Mori H. and Kangawa K. (2001a). Chronic administration of ghrelin improves left ventricular dysfunction and attenuates development of cardiac cachexia in rats with heart failure. Circulation, 104 (12), 1430-1435.

Nagaya N., Kojima M., Uematsu M., Yamagishi M., Hosoda H., Oya H., Hayashi Y. and Kangawa K. (2001b). Hemodynamic and hormonal effects of human ghrelin in healthy volunteers. Am J Physiol Regul Integr Comp Physiol, 280, R1483-R1487.

Nakazato M., Murakami N., Date Y., Kojima M., Matsuo H., Kangawa K. and Matsukura S. (2001). A role for ghrelin in the central regulation of feeding. Nature, 409 (6817), 194-198.

Obal F. Jr., Alt J., Taishi P., Gardi J. and Krueger J.M. (2002). Sleep in mice with non-functional growth hormone releasing hormone receptors. Am J Physiol Regul Integr Comp Physiol (in press).

Otto B., Cuntz U., Fruehauf E., Wawarta R., Folwaczny C., Riepl R.L., Heiman M.L., Lehnert P., Fichter M. and Tschop M. (2001). Weight gain decreases elevated plasma ghrelin concentrations of patients with anorexia nervosa. Eur J Endocrinol, 145 (5), 669-673.

Papotti M., Ghè C., Cassoni P., Catapano F., Deghenghi R., Ghigo E. and Muccioli G. (2000). Growth hormone secretagogue binding sites in peripheral human tissues. J Clin Endocrinol Metab, 85, 3803-3807.

Papotti M., Cassoni P., Volante M., Deghenghi R., Muccioli G. and Ghigo E. (2001). Ghrelin-producing endocrine tumors of the stomach and intestine. J Clin Endocrinol Metab, 86, 5052-5059.

Pong S.S., Chaung L-Y.P., Dean D., Nargund R.P., Patchett A.A. and Smith R.G. (1996). Identification of a new G-protein-linked receptor for growth hormone secretagogues. Mol Endocrinol, 10, 57-61.

Ravussin E., Tschop M., Morales S., Bouchard C. and Heiman M.L. (2001). Plasma ghrelin concentration and energy balance: overfeeding and negative energy balance studies in twins. J Clin Endocrinol Metab, 86(9), 4547-4551.

Rindi G., Necchi V., Savio A., Torsello A., Zoli M., Locatelli V., Raimondo F., Cocchi D., Solcia E. (2002). Characterisation of gastric ghrelin cells in man and other mammals. Studies in adult and foetal tissues. Histochem Cell Biol, 117(6), 511-519.

Rindi G., Savio A., Torsello A., Zoli M., Locatelli V., Cocchi D., Paolotti D. and Solcia E. (2002b). Ghrelin expression in gut endocrine growths. Histochem Cell Biol, 117(6), 521-525.

Rossoni G., De Gennaro Colonna V., Bernareggi M., Polvani G.L., Muller E.E. and Berti F. (1998). Protectant activity of hexarelin or growth hormone against postischemic ventricular dysfunction in hearts from aged rats. J Cardiovasc Pharmacol, 32 (2), 260-265.

Sakata I., Tanaka T., Matsubara M., Yamazaki M., Tani S., Hayashi Y., Kangawa K. and Sakai T. (2002). Postnatal changes in ghrelin mRNA expression and in ghrelin-producing cells in the rat stomach. J Endocrinol, 174 (3), 463-471.

Seoane L.M., Tovar S., Baldelli R., Arvat E., Ghigo E., Casanueva F.F. and Dieguez C. (2000). Ghrelin elicits a marked stimulatory effect on GH secretion in freely-moving rats. Eur J Endocrinol, 143, R7-R9.

Shiiya T., Nakazato M., Mizuta M., Date Y., Mondal M. S., Tanaka M., Nozoe S., Hosoda H., Kangawa K. and Matsukura S. (2002). Plasma ghrelin levels in lean and obese humans and the effect of glucose on ghrelin secretion. J Clin Endocrinol Metab, 87 (1), 240-244.

Shintani M., Ogawa Y., Ebihara K., Aizawa-Abe M., Miyanaga F., Takaya K., Hayashi T., Inoue G., Hosoda K., Kojima M., Kangawa K. and Nakao K. (2001). Ghrelin, an endogenous growth hormone secretagogue, is a novel orexigenic peptide that antagonizes leptin action through the activation of hypothalamic neuropeptide Y/Y1 receptor pathway. Diabetes, 50 (2), 227-232.

Sibilia V., Pagani F., Guidobono F., Locatelli V., Torsello A., Deghenghi R. and Netti C. (2002). Evidence for a central inhibitory role of growth hormone secretagogues and ghrelin on gastric acid secretion in conscious rats. Neuroendocrinology, 75, 92-97.

Sibilia V., Rindi G., Pagani F., Rapetti D., Locatelli V., Torsello A., Campanini N., Deghenghi R. and Netti C. (2003). Ghrelin protects against ethanol-induced gastric ulcers in rats: studies on the mechanisms of action. Endocrinology, 144(1), 353-359.

Smith R.G., Van der Ploegh L.H., Howard A.D., Feighner S.D., Cheng K., Hickey G.J., Wyvratt M.J. Jr., Fisher M.H., Nargund R.P. and Patchett A.A. (1997). Peptidomimetic regulation of growth hormone secretion. Endocr Rev, 18, 621-645.

Solcia E., Capella C., Vassallo G. and Buffa R. (1975). Endocrine cells of the gastric mucosa. Int Rev Cytol, 42, 223-286.

Solcia E., Capella C., Buffa R., Usellini L., Frigerio B. and Fontana P. (1979). Endocrine cells of the gastrointestinal tract and related tumors. Pathobiol Annu, 9, 163-204.

Svensson J., Lonn L., Jansson J.O., Murphy G., Wyss D., Krupa D., Cerchio K., Polvino W., Gertz B., Boseaus I., Sjostrom L. and Bengtsson B.A. (1998). Two-month treatment of obese subjects with the oral growth hormone (GH) secretagogue MK-677 increases GH secretion, fat-free mass, and energy expenditure. J Clin Endocrinol Metab, 83 (2), 362-369.

Takaya K., Ariyasu H., Kanamoto N., Iwakura H., Yoshimoto A., Harada M., Mori K., Komatsu Y., Usui T., Shimatsu A., Ogawa Y., Hosoda K., Akamizu T., Kojima M., Kangawa K. and Nakao K. (2000). Ghrelin strongly stimulates growth hormone release in humans. J Clin Endocrinol Metab, 85, 4908-4911.

Tamura H., Kamegai J., Shimizu T., Ishii S., Sugihara H. and Oikawa S. (2002). Ghrelin stimulates GH but not food intake in arcuate nucleus ablated rats. Endocrinology, 143(9), 3268-3275.

Thomas G.B., Fairhall K.M. and Robinson I.C. (1997). Activation of the hypothalamo-pituitary-adrenal axis by the growth hormone (GH) secretagogue, GH-releasing peptide -6, in rats. Endocrinology, 138 (4), 1585-1591.

Tolle V., Zizzari P., Tomasetto C., Rio M.C., Epelbaum J. and Bluet-Pajot M.T. (2001). In vivo and in vitro effects of ghrelin/motilin-related peptide on growth hormone secretion in the rat. Neuroendocrinology, 73, 54-61.

Tolle V., Bassant M.H., Zizzari P., Poindessous-Jazat F., Tomasetto C., Epelbaum J. and Bluet-Pajot M.T. (2002). Ultradian rhythmicity of ghrelin secretion in relation with GH, feeding behavior, and sleepwake patterns in rats. Endocrinology, 143, 1353-1361.

Tomasetto C., Karam S.M., Ribieras S., Masson R., Lefebvre O., Staub A., Alexander G., Chenard M.P. and Rio M.C. (2000). Identification and characterization of a novel gastric peptide hormone: the motilin-related peptide. Gastroenterology, 119, 395-405.
Torsello A., Luoni M., Schweiger F., Grilli R., Guidi M., Bresciani E., Deghenghi R., Muller E.E. and Locatelli V. (1998). Novel hexarelin analogs stimulate feeding in the rat through a mechanism not involving growth hormone release. Eur J Pharmacol, 360, 123-129.
Torsello A., Locatelli V., Melis M.R., Succu S., Spano M.S., Deghenghi R., Muller E.E. and Argiolas A. (2000). Differential orexigenic effects of hexarelin and its analogs in the rat hypothalamus: indication for multiple growth hormone secretagogue receptor subtypes. Neuroendocrinology, 72, 327-332.
Torsello A., Ghè C., Bresciani E., Catapano F., Ghigo E., Deghenghi R., Locatelli V. and Muccioli G. (2002). Short ghrelin peptides neither displace ghrelin binding in vitro nor stimulate GH release in vivo. Endocrinology 143,1968-1971.
Torsello A., Scibona B., Leo G., Bresciani E., Avallone R., Bulgarelli I., Luoni M., Zoli M., Rindi G., Cocchi D. and Locatelli V. (2003a). Ontogeny and tissue specific regulation of ghrelin mRNA expression in the rat strongly indicate that ghrelin is primarily involved in the control of extraendocrine functions. Neuroendocrinology, 77, 91-99.
Torsello A., Bresciani E., Rossoni G., Avallone R., Tulipano G., Cocchi D., Bulgarelli I., Deghenghi R., Berti F. and Locatelli V. (2003b). Ghrelin plays a minor role in the physiological control of cardiac function in the rat. Endocrinology, 144, 1787-1792.
Toshinai K., Mondal M.S., Nakazato M., Date Y., Murakami N., Kojima M., Kangawa K. and Matsukura S. (2001). Upregulation of Ghrelin expression in the stomach upon fasting, insulin-induced hypoglycemia, and leptin administration. Biochem Biophys Res Commun, 281 (5), 1220-1225.
Tschop M., Smiley D.L. and Heiman M.L. (2000). Ghrelin induces adiposity in rodents. Nature, 407, 908-913.
Tschop M., Weyer C., Tataranni P.A., Devanarayan V., Ravussin E. and Heiman M.L. (2001). Circulating ghrelin levels are decreased in human obesity. Diabetes, 50 (4), 707-709.
Tschop M., Statnick M.A., Suter T.M. and Heiman M.L. (2002). GH-releasing peptide-2 increases fat mass in mice lacking NPY: indication for a crucial mediating role of hypothalamic agouti-related protein. Endocrinology, 143 (2), 558-568.
Tullin S., Hansen B.S., Ankersen M., Moller J., von Cappelen K.A. and Thim L. (2000). Adenosine is an agonist of the growth hormone secretagogue receptor. Endocrinology, 141, 3397-3402.
Ukkola O., Ravussin E., Jacobson P., Snyder E.E., Chagnon M., Sjostrom L. and Bouchard C. (2001). Mutations in the preproghrelin/ghrelin gene associated with obesity in humans. J Clin Endocrinol Metab, 86 (8), 3996-3999.
Volante M., Fulcheri E., Allia E., Cerrato M., Pucci A. and Papotti M. (2002). Ghrelin expression in fetal, infant, and adult human lung. J Histochem Cytochem, 50 (8), 1013-1021.
Wierup N., Svensson H., Mulder H. and Sundler F. (2002). The ghrelin cell: a novel developmentally regulated islet cell in the human pancreas. Regul Peptides, 107 (1-3), 63-69.
Wiley K. E., Davenport A. P. (2002). Comparison of vasodilators in human internal mammary artery: ghrelin is a potent physiological antagonist of endothelin-1. Br J Pharmacol, 136 (8), 1146-1152.
Wren A.M., Small C.J., Abbott C.R., Dhillo W.S., Seal L.J., Cohen M.A., Batterham R.L., Taheri S., Stanley S.A., Ghatei M.A. and Bloom S.R. (2001). Ghrelin causes hyperphagia and obesity in rats. Diabetes, 50 (11), 2540-2547.
Yamazaki M., Nakamura K., Kobayashi H., Matsubara M., Hayashi Y., Kangawa K. and Sakai T. (2002). Regulational effect of ghrelin on growth hormone secretion from perifused rat anterior pituitary cells. J Neuroendocrinol, 14, 156-162.

CHAPTER 14

Endocrine and Nonendocrine Actions of Ghrelin and GHS: State of the Art in Clinic Research

A. BENSO, F. BROGLIO, C. GOTTERO, F. PRODAM, S. DESTEFANIS, M. VOLANTE, P. CASSONI, F. CATAPANO, E. TANABRA, L. FILTRI, R. DEGHENGHI, E. ARVAT, M. PAPOTTI, G. MUCCIOLI AND E. GHIGO

Introduction

Ghrelin, a 28-amino-acid peptide predominantly produced by the stomach, displays strong GH-releasing activity mediated by the activation of the GH secretagogue (GHS) receptor (GHS-R) 1a, which has been shown to be specific for a family of synthetic peptidyl and nonpeptidyl GHS (Smith et al., 1997; Kojima et al., 2001b; Muccioli et al., 2002). These synthetic molecules were invented more than 20 years ago and their strong GH-releasing activity even after oral administration suggested their potential usefulness as a new tool for the diagnosis and treatment of GH deficiency in childhood and somatopause in aging (Smith et al., 1997; Muccioli et al., 2002). The discovery of ghrelin as a natural ligand of the GHS-R1a represented a true turning point in our understanding the control of the GH/IGF-1 axis, but it is already clear that ghrelin is much more than simply a natural GHS.

Ghrelin and synthetic GHS act via receptors concentrated in the hypothalamus-pituitary unit but also distributed in other central and peripheral tissues (Smith et al., 1997; Muccioli et al., 2002). While hypothalamus-pituitary receptors explain their stimulatory effect on GH and also on PRL and ACTH secretion (Smith et al., 1997; Takaya et al., 2000; Kojima et al., 2001a; Arvat et al., 2001; Muccioli et al., 2002), other central and peripheral specific binding sites explain other activities such as the orexigenic effect coupled with control of energy expenditure, control of gastric motility and acid secretion as well as the influence on exocrine pancreatic function, influence on endocrine pancreatic function and glucose metabolism, influence on gonadal function, cardiovascular actions, modulation of cell proliferation and apoptosis, influence on behavior and influence on sleep (Muccioli et al., 2002; Yoshihara et al., 2002).

Historical Milestones: From GH-Releasing Peptides to Ghrelin

GH-releasing peptide-6 was the first hexapeptide that acted to release GH in vivo even after oral administration, though with low bioavailability and short-lasting effect (Smith et al., 1997). Further research led to synthesis of orally active nonpeptidyl molecules, the most representative of which is the spiroindoline MK-0677 (Smith et al., 1997). Notably, MK-0677 allowed the discovery and cloning of the GHS-R, the existence of which had been indicated by binding studies in the hypothalamus-pituitary area but also in other central nervous system areas and in peripheral, endocrine, and nonendocrine animal and human tissues (Smith et al., 1997; Muccioli et al., 2002).

Ghrelin is predominantly produced by the stomach, while substantially lower amounts derive from bowel, pancreas, kidney, placenta, pituitary, testis, ovary, and hypothalamus (Kojima et al., 2001a; Muccioli et al., 2002). Within the stomach ghrelin is produced by the enteroendocrine cells, probably by the X/A-like cells, which represent a major endocrine population in the oxyntic mucosa (Kojima et al., 2001a; Muccioli et al., 2002).

Ghrelin is the first peptide isolated from natural sources in which the hydroxyl group of one of its serine residues is acylated by *n*-octanoic acid (Kojima et al., 2001b). The acylation of the peptide has been supposed to be critical to crossing the blood-brain barrier, but it is also essential for binding the GHS-R1a and for its GH-releasing and other endocrine actions (Banks et al., 2002; Muccioli et al., 2002). However, nonacylated ghrelin, which circulates in amount far greater than the acylated form is not biologically inactive; it exerts some nonendocrine actions such as antiproliferative effects, probably binding nonclassical GHS-R1a (Muccioli et al., 2002).

There is also another endogenous ligand for the GHS-R1a isolated from the stomach. It has been named des-Gln14-ghrelin, has the same acylation in serine 3, and is homologous to ghrelin except for one missing glutamine; it is the result of an alternative splicing of the ghrelin gene and possesses the same activity as ghrelin (Kojima et al., 2001b).

Regarding the regulation of ghrelin secretion, it has been shown that the secretion of ghrelin, mostly represented in its acylated form, occurs in a pulsatile manner and, notably, there is no strict correlation between ghrelin and GH levels in rats; interestingly, ghrelin pulses are correlated with food intake episodes and sleep cycles (Tolle et al., 2002). Particularly in humans it has been shown that peaks in ghrelin levels anticipate food intake, suggesting the latter is triggered by ghrelin discharge (Cummings and Schwartz, 2003).

In concordance with the major influence of nutrition on ghrelin secretion, circulating ghrelin levels are increased in anorexia and cachexia but reduced in obesity and overfeeding (Cummings and Schwartz, 2003). In every condition ghrelin secretion is normalized by the recovery of ideal body weight (Cummings and Schwartz, 2003). These changes are opposite to those of leptin, suggesting that both ghrelin and leptin are hormones signaling the metabolic balance and managing the neuroendocrine and metabolic response to starvation (Muccioli et al., 2002; Yoshihara et al., 2002; Cummings and Schwartz, 2003).

Circulating ghrelin levels mostly reflect gastric secretion; in fact, they are reduced by 70% after gastrectomy (Kojima et al., 2001a; Muccioli et al., 2002). It had been reported that ghrelin secretion is not inhibited by simple gastric distension in animals but, more recently, it has been demonstrated that gastric bypass strongly inhibits it (Muccioli et al., 2002; Cummings and Schwartz, 2003). Either oral and intravenous glucose loads inhibit ghrelin secretion in humans as well as in animals; on the other hand, free fatty acid load as well as arginine load do not affect circulating ghrelin levels (Mohlig et al., 2002; Broglio et al., 2003).

In agreement with the negative association between ghrelin secretion and body mass, clear negative association between ghrelin and insulin secretion has been found in humans as well as in animals, suggesting inhibitory influence of insulin on ghrelin secretion (Broglio et al., 2003). Indeed, both euglycemic clamp steady state increase in insulin levels and insulin-induced hypoglycemia are associated to clear reduction in circulating ghrelin levels (Lucidi et al., 2002; Broglio et al., 2003). However, at present, the most remarkable inhibitory input on ghrelin secretion has been shown to be from somatostatin and its natural analogue cortistatin, both of which are also able to inhibit β-cell secretion (Broglio et al., 2002).

In all, evidence that insulin and somatostatin exert a critical inhibitory action on ghrelin secretion indicates that the latter is under major influence, mostly inhibitory, from the endocrine pancreas. A notable exception to the negative association between insulin and ghrelin secretion is represented by the Prader-Willi syndrome, which is generally connoted by obesity but nevertheless associated with ghrelin hypersecretion (Cummings and Schwartz, 2003).

Endocrine Activities of Ghrelin and GHS: Clinical Implications

GH-releasing Activity

Both ghrelin and synthetic GHS possess a strong and dose-related GH-releasing activity which is more marked is humans than in animals (Smith et al., 1997; Takaya et al., 2000; Kojima et al., 2001a; Arvat et al., 2001). Specifically, in rats, it has been demonstrated that, unlike GHRH, central ghrelin administration stimulates GH release but does not augment GH synthesis (Date et al., 2000).

Ghrelin, GHS, and GHRH have a synergetic effect, indicating that they act, at least partially, via different mechanisms (Smith et al., 1997; Arvat et al., 2001; Muccioli et al., 2002). Nevertheless, GHS need GHRH activity to fully express their GH-releasing effect, as has been shown in both in vitro and in vivo animal and human studies (Smith et al., 1997; Muccioli et al., 2002; Wren et al., 2002).

Both ghrelin and synthetic GHS have been reported to be ineffective in modifing hypothalamic somatostatin release, but there are data indicating that ghrelin and GHS might act as functional somatostatin antagonists at the pituitary and the hypothalamic level (Muccioli et al., 2002; Wren et al., 2002). In humans the GH response to both natural and synthetic GHS is not modified by substances acting via somatostatin inhibition and is partially refractory to the inhibitory effect of substances acting via stimulation of hypothalamic somatostatin and even of exogenous somatostatin (Muccioli et al., 2002).

The GH-releasing effect of ghrelin and synthetic GHS undergoes marked age-related variations, decreasing with age (Gottero et al., 2002; Muccioli et al., 2002; Broglio et al., 2003). The mechanisms underlying the age-related variations in the GH-releasing activity of GHS differ at different ages. For instance, the enhanced GH-releasing effect of GHS at puberty reflects a positive influence of estrogen, which could trigger an increase in GHS-R expression. However, estrogen insufficiency does not explain the reduced GH response to GHS in postmenopausal women. In concordance with the reduction in hypothalamic GHS-R in human aged brain, the GH response to hexarelin in elderly subjects is increased but not restored by supramaximal doses. The most important mechanism accounting for reduced GH-releasing activity of GHS in age is probably age-related variations in the neural control of somatotroph function, including GHRH hypoactivity and somatostatinergic hyperactivity (Muccioli et al., 2002). On the other hand, it has also been hypothesized that declining GH secretion reflects an age-related decrease in the activity of the endogenous GHS ligand, i.e., ghrelin. This hypothesis remains to be verified.

Regarding the clinical implications, particularly when combined with GHRH, GHS represent one of the most potent and reliable tests to evaluate the releasable pool of pituitary GH for the diagnosis of GH deficiency, at least in adulthood (Baldelli et al., 2001). The potential usefulness of GHS for treatment of short stature with isolated GH deficiency has been ruled out by a double-blind, placebo-controlled trial in short children with GH deficiency showing that the efficacy of chronic oral treatment with MK-0677 is not comparable with that of rhGH (Yu et al., 1998).

GHS could also represent anabolic treatment in frail elderly subjects with somatopause. To favor this hypothesis there is the following evidence: (1) the age-related reduction in the activity of the GH/IGF-1 axis probably accounts for changes in body composition and metabolism in normal elderly subjects which are remarkably similar to (but of lesser extent than) those in adults with GH deficiency (Corpas et al., 1993; Ghigo et al., 1996) and (2) the releasable pool of pituitary GH is still remarkable in aged subjects, indicating that GH-releasing substances would restore endogenous GH pulsatility more physiologically (Corpas et al., 1993; Ghigo et al., 1996). Clinical trials testing the effects of chronic treatment with MK-0677 as GH-mediated anabolic agent have shown that: (1) in elderly subjects it restores IGF-1 levels to the normal young range, indicating successful enhancement of somatotroph secretion (Chapman et al., 1996); (2) in elderly subjects it increases REM sleep while decreasing REM latency, thus counteracting alterations in sleep pattern that are hallmarks of brain aging (Copinschi et al., 1997); (3) it reverses diet-induced catabolism in young volunteers, indicating an anabolic effect (Murphy et al., 1998) while increasing fat-free mass and energy expenditure in obese patients (Svensson et al., 1998) and (4) in a large population of postmenopausal osteoporotic women, 1 year's treatment with MK-0677 alone and in combination with alendronate, a bisphosphonate, attenuates the indirect suppressive effect of alendronate on bone formation but does not translate into significant increases in bone mineral density at sites other than the femoral neck (Murphy et al., 2001). In all, there is no definitive evidence of the therapeutic efficacy of GHS as anabolic agents acting via rejuvenation of the GH/IGF-1 axis in elderly subjects.

PRL- and ACTH-releasing Activity

The stimulatory effect of ghrelin and synthetic GHS on PRL secretion in humans is slight, independent of both gender and age, and probably comes from direct stimulation of somatomammotroph cells (Muccioli et al., 2002).

The stimulatory effect of GHS on the activity of the hypothalamus-pituitary-adrenal axis in humans is remarkable and similar to that after naloxone, arginine-vasopressin, and even CRH, but is an acute neuroendocrine effect that probably vanishes during prolonged treatment (Muccioli et al., 2002). In physiological conditions, the ACTH-releasing activity of GHS totally depends on mechanisms mediated by the central nervous system, including actions mediated by arginine-vasopressin, neuropeptide Y (NPY), and/or GABA (Muccioli et al., 2002). The ACTH response to GHS is generally sensitive to the negative feedback action of cortisol, but it is surprisingly exaggerated (and higher than that to hCRH) in patients with pituitary ACTH-dependent Cushing's disease as well as in some patients with ectopic ACTH-dependent Cushing's syndrome (Muccioli et al., 2002). Interestingly, ghrelin and GHS-R are expressed in abnormal human pituitary as well as in other neuroendocrine tumors, including ACTH-secreting tumors, and GHS stimulate ACTH release from human ACTH-secreting pituitary adenomas but not from normal human pituitary (De Keyzer et al., 1997; Korbonits et al., 2001).

Influence on Gonadal Function

It has been shown that GHS-R are present in the testis as well as in the ovary (Muccioli et al., 2002). Moreover, Leydig cells have been reported to be able to synthesize ghrelin (Tena-Sempere et al., 2002). Notably, ghrelin was found to induce a significant inhibition of hCG- and cAMP-stimulated testosterone secretion in vitro coupled with a significant decrease in hCG-stimulated expression levels of the mRNAs encoding steroid acute regulatory protein and P450 cholesterol side-chain cleavage, 3β-hydroxysteroid dehydrogenase, and 17β-hydroxysteroid dehydrogenase type III enzymes (Tena-Sempere et al., 2002). These data, together with evidence that intracerebroventricularly injected ghrelin inhibits pulsatile LH secretions in rats (Furuta et al., 2001), provide evidence for a possible action of ghrelin in the regulation of gonadal axis and of testicular function.

Influence on Endocrine Pancreatic Function and Glucose Metabolism

Ghrelin and GHS-R1a mRNA are present in normal and neoplastic endocrine pancreas (Date et al., 2002; Gnanapavan et al., 2002; Volante et al., 2002; Wierup et al., 2002). Specifically, ghrelin has been demonstrated to be expressed by pancreatic endocrine α-cells, in rat and human tissue (Date et al. 2002) or by pancreatic β-cells (Volante et al., 2002). Studies in animals reported conflicting results regarding the influence of ghrelin on insulin secretion (Adeghate and Ponery, 2002; Date et al., 2002; Egido et al., 2002; Lee et al., 2002). In fact, ghrelin was able to stimulate insulin secretion from isolated rat pancreatic islets (Adeghate and Ponery, 2002; Date et al., 2002) and in rats in vivo as well (Lee et al., 2002). On the other hand, insulin secretion from isolated rat pancreas, perfused in situ after stimulation with glucose, arginine, and carbachol, was found to be blunted by exposure to ghrelin, which also reduced the somatostatin response to arginine (Egido et al., 2002).

In concordance with the possibility of a modulatory role of ghrelin on pancreatic function, a clear negative association between ghrelin and insulin secretion has been reported by the majority of authors in humans as well as in animals (Broglio et al., 2003). In humans, ghrelin has been reported to induce a significant increase in plasma glucose levels that is surprisingly followed by a reduction in insulin secretion (Broglio et al., 2003). Coupled with the observation that acute as well as chronic treatment with GHS, particularly nonpeptidyl derivatives, induced hyperglycemia and insulin resistance in a considerable number of elderly subjects and obese patients (Chapman et al., 1996; Svensson et al., 1998), these observations suggest that ghrelin is a gastroenteropancreatic hormone, exerting a significant role in the fine-tuning of insulin secretion and that in the mean time also affects glucose metabolism.

It is suggested that ghrelin might integrate the hormonal and metabolic response to fasting which, at least in humans, is connoted by a clear-cut increase in GH secretion coupled with inhibition of insulin secretion and activation of mechanisms devoted to maintain glucose levels.

Regarding glucose levels, it has been already shown that ghrelin probably blocks the inhibitory effects of insulin on gluconeogenesis (Murata et al., 2002).

In all, these data would agree with the hypothesis that ghrelin has major role in managing the neuroendocrine and metabolic response to variations in the energy balance but the potential clinical impact of this activity is, at present, far from defined.

Nonendocrine Activities of GHS: Potential Clinical Implications

GHS-R are concentrated in the hypothalamus-pituitary unit, but also distributed in other central and peripheral tissues, and this distribution explains other biological activities that could suggest potential clinical perspectives.

Orexigenic Activity

In concordance with previous reports addressing the effects of synthetic GHS, ghrelin is involved in the regulation of energy balance (Muccioli et al., 2002; Yoshihara et al., 2002). Exogenous ghrelin induces weight gain in rodents by increasing food intake and reducing fat utilization (Muccioli et al., 2002; Yoshihara et al., 2002). These activities are GH independent and are most likely mediated by a specific central network of neurons that is also modulated by leptin; ghrelin and leptin might really be complementary players of one regulatory system that has developed to inform the central nervous system about the status of the energy balance (Muccioli et al., 2002; Yoshihara et al., 2002). It is to be noted that in obesity leptin levels are elevated while ghrelin levels are decreased suggesting their adaptation to the positive energy balance rather than an involvement in the etiology of obesity (Muccioli et al., 2002; Yoshihara et al., 2002; Cummings and Schwartz, 2003).

Peripheral ghrelin is mainly produced in the gastrointestinal tract and could reach the GHS-R in the central nervous system, namely the hypothalamus, through the general circulation, to regulate food intake and energy homeostasis (Kojima et al., 2001a; Muccioli et al., 2002; Yoshihara et al., 2002). Ghrelin-containing cells are also present in the mediobasal hypothalamus, where GHRH-secreting neurons and the neuroendocrine network regulating energy balance are located (Kojima et al., 2001a; Muccioli et al., 2002). Indeed, NPY-receptor-1 antagonists as well as melanocortin agonists and antisera to both NPY and agouti-related peptide may interfere with the orexigenic effect of ghrelin, which is, however, preserved in NPY-knockout mice, suggesting a key role for agouti-related peptide (Muccioli et al., 2002).

The stimulatory effect of ghrelin and synthetic GHS on food intake is of obvious interest. Synthetic GHS analogues acting as agonists or antagonists on the appetite would have perspectives for drug intervention in eating disorders.

Gastroenteropancreatic and Metabolic Actions

It is not surprising that as a gastric hormone, ghrelin acts at the gastroenteropancreatic level, where GHS-R mRNA expression has been demonstrated (Gnanapavan et al., 2002; Muccioli et al., 2002). Ghrelin stimulates gastric contractility and modulates acid secretion in rats (Muccioli et al., 2002; Yoshihara et al., 2002). This action is mediated by the cholinergic system as it is abolished by muscarinic blockade; interestingly, the acetylcholine-mediated stimulatory effect of ghrelin on gastric acid secretion takes place, at least partially, at the central level (Muccioli et al., 2002).

Ghrelin is produced by about 20% of the rat and human neuroendocrine cell population of the stomach (A-like cells) (Kojima et al., 2001a; Muccioli et al., 2002). The endocrine cell population of the stomach may undergo proliferative phenomena of both hyperplastic and neoplastic nature, and it is noteworthy that gastric carcinoids (and also neuroendocrine cell hyperplastic conditions) often synthesize ghrelin. Thus, ghrelin could be the product of many apparently silent gastric carcinoids generally associated with atrophic gastritis (Papotti et al., 2001). These might represent conditions of ghrelin hypersecretion, while an obvious consequence of gastrectomy would be ghrelin insufficiency, but preliminary data indicate only a 50% reduction in circulating ghrelin levels after gastrectomy (Ariyasu et al., 2001). The clinical impact of ghrelin hyper- and hyposecretion is still unknown.

Cardiovascular Actions

Specific binding sites for GHS are present in the cardiovascular system (Muccioli et al., 2002). The presence of GHS-R1a mRNA has been demonstrated in both animal and human cardiac tissues (Kojima et al., 2001a). However, in ventricles, atria, aorta, coronaries, carotid, endocardium, and vena cava there are binding sites specific for peptidyl GHS only; the binding of labeled Tyr-Ala-hexarelin is inhibited by unlabeled peptidyl GHS such as hexarelin but not by MK-0677, a nonpeptidyl GHS, on even ghrelin (Muccioli et al., 2002). The functional action of these receptors is still unclear.

Prolonged treatment with peptidyl GHS markedly protects against cardiovascular ischemic damage and improves cardiac function in different animal models (Muccioli et al., 2000). In humans, peptidyl GHS and ghrelin have been reported to increase cardiac contractility in normal subjects and in patients with chronic heart failure although with different hemodynamic profiles (Muccioli et al., 2000, 2002).

Modulation of Cell Proliferation and Apoptosis

GHS binding sites have also been found in neoplastic endocrine and nonendocrine tissues; interestingly, GHS-R subtypes have been found in tumoral tissues from organs, such as breast, which do not express these receptor in physiological conditions (Muccioli et al., 2002).

Both physiological and neoplastic thyroid tissue expresses GHS-R (Cassoni et al., 2000). All follicular-derived thyroid tumors show specific GHS binding sites, even more than in the normal thyroid (Cassoni et al., 2000). Specific GHS binding sites are also present in thyroid tumor cell lines (follicular, papillary, and anaplastic tumoral cell lines) (Cassoni et al., 2000). Both ghrelin and synthetic GHS inhibit ^{3}H-thymidine incorporation and cell proliferation, at least at the earliest time of treatment in all cell lines (Muccioli et al., 2002).

Specific GHS-R have been shown in breast tumor but not fibroadenomas and normal breast parenchyma (Cassoni et al., 2001). In breast tumors the highest binding activity is present in well-differentiated invasive breast carcinomas, being progressively reduced in moderately to poorly differentiated tumors (Cassoni et al., 2001). Specific GHS binding sites are also present in different human breast (estrogen-dependent and estrogen-independent) carcinoma cell lines, in which acylated ghrelin as well as unacylated ghrelin and synthetic GHS inhibit cell proliferation (Cassoni et al., 2001).

Moreover, it has been recently reported that both nontumoral and tumoral lung tissue show the presence of a specific receptor that binds synthetic peptidyl GHS only (Ghè et al., 2002). In contrast, GHS-R1a mRNA expression is occasionally found only in endocrine lung neoplasms, but not in other nontumoral or tumoral lung tissues (Ghè et al., 2002). Accordingly, peptidyl but not nonpeptidyl GHS, as well as ghrelin, has been shown to inhibit DNA synthesis and proliferation of nonendocrine human lung carcinoma cell line (CALU-1) in vitro, suggesting that the growth-inhibitory effect of peptidyl GHS is likely to be mediated by a specific receptor other than GHS-R1a (Ghè et al., 2002).

The expression of ghrelin mRNA, the GHS-R1a and 1b mRNA isoforms, and ghrelin and GHS-R protein have also been reported in human prostate cancer cell lines (Jeffery et al., 2002). Interestingly, the same authors reported that ghrelin significantly increases the proliferation of prostate cancer cells in vitro, possibly either by the autocrine action of secreted prostatic GH or by some other more direct autocrine/paracrine signaling mechanism (Jeffery et al., 2002).

In all, evidence that ghrelin and synthetic GHS modulate cell proliferation in different experimental models further shows their multiple biological activities and suggests the possibility that GHS agonists or antagonists could exert an antineoplastic action; however, this possibility is not supported, at present, by any definite evidence.

Conclusions

GHS were born more than 20 years ago as synthetic molecule possessing strong GH-releasing activity and suggested the dream that GH deficiency could be treated by orally active GHS as an alternative to rhGH. History has shown this not to be the case, and their usefulness as an anabolic antiaging intervention in somatopause is also still unclear. Nevertheless, the GHS story went on to the discovery of ghrelin as a natural ligand of the specific receptors mediating the activities of synthetic GHS. It was not by chance that ghrelin was discovered by a group very active in the cardiovascular field. It had been already shown that synthetic GHS were more than simply molecules stimulating GH release, but that they had, for instance, cardiotropic actions. We now know that GHS were generally mimicking the activity of ghrelin, which is much more than a natural GHS. Other neuroendocrine, metabolic, and non-endocrine actions make up the profile of a new hormone that moves us from neuroendocrinology into the middle of internal medicine.

Acknowledgements. Studies by the authors mentioned in this paper were supported by MURST, CNR, Eureka (Peptido project 1923), SMEM Foundation and Europeptides.

References

Adeghate E. and Ponery A.S. (2002). Ghrelin stimulates insulin secretion from the pancreas of normal and diabetic rats. J Neuroendocrinol, 14, 555-560.

Ariyasu H., Takaya K., Tagami T., Ogawa Y., Hosoda K., Akamizu T., Suda M., Koh T., Natsui K., Toyooka S., Shirakami G., Usui T., Shimatsu A., Doi K., Hosoda H., Kojima M., Kangawa K. and Nakao K. (2001). Stomach is a major source of circulating ghrelin, and feeding state determines plasma ghrelin-like immunoreactivity levels in humans. J Clin Endocrinol Metab, 86, 4753-4758.

Arvat E., Maccario M., Di Vito L., Broglio F., Benso A., Gottero C., Papotti M., Muccioli G., Dieguez C., Casanueva F.F., Deghenghi R., Camanni F. and Ghigo E. (2001). Endocrine activities of ghrelin, a natural growth hormone secretagogue (GHS), in humans: comparison and interactions with hexarelin, a nonnatural peptidyl GHS, and GH-releasing hormone. J Clin Endocrinol Metab, 86, 1169-1174.

Baldelli R., Otero X.L., Camina J.P., Gualillo O., Popovic V., Dieguez C. and Casanueva F.F. (2001). Growth hormone secretagogues as diagnostic tools in disease states. Endocrine, 14, 95-99.

Banks W.A., Tschop M., Robinson S.M. and Heiman M.L. (2002). Extent and direction of ghrelin transport across the blood-brain barrier is determined by its unique primary structure. J Pharmacol Exp Ther, 302, 822-827.

Broglio F., Arvat E., Benso A., Gottero C., Prodam F., Grottoli S., Papotti M., Muccioli G., van der Lely A.J., Deghenghi R. and Ghigo E. (2002). Endocrine activities of cortistatin-14 and its interaction with GHRH and ghrelin in humans. J Clin Endocrinol Metab, 87, 3783-3790.

Broglio F., Benso A., Castiglioni C., Gottero C., Prodam F., Destefanis S., Gauna C., Filtri L., van der Lely A.J., Deghenghi R., Bo M., Arvat E. and Ghigo E. (2003). The endocrine response to ghrelin as function of gender in humans in young and elderly subjects. J Clin Endocrinol Metab, 88, 1537-1542.

Cassoni P., Papotti M., Catapano F., Ghe C., Deghenghi R., Ghigo E. and Muccioli G. (2000). Specific binding sites for synthetic growth hormone secretagogues in non-tumoral and neoplastic human thyroid tissue. J Endocrinol, 165, 139-146.

Cassoni P., Papotti M., Ghe C., Catapano F., Sapino A., Graziani A., Deghenghi R., Reissmann T., Ghigo E. and Muccioli G. (2001). Identification, characterization, and biological activity of specific receptors for natural (ghrelin) and synthetic growth hormone secretagogues and analogs in human breast carcinomas and cell lines. J Clin Endocrinol Metab, 86, 1738-1745.
Chapman I.M., Bach M.A., Van Cauter E., Farmer M., Krupa D., Taylor A.M., Schilling L.M., Cole K.Y., Skiles E.H., Pezzoli S.S., Hartman M.L., Veldhuis J.D., Gormley G.J. and Thorner M.O. (1996). Stimulation of the growth hormone (GH)-insulin-like growth factor I axis by daily oral administration of a GH secretogogue (MK-677) in healthy elderly subjects. J Clin Endocrinol Metab, 81, 4249-4257.
Copinschi G., Leproult R., Van Onderbergen A., Caufriez A., Cole K.Y., Schilling L.M., Mendel C.M., De Lepeleire I., Bolognese J.A. and Van Cauter E. (1997). Prolonged oral treatment with MK-677, a novel growth hormone secretagogue, improves sleep quality in man. Neuroendocrinology, 66, 278-286.
Corpas E., Harman S.M. and Blackman M.R. (1993). Human growth hormone and human ageing. Endocr Rev, 14, 20-39.
Cummings D.E. and Schwartz M.W. (2003). Genetics and pathophysiology of human obesity. Annu Rev Med, 54, 453-471.
Date Y., Murakami N., Kojima M., Kuroiwa T., Matsukura S., Kangawa K. and Nakazato M. (2000). Central effects of a novel acylated peptide, ghrelin, on growth hormone release in rats. Biochem Biophys Res Commun, 275, 477-480.
Date Y., Nakazato M., Hashiguchi S., Dezaki K., Mondal M.S., Hosoda H., Kojima M, Kangawa K., Arima T., Matsuo H., Yada T. and Matsukura S. (2002). Ghrelin is present in pancreatic alpha-cells of humans and rats and stimulates insulin secretion. Diabetes, 51, 124-129.
De Keyzer Y., Lenne F. and Bertagna X. (1997). Widespread transcription of the growth hormone-releasing peptide receptor gene in neuroendocrine human tumors. Eur J Endocrinol, 137, 715-718.
Egido E.M., Rodriguez-Gallardo J., Silvestre R.A. and Marco J. (2002). Inhibitory effect of ghrelin on insulin and pancreatic somatostatin secretion. Eur J Endocrinol, 146, 241-244.
Furuta M., Funabashi T. and Kimura F. (2001). Intracerebroventricular administration of ghrelin rapidly suppresses pulsatile luteinizing hormone secretion in ovariectomized rats. Biochem Biophys Res Commun, 288, 780-785.
Ghè C., Cassoni P., Catapano F., Marrocco T., Deghenghi R., Ghigo E., Muccioli G. and Papotti M. (2002). The antiproliferative effect of synthetic peptidyl GH secretagogues in human CALU-1 lung carcinoma cells. Endocrinology, 143, 484-491.
Ghigo E., Arvat E., Gianotti L., Ramunni J., DiVito L., Maccagno B., Grottoli S. and Camanni F. (1996). Human ageing and the GH-IGF-I axis. J Pediatr Endocrinol Metab, 9, 271-278.
Gnanapavan S., Kola B., Bustin S.A., Morris D.G., McGee P., Fairclough P., Bhattacharya S., Carpenter R., Grossman A.B. and Korbonits M. (2002). The tissue distribution of the mRNA of ghrelin and subtypes of its receptor, GHS-R, in humans. J Clin Endocrinol Metab, 87, 2988-2991.
Gottero C., Benso A., Prodam F., Broglio F., Castiglioni C., Bo M., Deghenghi R., Ghigo E. and Arvat E. (2002). Age-related variations of the GH response to GH secretagogues in humans. J Endocrinol Invest, 25, 42-43.
Jeffery P.L., Herington A.C. and Chopin L.K. (2002). Expression and action of the growth hormone releasing peptide ghrelin and its receptor in prostate cancer cell lines. J Endocrinol, 172, R7-11.
Kojima M., Hosoda H. and Kangawa K. (2001a). Purification and distribution of ghrelin: the natural endogenous ligand for the growth hormone secretagogue receptor. Horm Res, 56 (Suppl 1), 93-97.
Kojima M., Hosoda H., Matsuo H. and Kangawa K. (2001b). Ghrelin: discovery of the natural endogenous ligand for the growth hormone secretagogue receptor. Trends Endocrinol Metab, 12, 118-122.

Korbonits M., Bustin S.A., Kojima M., Jordan S., Adams E.F., Lowe D.G., Kangawa K. and Grossman A.B. (2001). The expression of the growth hormone secretagogue receptor ligand ghrelin in normal and abnormal human pituitary and other neuroendocrine tumors. J Clin Endocrinol Metab, 86, 881-887.

Lee H.M., Wang G., Englander E.W., Kojima M. and Greeley G.H. Jr. (2002). Ghrelin, a new gastrointestinal endocrine peptide that stimulates insulin secretion: enteric distribution, ontogeny, influence of endocrine, and dietary manipulations. Endocrinology, 143, 185-190.

Lucidi P., Murdolo G., Di Loreto C., De Cicco A., Parlanti N., Fanelli C., Santeusanio F., Bolli G.B. and De Feo P. (2002). Ghrelin is not necessary for adequate hormonal counterregulation of insulin-induced hypoglycemia. Diabetes, 51, 2911-2914.

Mohlig M., Spranger J., Otto B., Ristow M., Tschop M. and Pfeiffer A.F. (2002). Euglycemic hyperinsulinemia, but not lipid infusion, decreases circulating ghrelin levels in humans. J Endocrinol Invest, 25, RC36-38.

Muccioli G., Broglio F., Valetto M.R., Ghe C., Catapano F., Graziani A., Papotti M., Bisi G., Deghenghi R. and Ghigo E. (2000). Growth hormone-releasing peptides and the cardiovascular system. Ann Endocrinol, 61, 27-31.

Muccioli G., Tschop M., Papotti M., Deghenghi R., Hieman M. and Ghigo E. (2002). Neuroendocrine and peripheral activities of ghrelin: implications in metabolism and obesity. Eur J Pharmacol, 404, 235-254.

Murata M., Okimura Y., Iida K., Matsumoto M., Sowa H., Kaji H., Kojima M., Kangawa K. and Chihara K. (2002). Ghrelin modulates the downstream molecules of insulin signaling in hepatoma cells. J Biol Chem, 277, 5667-5674.

Murphy M.G., Plunkett L.M., Gertz B.J., He W., Wittreich J., Polvino W.M. and Clemmons D.R. (1998). MK-677, an orally active growth hormone secretagogue, reverses diet-induced catabolism. J Clin Endocrinol Metab, 83, 320-325.

Murphy M.G., Weiss S., McClung M., Schnitzer T., Cerchio K., Connor J., Krupa D. and Gertz B.J. (2001). Effect of alendronate and MK-677 (a growth hormone secretagogue), individually and in combination, on markers of bone turnover and bone mineral density in postmenopausal osteoporotic women. J Clin Endocrinol Metab, 86, 1116-1125.

Papotti M., Cassoni P., Volante M., Deghenghi R., Muccioli G. and Ghigo E.(2001). Ghrelin-producing endocrine tumors of the stomach and intestine. J Clin Endocrinol Metab, 86, 5052-5059.

Smith R.G., Van der Ploeg L.H., Howard A.D., Feighner S.D., Cheng K., Hickey G.J., Wyvratt M.J. Jr, Fisher M.H., Nargund R.P. and Patchett A.A. (1997). Peptidomimetic regulation of growth hormone secretion. Endocr Rev, 18, 621-645.

Svensson J., Lonn L., Jansson J.O., Murphy G., Wyss D., Krupa D., Cerchio K., Polvino W., Gertz B., Boseaus I., Sjostrom L. and Bengtsson B.A. (1998). Two-month treatment of obese subjects with the oral growth hormone (GH) secretagogue MK-677 increases GH secretion, fat-free mass, and energy expenditure. J Clin Endocrinol Metab, 83, 362-369.

Takaya K., Ariyasu H., Kanamoto N., Iwakura H., Yoshimoto A., Harada M., Mori K., Komatsu Y., Usui T., Shimatsu A., Ogawa Y., Hosoda K., Akamizu T., Kojima M., Kangawa K. and Nakao K. (2000). Ghrelin strongly stimulates growth hormone release in humans. J Clin Endocrinol Metab, 85, 4908-4911.

Tena-Sempere M., Barreiro M.L., Gonzalez L.C., Gaytan F., Zhang F.P., Caminos J.E., Pinilla L., Casanueva F.F., Dieguez C. and Aguilar E. (2002). Novel expression and functional role of ghrelin in rat testis. Endocrinology, 143, 717-725.

Tolle V., Bassant M.H., Zizzari P., Poindessous-Jazat F., Tomasetto C., Epelbaum J. and Bluet-Pajot M.T. (2002). Ultradian rhythmicity of ghrelin secretion in relation with GH, feeding behavior, and sleep-wake patterns in rats. Endocrinology, 143, 1353-1361.

Volante M., Allìa E., Gugliotta P., Funaro A., Broglio F., Deghenghi R., Muccioli G., Ghigo E. and Papotti M. (2002). Expression of ghrelin and of GH secretagogue receptor by pancreatic islet cells and related endocrine tumors. J Clin Endocrinol Metab, 87, 1300-1308.

Wierup N., Svensson H., Mulder H. and Sundler F. (2002). The ghrelin cell: a novel developmentally regulated islet cell in the human pancreas. Regul Pept, 107, 63-69.
Wren A.M., Small C.J., Fribbens C.V., Neary N.M., Ward H.L., Seal L.J., Ghatei M.A. and Bloom S.R. (2002). The hypothalamic mechanisms of the hypophysiotropic action of ghrelin. Neuroendocrinology, 76, 316-324.
Yoshihara F., Kojima M., Hosoda H., Nakazato M. and Kangawa K. (2002). Ghrelin: a novel peptide for growth hormone release and feeding regulation. Curr Opin Clin Nutr Metab Care, 5, 391-395.
Yu H., Cassorla F., Tiulpakov A., Shi Y.F., Setian N., Bercu B., Arango A., Kletter G., Pescovitz O., Di Martino J., Krupa D., Cambria M., Kanojia P. and Bach M.A. (1998). A double-blind placebo-controlled efficacy trial of an oral growth hormone (GH) secretagogue (MK-0677) in GH deficient (GHD) children. In: The Endocrine Society's 80th Annual Meeting; New Orleans, USA, OR24-6, p 84.

HORMONAL TREATMENTS FOR ENDOCRINE-DEPENDENT TUMORS

CHAPTER 15

Hormonal Treatments of Endocrine-Dependent Tumors: Preclinical Aspects

P. MAGNI AND M. MOTTA

Introduction

Breast and prostate carcinomas are the most frequently diagnosed diseases in the group of the so-called endocrine-dependent tumors. These diseases are given this name because their development and maintenance, and in several instances their progression, are sustained by the presence of gonadal hormones in the bloodstream, namely estrogens in females and androgens, particularly testosterone, the main testicular androgen, in males.

In most cases, these malignancies maintain the sensitivity to specific hormones that is present in the normal tissue of origin, and their growth is often initially dependent upon the action of these hormones. This characteristic forms the basis of several commonly employed hormonal treatments. The main goal of the different therapeutic options for the treatment of both breast and prostate cancer is to remove the gonadal hormones from the body or else to inactivate them. This can be achieved in two different ways: (1) inhibition of hormone production and secretion by the gonads; (2) inhibition of the action of circulating hormones, either by interference in their binding to the receptors or blocking their transformation to biologically more active compounds, through the inhibition of rate-limiting enzymes such as 5α-reductase and aromatase. A synopsis of the drug categories available is listed in Table 1. This paper describes both the physiological and the pharmacological profile of the different hormonal treatments available so far for both breast and prostate cancers.

Table 1. Categories of drugs available for the hormonal treatment of endocrine-dependent tumors

Inhibition of hormone production and secretion by the gonads:
GnRH agonists
GnRH antagonists
Inhibition of the action of circulating hormones by receptor antagonists:
Anti-androgens
Anti-estrogens/selective estrogen receptor modulators
Inhibition of the action of circulating hormones by inhibition of enzyme activity:
5α-Reductase inhibitors
Aromatase inhibitors

Role of Hormonal Steroids in Breast and Prostate Cancers

As mentioned before, normal as well as tumoral breast and prostate tissues are a target of sexual steroids. Several data have suggested that estrogens directly cause or contribute to the development of breast cancer (Zumoff, 1998). Estrogens reach the breast from three separate main sources: the ovaries, extraglandular tissues such as the adipose, and the breast stroma itself. Thus, these hormones may act by paracrine, autocrine, and intracrine mechanisms on cells in the breast (Mor et al., 1998). Moreover, the duration or the intensity of a woman's exposure to endogenous or exogenous estrogens appears relevant to the development of breast cancer (Mouridsen et al., 2001; Zhang et al., 1997). In this context, the degree of obesity and the consequent increase of fat mass seem to be important (Siiteri, 1987; Takayama et al., 1997), since the adipose tissue possesses aromatase activity and is able to convert circulating androgens of testicular and adrenal origin, such as androstenedione and dehydroepiandrosterone (DHEA), to different estrogenic compounds such as 17β-estradiol and estrone. Moreover, the administration of exogenous estrogens, such as oral contraceptives and the hormonal replacement therapy in the menopause, is a controversial and as yet unsolved issue as a risk factor for breast cancer.

Along with environmental, dietary, and genetic factors, hormonal factors, particularly circulating androgens, probably play a pivotal role in the initiation and promotion of another androgen-related tumor, the cancer of the prostate (Fradet et al., 1999). Testosterone, mainly secreted by the testis, is transformed in peripheral androgen-dependent tissues such as the prostate, to dihydrotestosterone (DHT) by the action of the enzyme 5α-reductase. DHT binds to androgen receptors with a 2.5-fold higher affinity than testosterone itself and represents the major intracellular regulator of prostatic tumor growth. In addition, the adrenal gland provides an additional 5% of the androgens produced in adult men (Sanford et al., 1977), including testosterone, androstenedione, DHEA, and DHEA sulfate. It has been shown that approximately 40% of prostatic DHT originates from steroids of adrenal origin (Sanford et al., 1977). Unlike the use of receptor status assessment in breast cancer, measurement of the androgen receptor does not provide predictive information regarding hormone responsiveness in prostate cancer. Mutations of the androgen receptor occur, but their frequency and their role in primary prostate cancer is a controversial issue (Taplin et al., 1995). At some point in the patient's course, the tumor becomes refractory to hormonally based therapies, thus losing its androgen dependence. Current evidence suggests that this phenomenon might be due to different mechanisms: ligand-independent activation of androgen receptors and upregulation of growth factor pathways are the main ones that have been considered (Denis and Griffiths, 2000).

GnRH Agonists and Antagonists in Hormone-Dependent Cancers

The above-reported considerations on the hormone dependence of some tumors offer the rationale for a therapy able to block the reproductive axis

Table 2. GnRH agonists and antagonists

GnRH agonists:	*GnRH antagonists*:
Triptorelin	Nal-Glu-LHRH
Leuprolide	Antide
Buserelin	Cetrorelix
Goserelin	Ganirelix
Nafarelin	Antarelix

and consequently the production of gonadal steroids. This category of treatments includes the use of gonadotropin-releasing hormone (GnRH) agonists and antagonists (Table 2) and surgical castration (Auclerc et al., 2000). GnRH agonists exert their antitumoral effect by inhibiting the pituitary-gonadal axis, with subsequent suppression of the production and secretion of gonadal hormones. GnRH is physiologically released by the hypothalamus in a pulsatile manner and, once it has reached the gonadotrophs in the anterior pituitary, stimulates the secretion of luteinizing hormone (LH) and follicle-stimulating hormone (FSH) via specific membrane receptors (Cook and Sheridan, 2000). Chronic administration of a GnRH agonist results, by contrast, in the downregulation/desensitization of GnRH receptors and thus in the blockade of LH/FSH release. As a consequence of this inhibitory action, gonadal steroids are no longer produced and secreted by the gonadal structures. The indirect suppression of the production of ovarian estrogen in females and of testicular androgen in males by GnRH analogues represents the pharmacological basis for the treatment of breast and prostate cancers with these synthetic hypothalamic hormones.

While GnRH agonists represent the currently most used therapeutical approach, GnRH antagonists have been introduced more recently. One major difference between the two classes of compounds is that GnRH antagonists are completely devoid of LH-releasing activity and consequently do not show the initial stimulation of testosterone normally observed with GnRH agonists. The so-called flare-up phenomenon observed at the beginning of treatment of prostate cancer with GnRH agonists is absent with GnRH antagonists. To counteract this phenomenon, an anti-androgen is added to GnRH agonist therapy. The treatment with both GnRH agonists and antagonists, however, does not take into consideration the contribution of adrenal steroids, which may be converted to androgens and estrogens by the action of specific enzymes present in the breast and the prostate. To overcome this additional direct proliferative effect, GnRH agonists are usually associated with anti-estrogens in the case of breast cancer and with anti-androgens in the case of prostate cancer, in order to achieve the so-called total blockade of the secretion and action of gonadal hormones (in males: CAB, complete androgen blockade). On the other hand, GnRH antagonists exhibit other drawbacks, such as some histamine-releasing activity and other adverse effects, although these have been improved with the most recent generation of GnRH antagonists. This pharmacological treatment has been successfully applied to the therapy of prostate cancer and is now also proposed for breast cancer.

Steroid Receptor Antagonists in Hormone-Dependent Cancers

Estrogens and androgens bind to specific nuclear receptors expressed in target cells to modulate the transcription of selected genes. The mechanism of action of compounds with anti-estrogenic and anti-androgenic properties mainly relies on their competition with native ligands in binding to the receptors. Therefore, both anti-estrogens and anti-androgens are receptor antagonists (Table 3). In this case, the plasma concentrations of gonadal hormones do not change, but the hormones cannot exert their action, since they cannot bind to the specific receptors, which are already occupied by the antihormone.

In the case of breast cancer, the blockade of estrogen action by anti-estrogens is a common approach: tamoxifen, the first compound of this class to be introduced, is still widely utilized. Together with the more recently developed raloxifene, tamoxifen has been defined as a selective estrogen receptor modulator (SERM). SERMs are compounds with anti-estrogenic actions on breast tissue, but with an estrogen agonist effect on uterus, vagina, bone, pituitary gland, and liver (Santen et al., 1990). This might be explained in part by the binding of SERMs to both estrogen receptor isoforms α and β and by the differential recruitment of corepressors and coactivators in the various cell types (Petterson and Gustafsson, 2001). Additional estrogenic effects are mediated by nongenomic actions at the cell membrane as well as by protein-protein interactions with several transcription factors and components of some intracellular signaling pathways (Filardo et al., 2000; Paech et al., 1997; Porter et al., 1997). In addition to treating breast cancer, tamoxifen and raloxifene have also been proposed for and introduced in to protocols for prevention of the disease in selected women at high risk (Cummings et al., 1999; Fisher et al., 1998, 1999; Powles et al., 1998; Veronesi et al., 1998). An additional category of pure estrogen antagonists, such as faslodex, is currently under investigation, but the available data are still preliminary.

In prostate cancer, monotherapy with anti-androgens provides an alternative to surgical or medical castration. These agents can be subclassified as steroidal and nonsteroidal compounds, according to their chemical structure. The steroidal anti-androgen cyproterone acetate also possesses progestational and glucocorticoid activity, and its long-term administration has been associated with hepatotoxicity. The most frequently used anti-androgens are the

Table 3. Estrogen and androgen receptor antagonists

Estrogen receptor antagonists:	Androgen receptor antagonists:
Tamoxifen	Steroidal:
Raxolifene	Cyproterone acetate
	Megestrol acetate
	Nonsteroidal:
	Flutamide
	Nilutamide
	Bicalutamide

nonsteroidal agents flutamide and bicalutamide, which differ from their steroidal counterpart in acting only at the androgen receptor, thus blocking the cellular effects of circulating testosterone and DHT on cell proliferation. Interruption of the androgen negative feedback system results in reflex increments in serum LH, testosterone, and DHT levels. Side effects include hot flashes and diarrhea, particularly with flutamide (Buzdar and Hortobagyi, 1998). Several studies have led to the conclusion that anti-androgens as monotherapy may not block androgen effects as effectively as medical or surgical castration. For these reasons, the use of anti-androgens appears more effective in combination with GnRH analogues, to achieve complete or maximum androgen blockade (CAB and MAB, respectively), as already mentioned in the preceding section.

An anti-androgen withdrawal syndrome is observed in a proportion of patients after prolonged treatment with anti-androgens (flutamide) has been stopped; this consists in a paradoxical tumor regression. Some studies suggest that, due to mutated androgen receptors, in these cases flutamide works as a receptor agonist and stimulates cell proliferation (Small and Srinivas, 1995).

Enzyme Inhibitors in Hormone-Dependent Cancers

As estrogens and androgens are produced by the gonads and to a lesser extent by other tissues, the use of inhibitors of these enzymes has a strong rationale in the treatment of breast and prostate cancers. Both aromatase inhibitors and 5α-reductase inhibitors are used within the context of the therapy of these tumors (Table 4). Aromatase catalyzes the rate-limiting step in the conversion of androgens to estrogens (Santen and Harvey, 1999) and has been a key target for the development of inhibitors over the past 25 years (Santen et al., 1990). The first-generation inhibitor, aminoglutethimide, inhibits aromatase by 90% in postmenopausal women and is as effective as tamoxifen in causing breast tumor regression (Gale et al., 1994; Smith et al., 1982). However, it is nonselective, blocks cortisol production, and induces significant side effects. Nevertheless, the efficacy of aminoglutethimide in postmenopausal patients prompted the further development of second- and third-generation aro-

Table 4. Inhibitors of androgen metabolizing enzymes

Aromatase inhibitors:	*5α-Reductase inhibitors*:
First generation:	Finasteride
Aminoglutethimide	Episteride
Second generation:	
Formestane (4-OHA)	
Arimidex	
Third generation (selective aromatase inhibitors):	
Anastrozole	
Letrozole	
Exemestane	
Vorozole	

matase inhibitors. The latter compounds (anastrozole, letrozole, exemestane), now approved in Europe and the United States, are 100-fold to 10 000-fold more potent than aminoglutethimide, and are called selective aromatase inhibitors, because they do not inhibit other enzymatic steps (Bonneterre et al., 2000; Ingle et al., 1999; Nabholtz et al., 2000; Santen and Harvey, 1999). The two major subclasses are nonsteroidal competitive inhibitors (anastrozole, letrozole, vorozole), and steroidal enzyme inactivators (exemestane), which bind covalently to the enzyme and permanently block its activity (Santen and Harvey, 1999). Both classes of drugs reduce aromatase to 1%-10% of baseline activity (Dowsett et al., 1995; MacNeill et al., 1992), substantially reduce plasma estradiol levels, and suppress tissue concentrations of this steroid in breast tumors. Several studies have compared the efficacy and toxicity of these aromatase inhibitors and found that, at least in the advanced disease setting, they are superior to tamoxifen (Bonneterre et al., 2000; Mouridsen et al., 2001).

At present, the choice of aromatase inhibitors over tamoxifen as first-line therapy for advanced disease seems correct, but it is still based on incomplete data. Because they lack estrogen-agonistic properties, aromatase inhibitors do not increase the incidence of endometrial cancer, as may occur with tamoxifen and related compounds. If they are used for long periods, one would expect acceleration of bone loss and perhaps cardiovascular disease as a result of total body aromatase inhibition. Studies on these issues are ongoing. Adverse effects on lipid concentrations have not been found in preliminary studies.

The important role of the 5α-reductase enzyme system (type 1 and type 2 isoenzymes) in prostate physiology is well recognized. Recent efforts have led to the development of specific 5α-reductase inhibitors aimed at the treatment of both benign and malignant diseases of the prostate. The first inhibitor to be developed was finasteride, a structural analogue of testosterone which selectively inhibits the type 2 isoenzyme without inhibiting the type 1 or interfering with androgen receptor binding. Finasteride treatment results in a reduction of serum and intraprostatic DHT and prostate-specific antigen and an increase of intraprostatic testosterone (Gormley, 1996). Finasteride represents a treatment option for benign prostatic hyperplasia. In addition, some experimental evidence suggests that type 2 5α-reductase inhibitors may have a significant role in the treatment of prostate cancer (Bologna et al., 1992 1995). However, the real effectiveness of 5α-reductase inhibitors in the clinical setting of prostate cancer still remains to be established. Due to their low toxicity, an interesting application of these compounds may be in the possible chemoprevention of prostate cancer (Coltman et al., 1999).

Conclusions

The hormonal treatment of endocrine-dependent tumors is a nondefinitive (noncurative) therapeutic option and includes a series of different approaches which in several instances are combined to achieve greater efficacy. The future lines of research in this field should lead to the development of more effective drugs targeting the specific mechanisms of gonadal secretion of steroid hormones and of their gonadal and extragonadal enzymatic conversion to active metabolites, and interference with the action of these hormones at the receptor level, in order to optimize this therapeutic approach. Moreover, it appears necessary to better understand the role played in the progression of endocrine-dependent tumors by other biological systems (cytokines and growth factors), which may be particularly relevant when the dependence on gonadal steroids is lost. These systems may represent a target for future drug treatments.

References

Auclerc G., Antoine E.C., Cajfinger F., Brunet-Pommeyrol A., Agazia C., Khayat D. (2000). Management of advanced prostate cancer. Oncologist, 5, 36-44.

Bologna M., et al. (1992). Anti-androgens and 5alpha-reductase inhibition of the proliferation rate in PC3 and DU145 human prostatic cancer cell line. Curr Ther Res, 51, 799-813.

Bologna M., et al. (1995). Finasteride dose-dependently reduces the proliferation rate of the LnCAP human prostatic cancer cell line in vitro. Urology, 45, 282-290.

Bonneterre J., et al. (2000). Anastrozole versus tamoxifen as first-line therapy for advanced breast cancer in 668 postmenopausal women: results of the Tamoxifen or Arimidex Randomized Group Efficacy and Tolerability Study. J Clin Oncol, 18, 3748-3757.

Buzdar A. and Hortobagyi G. (1998). Tamoxifen and toremifene in breast cancer: comparison of safety and efficacy. J Clin Oncol, 16, 348-353.

Coltman C.A., et al. (1999). Prostate cancer prevention trial (PCPT) update. Eur Urol, 35, 544-547.

Cook T., Sheridan W.P. (2000). Development of GnRH antagonists for prostate cancer: new approaches to treatment. Oncologist, 5, 162-168.

Cummings S., et al. (1999). The effect of raloxifene on risk of breast cancer in postmenopausal women: results from the MORE randomised trial. Multiple Outcomes of Raloxifene Evaluation. JAMA, 281, 2189-2197.

Denis L. and Griffiths K. (2000). Endocrine treatment in prostate cancer. Semin Surg Oncol, 18, 52-74.

Dowsett M., et al. (1995). In vivo measurement of aromatase inhibition by letrozole (CGS 20267) in post-menopausal patients with breast cancer. Clin Cancer Res, 1, 1511-1515.

Filardo E., et al. (2000). Estrogen-induced activation of Erk-1 and Erk-2 requires the G protein-coupled receptor homolog, GPR30, and occurs via *trans*-activation of the epidermal growth factor receptor through release of HB-EGF. Mol Endocrinol, 14, 1649-1660.

Fisher B., et al. (1998). Tamoxifen for prevention of breast cancer: report of the National Surgical Adjuvant Breast and Bowel Project P-1 Study. J Natl Cancer Inst, 90, 1371-1388.

Fisher B., et al. (1999). Tamoxifen in treatment of intraductal breast cancer: National Surgical Adjuvant Breast and Bowel Project B-24 randomised controlled trial. Lancet, 353, 1993-2000.

Fradet Y., et al. (1999). Dietary fat and prostate cancer progression and survival. Eur Urol, 35, 388-391.

Gale K., et al. (1994). Hormonal treatment for metastatic breast cancer: an Eastern Cooperative Oncology Group Phase III trial comparing aminogluthetimide to tamoxifen. Cancer, 73, 354-361.

Gormley G. (1996). 5alpha-reductase inhibitors in prostate cancer. Endocrine-Related Cancer, 3, 57-63.

Ingle J., et al. (1999). Evaluation of tamoxifen plus letrozole with assessment of pharma-

cokinetic interaction in postmenopausal women with metastatic breast cancer. Clin Cancer Res, 5, 1642-1649.
MacNeill F., et al. (1992). The influence of aminoglutethimide and its analogue rogletimide on peripheral aromatisation in breast cancer. Br J Cancer, 66, 692-697.
Mor G., et al. (1998). Macrophages, estrogen and the microenvironment of breast cancer. The steroidal antiestrogen ICI 182,780 is an inhibitor of cellular aromatase activity. J Steroid Biochem Mole Biol, 67, 403-411.
Mouridsen H., et al. (2001). Superior efficacy of letrozole versus tamoxifen as first-line therapy for postmenopausal women with advanced breast cancer: results of a phase III study of the International Letrozole Breast Cancer Group. J Clin Oncol, 19, 2596-2606.
Nabholtz J., et al. (2000). Anastrozole is superior to tamoxifen as first-line therapy for advanced breast cancer in postmenopausal women: results of a North American multicenter randomized trial. J Clin Oncol, 18, 3758-3767.
Paech K. et al. (1997). Differential ligand activation of estrogen receptors ERalpha and ERbeta at AP1 sites. Science, 277, 1508-1510.
Petterson K. and Gustafsson J. (2001). Role of estrogen receptor beta in estrogen action. Annu Rev Physiol, 63, 165-192.
Porter W., et al. (1997). Functional synergy between the transcription factor Sp1 and the estrogen receptor. Mol Endocrinol, 11, 1569-1580.
Powles T., et al. (1998). Interim analysis of the incidence of breast cancer in the Royal Marsden Hospital tamoxifen randomised chemoprevention trial. Lancet, 352, 98-101.
Sanford E.J., et al. (1977). The effects of castration on adrenal testosterone secretion in men with prostatic carcinoma. J Urol, 118, 1019-1021.
Santen R. and Harvey H. (1999). Use of aromatase inhibitors in breast carcinoma. Endocr Relat Cancer, 6, 75-92.
Santen R., et al. (1990). Endocrine treatment of breast cancer in women. Endocr Rev, 11, 221-265.
Siiteri P.K. (1987). Adipose tissue as a source of hormones. Am J Clin Nutr, 45, 277-82.
Small E. and Srinivas S. (1995). The anti-androgen withdrawal syndrome: experience in a large cohort of unselected patients with advanced prostate cancer. Cancer, 76, 1428-1434.
Smith I., et al. (1982). Tamoxifen versus aminoglutethimide versus combined tamoxifen and aminoglutethimide in the treatment of advanced breast carcinoma. Cancer Res, 42 (8 Suppl), 3430s-3433s.
Takayama K., et al. (1997). Transcriptional regulation of CYP19 gene (aromatase) expression in adipose stromal cells in primary culture. J Clin Endocrinol Metab, 82, 600-606.
Taplin M., et al. (1995). Mutation of the androgen-receptor gene in metastatic androgen-independent prostate cancer. N Engl J Med, 332, 1393-1398.
Veronesi U., et al. (1998). Prevention of breast cancer with tamoxifen: preliminary findings from the Italian randomised trial among hysterectomised women. Italian Tamoxifen Prevention Study. Lancet, 352, 93-97.
Zhang Y., et al. (1997). Bone mass and the risk of breast cancer among postmenopausal women. N Engl J Med, 336, 661-617.
Zumoff B. (1998). Does postmenopausal estrogen administration increase the risk of breast cancer? Contributions of animal, biochemical, and clinical investigative studies to a resolution of the controversy. Proc Soc Exp Biol Med, 217, 30-37.

CHAPTER 16

Hormonal Treatment of Endocrine-Dependent Tumours: Clinical Considerations

F. BOCCARDO, E. VERRI AND P. GUGLIELMINI

Aims and Modalities of Hormone Treatment

Today hormone therapies still aim at interfering with the mitogenic action of sexual hormones. Basically this aim can be attained through the inhibition of the synthesis of steroid hormones. In this way target cells are spared the trophic stimulus represented by those hormones ("ablative hormone therapy"). Otherwise, it is possible to affect the link between sexual hormones and their receptors, and to interfere with one or more stages of the transcription process ("competitive hormone therapy").

Ablative Hormone Treatments

Steroid hormone synthesis can be inhibited by surgical removal of the gonads or by inducing interstitial cell atrophy by means of irradiation. It can also be obtained by long-term administration of Gn-RH analogues. Obviously these molecules have some analogy with the amino acid structure of native Gn-RH, but they differ from it in some modifications in the 6 or 9 position, which imply an agonistic (super-agonistic analogues) or antagonistic activity (antagonistic analogues) (Kirby, 1996; McLeod et al., 2001; Trachtenberg et al., 2002).

Unavoidably, the clinical use of the former class of drugs causes first a stimulation of sexual hormone synthesis. Initially this can cause a worsening of the symptomatology ("disease flare"), especially in patients suffering from prostate cancer. This effect virtually disappears after the use of antagonistic analogues (Trachtenberg et al., 2002).

The Gn-RH analogues are mainly employed in the treatment of prostate cancer, either alone or in association with pure anti-androgens (total androgenic blockade) (Boccardo et al., 1993; No authors, 1995) and in the treatment of pre-menopausal breast cancer (Boccardo et al., 1994). Even in the latter, some studies appear to suggest the potential superiority of the combination with anti-estrogens (Michaud and Buzdar, 2000; Klijn et al., 2001). Several trials have indicated some therapeutic activity of these compounds, even in post-menopausal breast cancer patients (Waxman et al., 1985; Plowman et al., 1986; Vici et al., 1991). This therapeutic activity can be explained through the anti-gonadotrophic action of these drugs, and consequently through their effect on ovarian interstitial cells. In fact, these cells keep on working for several years after the menopause. Many trials have shown a further reduction of oestradiol and oestrone circulating levels in post-menopausal patients treated with Gn-RH agonists (Waxman et al., 1985). However, aromatase inhibition represents the most appropriate ablative treatment for post-menopausal women. These drugs can inhibit oestradiol and oestrone synthesis in a more selective way, interfering with the aromatase system, either in the peripheral or in the tumour tissues (Bonneterre et al., 2000; Nabholtz et al., 2000).

Competitive Hormone Treatments

Competitive hormone treatments consist in the administration of compounds able to link up, with high affinity, with the sexual hormone receptors. Tamoxifen is the first of a family of non-steroidal anti-estrogens derived from triphenylethylene. These compounds have a stilbene structure and their link with the receptor can inhibit the transcription of only one of the two transcriptional domains of the receptor. This is the reason why these compounds have also agonistic effects, beyond the antagonistic ones, and show a substantial cross-resistance each other (Howell, 2001). Nowadays tamoxifen is still the most used drug, being superior to all the other compounds of this group, such as toremifene and raloxifene, the latter of which is used only in the management of osteoporosis (Cranney et al., 2002; Holli, 2002; Pukkala et al., 2002).

Unlike the triphenylethylene derivatives, steroid anti-estrogens have the same structure as oestradiol-17β. However, the presence of a long chain in position 7 enables these compounds to bind the oestrogen receptor, preventing its dimerisation and activation, and thus interfering with the transcriptional process in both domains. Lack of receptor activation induces its fast degradation by the endocellular proteases, and therefore a premature "down-regulation" (Robertson, 2002). Due to these peculiarities, the activity of these compounds is exclusively antagonistic, and they only partially cross-react with non-steroidal anti-estrogens (Robertson, 2002). The studies carried out so far in breast cancer have demonstrated that Fulvestran (the first of these compounds to go into clinical experimentation) is as effective as anti-aromatase agents in the second-line treatment and as tamoxifen in the first-line treatment (Jones, 2002).

Pure anti-androgens are compounds able to bind, with high affinity to the androgenic receptor, stopping its activation, probably through a mechanism similar to that of anti-estrogens. These drugs have an antagonistic effect (Neri and Kassem, 1984). However, some mutations of the androgenic receptor have been proven to allow these compounds to activate the transcriptional processes, and thus to develop agonist effects (Hara et al., 2003). Knowledge of these biological mechanisms has allowed documentation of the "anti-androgen withdrawal syndrome", characterized by a clinical response on the discontinuation of the anti-androgen treatment, in patients treated with pure anti-androgens and LH-RH analogues (Kelly and Scher, 1993; Kelly, 1998; Paul and Breul, 2000). Moreover, this knowledge allows us to explain the lack of cross-resistance among the different drugs of this group. This lack is what underlies the therapeutic responses sometimes observed in patients suffering from prostate cancer when the type of anti-androgen is changed (Fujikawa et al., 2000; Desai et al., 2001). Flutamide and bicalutamide are the most commonly used drugs. Nilutamide is also an active drug, but it is less commonly used because of its significant side effects which include visual disturbances (hemeralopia) and gastrointestinal toxicity (diarrhoea, transaminase increase) (Decensi et al., 1991). The efficacy of all previous compounds is almost comparable. However, a controlled trial comparing bicalutamide and flutamide, both associated with castration, has shown a better tolerability and, in some patient subsets, greater efficacy of bicalutamide (Schellhammer et al., 1997).

Pure anti-androgens can be given as monotherapy in the attempt to avoid the side effects caused by androgen-suppressive therapies (loss of libido, impotency, osteoporosis, pathological fractures, decrease of muscle mass and tone, progressive anaemia, asthenia, and depression) (Tyrrell, 1992). The use of these compounds in patients with intact gonads induces a condition of hypergonadotrophic hypergonadism, which allows high circulating levels of testosterone to be maintained. According to the controlled clinical trials available so far, monotherapy with pure anti-androgens is as effective as castration or as total androgenic blockade in only some categories of patients, such as M_0 patients, and in those with more differentiated neoplasms (Iversen et al., 1998; Tyrrell et al., 1998; Boccardo et al., 1999; Iversen et al., 2000; Boccardo et al., 2002). In these patients, therefore, monotherapy can be quite a safe alternative to the more common androgen-suppressive treatments, especially if the patient is determined to maintain his virility and to tolerate a side effect such as gynaecomastia, which is a nearly unavoidable complication of this therapeutic approach and causes it to be interrupted in a substantial proportion of patients (Kelly, 1998).

Unlikely pure anti-androgens, cyproterone acetate is a progestin compound able to interfere not only with the binding of dihydrotestosterone to its receptor, but also with the synthesis of dihydrotestosterone itself, through the inhibition of 5α-reductase (Jacobi et al., 1980). At the highest dosages, cyproterone acetate is also able to interfere with the release of gonadotrophins at the pituitary level (Isurugi et al., 1980). Therefore, even when used as monotherapy, cyproterone acetate causes hypogonadism with all its consequences (Isurugi et al., 1980). An old study of the EORTC urologic group showed that cyproterone acetate is as effective as diethylstilbestrol (Pavone-Macaluso et al., 1986). Although there are no comparative studies, this drug is likely to be as effective as castration. However, this compound induces relevant effects on the coagulative system. A recent meta-analysis relating to total androgenic blockade has shown that cyproterone acetate when combined with castration reduces the long-term efficacy of androgen-suppressive treatments. In fact, it causes an increase in treatment-related mortality, mainly due to cardiovascular complications (No authors, 2000).

By contrast, according to the same meta-analysis, total androgenic blockade obtained by combining castration with a pure anti-androgen can increase the efficacy of treatment in comparison to androgen-suppressive therapy alone. This increase is moderate, but statistically significant (No authors, 2000).

Clinical Indications and Results of Hormone Treatments

Palliative Therapy of Hormone-Dependent Tumours

As mentioned above, nowadays hormonal treatments are still widely used in the palliative treatment of breast and endometrial cancer in women and of prostate cancer in men. Nearly 50% of the patients suffering from breast or endometrial cancer may obtain therapeutic, often durable benefit, if their tumours express adequate amounts of steroid hormone receptors (Buzdar, 2001).

In addition to receptor positivity, some other clinical parameters (number and site of metastases, duration of disease-free interval, response to previous hormone therapy) or morpho-biological parameters (differentiation grade, hyperexpression of the oncoprotein erb-b2) may allow identification of the patients who are most likely to respond to hormone therapy and, in particular, to specific compounds such as the non-steroidal anti-estrogens (Buzdar, 2001).

In breast cancer patients, basically, the probabilities of response are nearly identical for all the drugs of the hormonal system. However, some controlled trials have shown that:

1. The new generation anti-aromatase agents such as examestane, anastrozole, and letrozole are more effective than first-generation anti-aromatase agents such as aminoglutethimide, or progestins, when used as second-line treatment for breast cancer (Thurlimann et al., 1997; Buzdar et al., 1998; Dombernowsky et al., 1998).
2. The new generation anti-aromatase agents such as anastrozole and letrozole are also at least as effective as tamoxifen in the first line of treatment, and probably more effective in patients previously treated with this kind of therapy in the adjuvant setting (Bonneterre et al., 2000; Nabholtz et al., 2000; Buzdar, 2002).
3. Patients who have previously responded to non-steroidal anti-aromatase agents treatment can further respond to steroidal anti-aromatase agents, and vice versa (Murray and Pitt, 1995; Lonning et al., 2000).
4. Fulvestran is as effective as anastrazole as second-line treatment and as effective as tamoxifen as front-line treatment (Morris and Wakeling, 2002).
5. In pre-menopausal patients comparable results can be obtained by surgical castration or by treatment with LH-RH analogues (Boccardo et al., 1994). Comparable results were also achieved by tamoxifen and LH-RH analogues in one study (Klijn et al., 2000). However, some studies, including the previous one, and a recent meta-analysis seem to identify the combination of LH-RH analogues with tamoxifen as the most adequate treatment for pre-menopausal breast cancer patients (Klijn et al., 2001).

Therefore, in relation to breast cancer we can reasonably formulate the following guidelines, taking into account the data on efficacy, tolerability, and economic costs too (Blamey, 2002). These guidelines must be adapted to the preferences and the requirements of each patient.

1. In pre-menopausal patients who are still regularly menstruating, the combination of an LH-RH analogue and tamoxifen is probably the treatment of

choice. If this treatment leads to satisfactory results, tamoxifen can be replaced with a new-generation anti-aromatase agent when progression occurs. In patients pre-treated with tamoxifen in the adjuvant setting, treatment with LH-RH analogues alone or with these drugs in combination with an anti-aromatase agent can be considered adequate.

2. In post-menopausal patients, front-line treatment could be either tamoxifen or a new-generation anti-aromatase agent. The latter type of drug is preferable for patients pre-treated with tamoxifen in the adjuvant setting. Anti-aromatase agents are also a rational choice for women whose disease progresses after first-line tamoxifen treatment. Progestins are still used in particular situations (neoplastic cachexia, hyporexic patients, etc.) or as a further therapeutic attempt in patients responsive to previous hormonal lines.

Comparable results can be obtained in the treatment of endometrial cancer with progestins or tamoxifen: the choice is restrained by the possible contraindications for each treatment (obesity, hypertension, etc.) (Imai et al., 2001; Podczaski and Mortel, 2001; Baekelandt, 2002). Interesting results have also been obtained with Gn-RH analogues and anti-aromatase agents, but they are not yet applicable to clinical practice (Asbury et al., 2002).

With regard to the palliative treatment of prostate cancer, castration is still the treatment of choice (Kirby, 1996). Basically, all the Gn-RH analogues currently marketed (buserelin, goserelin, triptorelin, leuprorelin) have comparable therapeutic activities and are available in depot formulations, to be administered every 2 or 3 months. This therapy is preferable for elderly patients and for those with indolent disease. Patients with more extensive disease, or those who need a faster response (if only from a subjective point of view), should reasonably be seen as candidates for total androgen blockade (Boccardo et al., 1993; No authors, 1995). These men should preferably start treatment with pure anti-androgens (to avoid the possible consequences of tumour flare-up). The intermittent use of Gn-RH analogues (alone or combined with a pure anti-androgen) is based on a solid biological rationale (Gleave et al., 1994), and can bring potential advantages in both efficacy and quality of life compared to continuous androgen-suppressive therapy (Goldenberg et al., 1995). However, no study has yet shown the real superiority of this approach, which should be avoided in daily practice. Finally, in patients who wish to maintain their sexual potency, and, more generally speaking, to avoid the effects caused by androgen suppression, the therapeutic option of monotherapy with pure anti-androgens may be considered. This option should anyway be proposed only to patients with minimal tumour burden or to those suffering from less aggressive disease (Boccardo et al., 1999; Iversen et al., 2000; Boccardo et al., 2002).

Primary and Neoadjuvant Therapy of Endocrine-Dependent Tumours

Hormonal therapy has been successfully used even in patients with organ-confined disease who otherwise are candidates for local treatment with radical intent.

Several studies have evaluated the potential utility of tamoxifen in postmenopausal patients with neoplasms which could in theory be surgically removed. These studies have shown a high therapeutic activity of tamoxifen at the primary tumour level (Foudraine et al., 1992; Ciatto et al., 1996). However, randomised studies have shown the superiority of combined treatment with surgery (or radiotherapy). These studies have also shown that most of the patients initially treated with tamoxifen alone have later on needed surgery because of local progression (Mustacchi et al., 1994; Willsher et al., 1996). Therefore, at present it is thought that anti-estrogenic treatment alone should be restricted just to frail patients and elderly women who refuse to undergo surgery.

Hormonal therapy with anti-estrogens or third-generation anti-aromatase inhibitors can represent the treatment of choice to achieve tumour debulking in patients with locally advanced receptor-positive breast tumours who are not suitable for immediate surgery (Dixon et al., 2001).

With regard to prostate cancer, front-line hormonal therapy is an accepted therapeutic option for patients with locally advanced neoplasms who are not suitable for or who refuse local-regional treatments with radical intent. There are no comparative studies on this subject, but several retrospective studies show that 5- and 10-year results obtainable with hormonal therapy alone in these patients are almost identical to the results obtainable with radiation (or surgery) (Fowler et al., 2002; Labrie, 2002; Akaza et al., 2003).

The high therapeutic activity of LH-RH analogues, either alone or combined with pure anti-androgens, against primary prostate cancer has already been demonstrated. However, no study has yet proved that hormonal therapy can prolong the survival of patients with T_2 or T_3 tumours when this therapy is used in the neoadjuvant setting, although a statistically significant reduction in the incidence of positive surgical margins has been demonstrated in several series, particularly when neoadjuvant treatment has been prolonged for more than 6 months (Gleave et al., 2001; Aus et al., 2002; Meng et al., 2002). Therefore, at present, neoadjuvant hormonal therapy is not advisable in daily clinical practice, though it may be a choice for patients with "large" T_3 tumours who are candidates for definitive radiotherapy (Shipley et al., 2002).

Primary or neoadjuvant therapy with progestins has almost no indications in patients suffering from endometrial cancer. This therapeutic option can be considered only for the patients of child-bearing age with well-differentiated neoplasms confined to the endometrium. In fact, it has been proved that in these patients a complete tumour response can be achieved without compromising the possibility of a subsequent pregnancy (Kim et al., 1997; Imai et al., 2001).

Adjuvant Hormone Therapy

Hormone therapy is currently an additional treatment almost unavoidable for all patients surgically treated for receptor-positive breast cancer, who can be considered at intermediate or high risk of relapse on the basis of their age, the size of their tumour, or the degree of tumour differentiation

(Goldhirsch et al., 2001). In fact, all patients with positive lymph-nodes can be considered at high risk, irrespective of their age or any other phenotypic characteristics of aggressiveness (Goldhirsch et al., 2001). The 2001 St Gallen Conference recommended that all these patients must be treated with tamoxifen for almost 5 years, combined or not (according to risk) with chemotherapy (Goldhirsch et al., 2001). In premenopausal patients tamoxifen can be replaced by or combined with castration (especially with LH-RH analogues) (Goldhirsch et al., 2001). Gonadal suppression is particularly advisable for patients previously treated with chemotherapy and still regularly menstruating. In fact, some retrospective studies have demonstrated the importance of chemically induced amenorrhoea in reducing the risk of relapse or death (Pagani et al., 1998).

Several studies are currently exploring the superiority of alternative treatments to anti-estrogenic treatment, as is the case of anti-aromatase treatment (Ragaz, 2001). One study has recently shown that anastrozole treatment can considerably reduce the risk of relapse at 5 years compared to tamoxifen (Baum, 2001). This study has also demonstrated that anastrozole treatment is more effective than tamoxifen in preventing the development of contralateral breast cancer, and has no appreciable effects on endometrium or on the incidence of cardiovascular events (Baum, 2001). However, the results regarding mortality and the long-term safety of anti-aromatase treatment, particularly in respect to the effects on lipidic state, osteoporosis (as a matter of fact, the preliminary results point towards an increase in the occurrence of pathological fractures in the patients assigned to anastrozole), and cognitive function, are not yet available. For these reasons, adjuvant treatment with anti-aromatase agents cannot yet be considered a valid alternative to tamoxifen treatment - also because of the higher costs. However, the results of the above-mentioned study, and of some other studies in which the anti-aromatase agent has been used sequentially to tamoxifen (Boccardo et al., 2001), seem quite promising and allow the use of these compounds to be considered in patients who are not candidates for or who become intolerant to anti-estrogenic treatment.

While hormone therapy has a definite role in the adjuvant treatment of breast cancer, its role in the adjuvant therapy of prostate cancer has yet to be defined. Only a few studies have shown that hormone therapy can prolong overall and cancer-specific survival of patients subjected to radical prostatectomy or definitive radiotherapy (Pilepich et al., 1997, 2001; Messing et al., 1999; Lawton et al., 2001; Bolla et al., 2002). In particular, only one small prospective study has shown RH-LH analogue treatment to prolong the survival of patients with demostrated lymph node metastasis after radical prostatectomy (Messing et al., 1999). The results of this study are in agreement with those of previous retrospective studies carried out by the Mayo Clinic Group (Zincke et al., 2001) and legitimate the use of adjuvant hormone therapy in patients with microscopic metastases in the pelvic lymph nodes. The results of the studies of the RTOG group in the USA (Pilepich et al., 1997, 2001; Lawton et al., 2001) and the EORTC urological group in Europe (Bolla et al., 2002) appear to be more convincing: they evaluated the efficacy of adjuvant hormone therapy (combined or not with neoadjuvant hormone therapy) after definitive radiotherapy. These studies suport the use of adjuvant hormone therapy in patients with locally advanced tumours (T_3-T_4), especially in those with poorly differentiated high "Gleason" neoplasms.

Anyway, the problems of which treatment modality might be most appropriate and how long it should be given are still open, partly in view of the effects of androgen deprivation when prolonged over time.

Recently the preliminary results of the so-called EPC studies have been published. These studies have involved more than 8000 patients suffering from intraprostatic or locally advanced tumours, who have been randomly allocated to be treated with bicalutamide monotherapy (Wirth, 2001; Carswell and Figgitt, 2002). Preliminary results indicate a considerable advantage for the patients treated with bicalutamide, who showed a nearly 30% reduced risk of relapse compared to the patients treated with the placebo. However, these are still early results, and overall survival figures are not available yet. Therefore, even in this case, it is difficult to formulate recommendations, bearing in mind the possible side effects of protracted anti-androgen monotherapy, such as gynaecomastia.

Finally, no hormone therapy is advisable, at the present state of the knowledge, in patients treated by hysterectomy for endometrial carcinoma. Most of the studies and a recent meta-analysis have shown the absence of a definite advantage, particularly for patients treated with progestins at the highest dosage and for the longest periods of time (Martin-Hirsch et al., 1996; Loibl et al., 2002).

Conclusions

Hormone therapy represents a formidable therapeutic tool for some of the most frequent and lethal tumours, being able to strike tumour cells selectively, often without evident side effects. In a sense, hormone therapies represent biological therapies able to strike the intracellular signal track selectively, causing apoptosis of cancer cells without destroying their DNA. These treatments, alone or in combination with chemotherapy, have prolonged the clinical course of disease in the advanced phase and increased the chance of cure for patients with early-stage disease. These treatments offer themselves as effective instruments in the chemoprevention of cancer and in the treatment of pre-neoplastic lesions (van der Kwast et al., 1999; Alberts and Blute, 2001; Steiner et al., 2001; Powles, 2002; Veronesi et al., 2003). The possibility of using these treatments in a more selective way is particularly interesting, thanks to the progress achieved by post-genomic research and to the set-up of new therapeutic strategies based on the use of other "biologicals" that interfere with the different stages of cancerogenesis and neoplastic progression.

References

No authors (1995). Maximum androgen blockade in advanced prostate cancer: an overview of 22 randomised trials with 3283 deaths in 5710 patients. Prostate Cancer Trialists' Collaborative Group. Lancet, 346, 265-269.

No authors (2000). Maximum androgen blockade in advanced prostate cancer: an overview of the randomised trials. Prostate Cancer Trialists' Collaborative Group. Lancet, 355, 1491-1498.

Akaza H., Homma Y., Okada K., Yokoyama M., Usami M., Hirao Y., Tsushima T., Ohashi Y. and Aso Y. (2003). A prospective and randomized study of primary hormonal therapy for patients with localized or locally advanced prostate cancer unsuitable for radical prostatectomy: results of the 5-year follow-up. BJU Int, 91, 33-36.

Alberts S.R. and Blute M.L. (2001). Chemoprevention for prostatic carcinoma: the role of flutamide in patients with prostatic intraepithelial neoplasia. Urology, 57, 188-190.

Asbury R.F., Brunetto V.L., Lee R.B., Reid G. and Rocereto T.F. (2002). Goserelin acetate as treatment for recurrent endometrial carcinoma: a Gynecologic Oncology Group study. Am J Clin Oncol, 25, 557-560.

Aus G., Abrahamsson P.A., Ahlgren G., Hugosson J., Lundberg S., Schain M., Schelin S. and Pedersen K. (2002). Three-month neoadjuvant hormonal therapy before radical prostatectomy: a 7-year follow-up of a randomized controlled trial. BJU Int, 90, 561-566.

Baekelandt M. (2002). Hormonal treatment of endometrial carcinoma. Expert Rev Anticancer Ther, 2, 106-112.

Baum M. (2001). The ATAC (Arimidex, tamoxifen, alone or in combination) adjuvant breast cancer trial in postmenopausal women. Breast Cancer Res Treat, 69, 210.

Blamey R.W. (2002). Guidelines on endocrine therapy of breast cancer. EUSOMA. Eur J Cancer, 38, 615-634.

Boccardo F., Barichello M., Battaglia M., Carmignani G., Comeri G., Ferraris V., Lilliu S., Montefiore F., Portoghese F., Cortellini P., Rigatti P., Usai E. and Rubagotti A. (2002). Bicalutamide monotherapy versus flutamide plus goserelin in prostate cancer: updated results of a multicentric Trial. Eur Urol, 42, 481-490.

Boccardo F., Pace M., Rubagotti A., Guarneri D., Decensi A., Oneto F., Martorana G., Giuliani L., Selvaggi F., Battaglia M. et al. (1993). Goserelin acetate with or without flutamide in the treatment of patients with locally advanced or metastatic prostate cancer. The Italian Prostatic Cancer Project (PONCAP) Study Group. Eur J Cancer, 29A, 1088-1093.

Boccardo F., Rubagotti A., Amoroso D., Mesiti M., Romeo D., Caroti C., Farris A., Cruciani G., Villa E., Schieppati G. and Mustacchi G. (2001). Sequential tamoxifen and aminoglutethimide versus tamoxifen alone in the adjuvant treatment of postmenopausal breast cancer patients: results of an Italian cooperative study. J Clin Oncol, 19, 4209-4215.

Boccardo F., Rubagotti A., Barichello M., Battaglia M., Carmignani G., Comeri G., Conti G., Cruciani G., Dammino S., Delliponti U., Ditonno P., Ferraris V., Lilliu S., Montefiore F., Portoghese F. and Spano G. (1999). Bicalutamide monotherapy versus flutamide plus goserelin in prostate cancer patients: results of an Italian Prostate Cancer Project study. J Clin Oncol, 17, 2027-2038.

Boccardo F., Rubagotti A., Perrotta A., Amoroso D., Balestrero M., De Matteis A., Zola P., Sismondi P., Francini G., Petrioli R. et al. (1994). Ovarian ablation versus goserelin with or without tamoxifen in pre-perimenopausal patients with advanced breast cancer: results of a multicentric Italian study. Ann Oncol, 5, 337-342.

Bolla M., de Reijke T.M., Zurlo A. and Collette L. (2002). Adjuvant hormone therapy in locally advanced and localized prostate cancer: three EORTC trials. Front Radiat Ther Oncol, 36, 81-86.

Bonneterre J., Thurlimann B., Robertson J. F., Krzakowski M., Mauriac L., Koralewski P., Vergote I., Webster A., Steinberg M. and von Euler M. (2000). Anastrozole versus tamoxifen as first-line therapy for advanced breast cancer in 668 postmenopausal women: results of the Tamoxifen or Arimidex Randomized Group Efficacy and Tolerability study. J Clin Oncol, 18, 3748-3759.

Buzdar A.U. (2001). Endocrine therapy in the treatment of metastatic breast cancer. Semin Oncol, 28, 291-304.

Buzdar A.U. (2002). Superior efficacy of letrozole versus tamoxifen as first-line therapy. J Clin Oncol, 20, 876-878.
Buzdar A.U., Jonat W., Howell A., Jones S.E., Blomqvist C.P., Vogel C.L., Eiermann W., Wolter J.M., Steinberg M., Webster A. and Lee D. (1998). Anastrozole versus megestrol acetate in the treatment of postmenopausal women with advanced breast carcinoma: results of a survival update based on a combined analysis of data from two mature phase III trials. Arimidex Study Group. Cancer, 83, 1142-1152.
Carswell C.I. and Figgitt D.P. (2002). Bicalutamide: in early-stage prostate cancer. Drugs, 62, 2471-2479; discussion 2480-2481.
Ciatto S., Cirillo A., Confortini M. and Cardillo Cde L. (1996). Tamoxifen as primary treatment of breast cancer in elderly patients. Neoplasma, 43, 43-45.
Cranney A., Tugwell P., Zytaruk N., Robinson V., Weaver B., Adachi J., Wells G., Shea B. and Guyatt G. (2002). Meta-analyses of therapies for postmenopausal osteoporosis. IV. Meta-analysis of raloxifene for the prevention and treatment of postmenopausal osteoporosis. Endocr Rev, 23, 524-528.
Decensi A.U., Boccardo F., Guarneri D., Positano N., Paoletti M.C., Costantini M., Martorana G. and Giuliani L. (1991). Monotherapy with nilutamide, a pure nonsteroidal anti-androgen, in untreated patients with metastatic carcinoma of the prostate. The Italian Prostatic Cancer Project. J Urol, 146, 377-381.
Desai A., Stadler W.M. and Vogelzang N.J. (2001). Nilutamide: possible utility as a second-line hormonal agent. Urology, 58, 1016-1020.
Dixon J.M., Love C.D., Bellamy C.O., Cameron D.A., Leonard R.C., Smith H. and Miller W.R. (2001). Letrozole as primary medical therapy for locally advanced and large operable breast cancer. Breast Cancer Res Treat, 66, 191-199.
Dombernowsky P., Smith I., Falkson G., Leonard R., Panasci L., Bellmunt J., Bezwoda W., Gardin G., Gudgeon A., Morgan M., Fornasiero A., Hoffmann W., Michel J., Hatschek T., Tjabbes T., Chaudri H.A., Hornberger U. and Trunet P.F. (1998). Letrozole, a new oral aromatase inhibitor for advanced breast cancer: double-blind randomized trial showing a dose effect and improved efficacy and tolerability compared with megestrol acetate. J Clin Oncol, 16, 453-461.
Foudraine N.A., Verhoef L.C. and Burghouts J.T. (1992). Tamoxifen as sole therapy for primary breast cancer in the elderly patient. Eur J Cancer, 28A, 900-903.
Fowler J.E. Jr, Bigler S.A., White P.C. and Duncan W.L. (2002). Hormone therapy for locally advanced prostate cancer. J Urol, 168, 546-549.
Fujikawa K., Matsui Y., Fukuzawa S. and Takeuchi H. (2000). Prostate-specific antigen levels and clinical response to flutamide as the second hormone therapy for hormone-refractory prostate carcinoma. Eur Urol, 37, 218-222.
Gleave M., Bruchovsky N., Bowden M., Goldenberg S.L. and Sullivan L.D. (1994). Intermittent androgen suppression prolongs time to androgen-independent progression in the LNCaP prostate tumor model. J Urol, 151, 457A.
Gleave M.E., Goldenberg S.L., Chin J.L., Warner J., Saad F., Klotz L.H., Jewett M., Kassabian V., Chetner M., Dupont C. and Van Rensselaer S. (2001). Randomized comparative study of 3 versus 8-month neoadjuvant hormonal therapy before radical prostatectomy: biochemical and pathological effects. J Urol, 166, 500-506; discussion 506-507.
Goldenberg S.L., Bruchovsky N., Gleave M.E., Sullivan L.D. and Akakura K. (1995). Intermittent androgen suppression in the treatment of prostate cancer: a preliminary report. Urology, 45, 839-844; discussion 844-845.
Goldhirsch A., Glick J.H., Gelber R.D., Coates A.S. and Senn H.J. (2001). Meeting highlights: International Consensus Panel on the Treatment of Primary Breast Cancer. Seventh International Conference on Adjuvant Therapy of Primary Breast Cancer. J Clin Oncol, 19, 3817-3827.
Hara T., Miyazaki J., Araki H., Yamaoka M., Kanzaki N., Kusaka M. and Miyamoto M. (2003). Novel mutations of androgen receptor: a possible mechanism of bicalutamide withdrawal syndrome. Cancer Res, 63, 149-153.

Holli K. (2002). Tamoxifen versus toremifene in the adjuvant treatment of breast cancer. Eur J Cancer, 38 (Suppl 6), S37-S38.

Howell A. (2001). Future use of selective estrogen receptor modulators and aromatase inhibitors. Clin Cancer Res, 7, 4402s-4410s; discussion 4411s-4412s.

Imai M., Jobo T., Sato R., Kawaguchi M. and Kuramoto H. (2001). Medroxyprogesterone acetate therapy for patients with adenocarcinoma of the endometrium who wish to preserve the uterus-usefulness and limitations. Eur J Gynaecol Oncol, 22, 217-220.

Isurugi K., Fukutani K., Ishida H. and Hosoi Y. (1980). Endocrine effects of cyproterone acetate in patients with prostatic cancer. J Urol, 123, 180-183.

Iversen P., Tyrrell C.J., Kaisary A.V., Anderson J.B., Baert L., Tammela T., Chamberlain M., Carroll K., Gotting-Smith K. and Blackledge G.R. (1998). Casodex (bicalutamide) 150-mg monotherapy compared with castration in patients with previously untreated nonmetastatic prostate cancer: results from two multicenter randomized trials at a median follow-up of 4 years. Urology, 51, 389-396.

Iversen P., Tyrrell C.J., Kaisary A.V., Anderson J.B., Van Poppel H., Tammela T.L., Chamberlain M., Carroll K. and Melezinek I. (2000). Bicalutamide monotherapy compared with castration in patients with nonmetastatic locally advanced prostate cancer: 6.3 years of followup. J Urol, 164, 1579-1582.

Jacobi G.H., Altwein J.E., Kurth K.H., Basting R. and Hohenfellner R. (1980). Treatment of advanced prostatic cancer with parenteral cyproterone acetate: a phase III randomised trial. Br J Urol, 52, 208-215.

Jones S.E. (2002). A new estrogen receptor antagonist--an overview of available data. Breast Cancer Res Treat, 75 (Suppl 1), S19-S21; discussion S33-S35.

Kelly W.K. (1998). Endocrine withdrawal syndrome and its relevance to the management of hormone refractory prostate cancer. Eur Urol, 34 (Suppl 3), 18-23.

Kelly W.K. and Scher H.I. (1993). Prostate specific antigen decline after anti-androgen withdrawal: the flutamide withdrawal syndrome. J Urol, 149, 607-609.

Kim Y.B., Holschneider C.H., Ghosh K., Nieberg R.K. and Montz F.J. (1997). Progestin alone as primary treatment of endometrial carcinoma in premenopausal women. Report of seven cases and review of the literature. Cancer, 79, 320-327.

Kirby R.S. (1996). Recent advances in the medical management of prostate cancer. Br J Clin Pract, 50, 88-93.

Klijn J.G., Beex L.V. Mauriac L., van Zijl J.A., Veyret C., Wildiers J., Jassem J., Piccart M., Burghouts J., Becquart D., Seynaeve C., Mignolet F. and Duchateau L. (2000). Combined treatment with buserelin and tamoxifen in premenopausal metastatic breast cancer: a randomized study. J Natl Cancer Inst, 92, 903-911.

Klijn J.G., Blamey R.W., Boccardo F., Tominaga T., Duchateau L. and Sylvester R. (2001). Combined tamoxifen and luteinizing hormone-releasing hormone (LHRH) agonist versus LHRH agonist alone in premenopausal advanced breast cancer: a meta-analysis of four randomized trials. J Clin Oncol, 19, 343-353.

Labrie F. (2002). Androgen blockade in prostate cancer in 2002: major benefits on survival in localized disease. Mol Cell Endocrinol, 198, 77-87.

Lawton C.A., Winter K., Murray K., Machtay M., Mesic J.B., Hanks G.E., Coughlin C.T. and Pilepich M.V. (2001). Updated results of the phase III Radiation Therapy Oncology Group (RTOG) trial 85-31 evaluating the potential benefit of androgen suppression following standard radiation therapy for unfavorable prognosis carcinoma of the prostate. Int J Radiat Oncol Biol Phys, 49, 937-946.

Loibl S., von Minckwitz G. and Kaufmann M. (2002). Adjuvant hormone therapy following primary therapy for endometrial cancer. Eur J Cancer, 38 (Suppl 6), S41-S43.

Lonning P.E., Bajetta E., Murray R., Tubiana-Hulin M., Eisenberg P.D., Mickiewicz E., Celio L., Pitt P., Mita M., Aaronson N.K., Fowst C., Arkhipov A., di Salle E., Polli A. and Massimini G. (2000). Activity of exemestane in metastatic breast cancer after failure of nonsteroidal aromatase inhibitors: a phase II trial. J Clin Oncol, 18, 2234-2244.

Martin-Hirsch P.L., Lilford R.J. and Jarvis G.J. (1996). Adjuvant progestagen therapy for the treatment of endometrial cancer: review and meta-analyses of published randomised controlled trials. Eur J Obstet Gynecol Reprod Biol, 65, 201-207.
McLeod D., Zinner N., Tomera K., Gleason D., Fotheringham N., Campion M. and Garnick M.B. (2001). A phase 3, multicenter, open-label, randomized study of abarelix versus leuprolide acetate in men with prostate cancer. Urology, 58, 756-761.
Meng M.V., Grossfeld G.D., Carroll P.R. and Small E.J. (2002). Neoadjuvant strategies for prostate cancer prior to radical prostatectomy. Semin Urol Oncol, 20, 10-18.
Messing E.M., Manola J., Sarosdy M., Wilding G., Crawford E.D. and Trump D. (1999). Immediate hormonal therapy compared with observation after radical prostatectomy and pelvic lymphadenectomy in men with node-positive prostate cancer. N Engl J Med, 341, 1781-1788.
Michaud L.B. and Buzdar A.U. (2000). Complete estrogen blockade for the treatment of metastatic and early stage breast cancer. Drugs Aging, 16, 261-271.
Morris C. and Wakeling A. (2002). Fulvestrant ('Faslodex')-a new treatment option for patients progressing on prior endocrine therapy. Endocr Relat Cancer, 9, 267-276.
Murray R. and Pitt P. (1995). Aromatase inhibition with 4-OHAndrostenedione after prior aromatase inhibition with aminoglutethimide in women with advanced breast cancer. Breast Cancer Res Treat, 35, 249-253.
Mustacchi G., Milani S., Pluchinotta A., De Matteis A., Rubagotti A. and Perrota A. (1994). Tamoxifen or surgery plus tamoxifen as primary treatment for elderly patients with operable breast cancer: The GRETA Trial. Group for Research on Endocrine Therapy in the Elderly. Anticancer Res, 14, 2197-2200.
Nabholtz J.M., Buzdar A., Pollak M., Harwin W., Burton G., Mangalik A., Steinberg M., Webster A. and von Euler M. (2000). Anastrozole is superior to tamoxifen as first-line therapy for advanced breast cancer in postmenopausal women: results of a North American multicenter randomized trial. Arimidex Study Group. J Clin Oncol, 18, 3758-3767.
Neri R. and Kassem N. (1984). Biological and clinical properties of anti-androgens. In Progress in Cancer Research and Therapy, eds. Bresciani F et al, 31, pp. 507-518, New York, Raven Press.
Pagani O., O'Neill A., Castiglione M., Gelber R.D., Goldhirsch A., Rudenstam C.M., Lindtner J., Collins J., Crivellari D., Coates A., Cavalli F., Thurlimann B., Simoncini E., Fey M., Price K. and Senn H.J. (1998). Prognostic impact of amenorrhoea after adjuvant chemotherapy in premenopausal breast cancer patients with axillary node involvement: results of the International Breast Cancer Study Group (IBCSG) Trial VI. Eur J Cancer, 34, 632-640.
Paul R. and Breul J. (2000). Anti-androgen withdrawal syndrome associated with prostate cancer therapies: incidence and clinical significance. Drug Saf, 23, 381-390.
Pavone-Macaluso M., de Voogt H.J., Viggiano G., Barasolo E., Lardennois B., de Pauw M. and Sylvester R. (1986). Comparison of diethylstilbestrol, cyproterone acetate and medroxyprogesterone acetate in the treatment of advanced prostatic cancer: final analysis of a randomized phase III trial of the European Organization for Research on Treatment of Cancer Urological Group. J Urol, 136, 624-631.
Pilepich M.V., Caplan R., Byhardt R.W., Lawton C.A., Gallagher M.J., Mesic J.B., Hanks G.E., Coughlin C.T., Porter A., Shipley W.U. and Grignon D. (1997). Phase III trial of androgen suppression using goserelin in unfavorable-prognosis carcinoma of the prostate treated with definitive radiotherapy: report of Radiation Therapy Oncology Group Protocol, 85-31. J Clin Oncol, 15, 1013-1021.
Pilepich M.V., Winter K., John M.J., Mesic J.B., Sause W., Rubin P., Lawton C., Machtay M. and Grignon D. (2001). Phase III radiation therapy oncology group (RTOG) trial 86-10 of androgen deprivation adjuvant to definitive radiotherapy in locally advanced carcinoma of the prostate. Int J Radiat Oncol Biol Phys, 50, 1243-1252.

Plowman P.N., Nicholson R.I. and Walker K.J. (1986). Remission of postmenopausal breast cancer during treatment with the luteinising hormone releasing hormone agonist ICI 118630. Br J Cancer, 54, 903-909.
Podczaski E. and Mortel R. (2001). Hormonal treatment of endometrial cancer: past, present and future. Best Pract Res Clin Obstet Gynaecol, 15, 469-489.
Powles T.J. (2002). Anti-oestrogenic prevention of breast cancer--the make or break point. Nat Rev Cancer, 2, 787-794.
Pukkala E., Kyyronen P., Sankila R. and Holli K. (2002). Tamoxifen and toremifene treatment of breast cancer and risk of subsequent endometrial cancer: a population-based case-control study. Int J Cancer, 100, 337-341.
Ragaz J. (2001). Adjuvant trials of aromatase inhibitors: determining the future landscape of adjuvant endocrine therapy. J Steroid Biochem Mol Biol, 79, 133-141.
Robertson, J. F. (2002). Estrogen receptor downregulators: new antihormonal therapy for advanced breast cancer. Clin Ther, 24 (Suppl A), A17-A30.
Schellhammer P.F., Sharifi R., Block N.L., Soloway M.S., Venner P.M., Patterson A.L., Sarosdy M.F., Vogelzang N.J., Schellenger J.J. and Kolvenbag G.J. (1997). Clinical benefits of bicalutamide compared with flutamide in combined androgen blockade for patients with advanced prostatic carcinoma: final report of a double-blind, randomized, multicenter trial. Casodex Combination Study Group. Urology, 50, 330-336.
Shipley W.U., Lu J.D., Pilepich M.V., Heydon K., Roach M., Wolkov H.B., Sause W.T., Rubin P., Lawton C.A. and Machtay M. (2002). Effect of a short course of neoadjuvant hormonal therapy on the response to subsequent androgen suppression in prostate cancer patients with relapse after radiotherapy: a secondary analysis of the randomized protocol RTOG 86-10. Int J Radiat Oncol Biol Phys, 54, 1302-1310.
Steiner M.S., Raghow S. and Neubauer B.L. (2001). Selective estrogen receptor modulators for the chemoprevention of prostate cancer. Urology, 57, 68-72.
Thurlimann B., Paridaens R., Serin D., Bonneterre J., Roche H., Murray R., di Salle E., Lanzalone S., Zurlo M.G. and Piscitelli G. (1997). Third-line hormonal treatment with exemestane in postmenopausal patients with advanced breast cancer progressing on aminoglutethimide: a phase II multicentre multinational study. Exemestane Study Group. Eur J Cancer, 33, 1767-1773.
Trachtenberg J., Gittleman M., Steidle C., Barzell W., Friedel W., Pessis D., Fotheringham N., Campion M. and Garnick M.B. (2002). A phase 3, multicenter, open label, randomized study of abarelix versus leuprolide plus daily anti-androgen in men with prostate cancer. J Urol, 167, 1670-1674.
Tyrrell C.J. (1992). Casodex: a pure non-steroidal anti-androgen used as monotherapy in advanced prostate cancer. Prostate Suppl, 4, 97-104.
Tyrrell C.J., Kaisary A.V., Iversen P., Anderson J.B., Baert L., Tammela T., Chamberlain M., Webster A. and Blackledge G. (1998). A randomised comparison of 'Casodex' (bicalutamide) 150 mg monotherapy versus castration in the treatment of metastatic and locally advanced prostate cancer. Eur Urol, 33, 447-456.
van der Kwast T. H., Labrie F. and Tetu B. (1999). Prostatic intraepithelial neoplasia and endocrine manipulation. Eur Urol, 35, 508-510.
Veronesi U., Maisonneuve P., Rotmensz N., Costa A., Sacchini V., Travaglini R., D'Aiuto G., Lovison F., Gucciardo G., Muraca M.G., Pizzichetta M.A., Conforti S., Decensi A., Robertson C. and Boyle P. (2003). Italian randomized trial among women with hysterectomy: tamoxifen and hormone-dependent breast cancer in high-risk women. J Natl Cancer Inst, 95, 160-165.
Vici P., Veltri E., Carpano S., Di Lauro L. and Lopez M. (1991). [Buserelin therapy in postmenopausal patients with advanced breast carcinoma]. Clin Ter, 136, 195-199.
Waxman J.H., Harland S.J., Coombes R.C., Wrigley P.F., Malpas J.S., Powles T. and Lister T.A. (1985). The treatment of postmenopausal women with advanced breast cancer with buserelin. Cancer Chemother Pharmacol, 15, 171-173.

Willsher P.C., Robertson J.F., Armitage N.C., Morgan D.A., Nicholson R.I. and Blamey R.W. (1996). Locally advanced breast cancer: long-term results of a randomized trial comparing primary treatment with tamoxifen or radiotherapy in post-menopausal women. Eur J Surg Oncol, 22, 34-37.
Wirth M. (2001). Delaying/reducing the risk of clinical tumour progression after primary curative procedures. Eur Urol, 40 (Suppl 2), 17-23.
Zincke H., Lau W., Bergstralh E. and Blute M.L. (2001). Role of early adjuvant hormonal therapy after radical prostatectomy for prostate cancer. J Urol, 166, 2208-2215.

CHAPTER 17

Letrozole in the Treatment of Advanced Breast Cancer

P. PRONZATO AND A. TOGNONI

Hormonotherapy of Advanced Breast Cancer

Hormones and Breast Cancer

Advanced metastatic breast cancer is commonly considered as an incurable disease. In spite of the high rate of objective remissions achieved with the most recent polychemotherapy regimens or hormonal manipulations, the duration of response is limited, the disease progresses and, after a median interval of 24-36 months from the appearance of clinically detectable metastases, the patients inexorably die from cancer. Currently, there are two broad categories of treatment for metastatic breast cancer: cytotoxic chemotherapy and hormonal treatment. Women who are known to have a hormone-dependent tumor usually receive hormonal therapies, as these are better tolerated than chemotherapy.

The basis for hormonal treatment of metastatic breast cancer is the hormonodependence of breast cancer cells (Gruber et al., 2002): at least in part they grow only in the presence of estradiol and estrogens (hormonopendence) or their growth is made easier by these hormones (hormonosensitivity). This fact represents the basis for explaining several epidemiological observations, e.g. it is well known that hormones play a major role in the risk of developing breast cancer. The risk of breast cancer is related to the cumulative exposure of the breast to estrogens and possibly to progestins (as in the cases of early menarche, nulliparity, late age at first pregnancy, late menopause). Furthermore, the effects of exogeously administered estrogens and progestins have been extensively studied, both in the setting of contraception and in the setting of hormone replacement therapy, often reaching the conclusion of a small increase in risk of breast cancer with prolonged exposure to estrogens.

During both the cancerogenetic process and neoplastic progression, estrogens may stimulate breast cancer cell proliferation; this action is mediated by the peptydic autocrine and paracrine growth factors produced by the breast cancer cells themselves. In particular, estradiol links to the cytoplasmatic estrogen receptor (ER), resulting in dimerization of receptor with full activation of the two domains, AF1 and AF2; subsequently, the nuclear localization of the fully active ER results in a link with nuclear receptor (DNA) and in the fully activated transcription of genes coding for proteins acting as autocrine or paracrine factors in stimulating cell growth.

Basically, two ways have been explored to block estrogenic actions on the cancer cells: to inhibit the synthesis of hormones (ovariectomy, aromatase inhibitors) and to prevent interaction between the hormone and its receptor (anti-estrogens). Hormonal manipulations attempt to slow or block cell growth and are accompanied by modulation of the growth factors involved in breast cancer growth, such as transforming growth factor-α, insulin-like growth factor-β and transforming growth factor-β.

Therefore, the presence and the functional integrity of ERs represents the basis for hormonal manipulation. Among the long and ever-increasing list of potential prognostic and predictive factors for breast cancer, the hormone receptors (ER and progesterone receptors, PgR) are well established in predicting a better prognosis and reponsiveness to hormonotherapy. Patients whose tumors express ER and/or PgR have a higher response rate and a prolonged disease-free interval and overall survival when treated with endocrine therapies.

Considering that about 50% of tumors containing large amounts of ER and PgR fail to respond to hormonotherapy, more sensitive markers are needed. Explanations for the hormonoresistance of ER positive tumors are many: tamoxifen-stimulated growth (selection of clones for which the tamoxifen receptor complex acts as a stimulator rather than an inhibitor); expression of epidermal growth factor receptor (EGFR) and c-erbB-2 (HER2/neu); absence of PgR; high proliferative activity (Lipton et al., 2002; Yamauchi et al., 2001).

Classical Hormonal Treatments

Tamoxifen has been the hormonal agent of choice in adjuvant and first-line treatment of patients with hormone-sensitive metastatic breast cancer for many years, because it provided higher efficacy and lower toxicity than other ablative, additive or inhibitory endocrine treatments. Nevertheless, new agents and modalities of hormonal manipulation are now available and in some cases they are superior to tamoxifen in terms of toxicity and antitumor activity (Goss and Strasser, 2001; Hamilton and Piccart, 1999).

Premeopause

Advanced breast cancer patients in premenopause may theoretically be treated by the suppression of estrogenic production in the ovaries or by receptor inhibition by anti-estrogens (tamoxifen and others). The former modality is based on the administration of synthetic agonist analogs of the naturally occurring decapeptide, luteinizing hormone releasing hormone (LHRH). The so-called LHRH analogs act on the hypotalamic-pituitary axis by a process of receptor downregulation. The normal stimulus for the release of gonadotrophins from the pituitary gland is the pulsatile secretion of LHRH by the hypothalamus. Following the initial administration of an LHRH analog, all the LHRH receptors on the pituitary cell become occupied, with a transient increase in serum LH; then the receptors gradually disappear and a profound suppression of LH and estradiol occurs. Goserelin and other LHRH analogs have been studied in advanced breast cancer and have response rates of 20-35%, according to pretreatment characteristics. The combination of the suppression of ovarian production of estradiol by an LHRH analog plus the anti-estrogenic effect of tamoxifen might be expected to provide additional antitumor activity, in comparison with each modality alone. Several clinical studies have investigated the comparison between goserelin plus tamoxifen with goserelin alone. Recently, a meta-analysis of randomized studies of an LHRH analog with or without tamoxifen has been performed by the EORTC Group, showing that the so-called complete estrogen blockade (LHRH analogue plus tamoxifen) results in better outcome in terms of response rate and overall survival.

Postmenopause

For many years tamoxifen has represented the mainstay of hormonotherapy for advanced breast cancer in postmenopause. Between the early 1970s and the 1980s many randomised trials have been carried out comparing tamoxifen and other classical hormonal agents, such as progestins (megestrol acetate, medroxiprogesterone acetate), androgens, high-dose estrogens and the first-generation aromatase inhibitor aminoglutethimide. Invariably, tamoxifen was found to be superior, at least in terms of toxicity, with a response rate of 30-35%. In these studies much has been learned about the prognostic factors for response to tamoxifen and hormonotherapy. ER and/or PgR positivity, a long interval between diagnosis and relapse, the absence of visceral metastasis and a previous response to hormonotherapy were found to predict a likelihood of response to tamoxifen. Combinations of different traditional hormonal agents have not resulted in superior outcome in comparison with each agent alone.

New Aromatase Inhibitors

In postmenopause the estrogens are produced mainly through the aromatization of androgens by a peripheral aromatase present in the peripheral tissues and at high concentration in the tumor itself. The aromatase inhibitors notably reduce circulating estrogens. Two classes of agents exist: non-steroidal antiaromatases, also called aromatase inhibitors and steroidal antiaromatases, also called aromatase inactivators. Among the non-steroidal antiaromatases, first generation aminoglutethimide was the first to be introduced: the drug is not specific and all steroidogenesis is affected, resulting in the need for association with a corticosteroid. Two newer agents, anastrozole and letrozole, are more specific and act only on the aromatase.

Letrozole is a third generation non-steroidal aromatase inhibitor. Its high selectivity of action with respect to first- and second-generation aromatase inhibitors represents the basis for the profound endocrine effect, in terms of both peripheral and intratumor estrogen reduction and tolerability. In a study evaluating inhibition of total body aromatization vs. total body and plasma estrogen suppression, letrozole proved to be significantly more potent than the other third-generation non-steroidal aromatase inhibitor, anastrozole.

As second-line hormonal treatment in patients progressing on tamoxifen, letrozole was shown to be superior to the first-generation aromatase inhibitor aminoglutethimide (Gershanovich, 1998) and to the progestin megestrol acetate (Buzdar, 2001; Dombernowsky, 1998) as well to the third-generation aromatase inhibitor, anastrozole (Rose, 2002).

Recently, a study (Mouridsen et al., 2001) comparing tamoxifen with letrozole in first-line treatment of postmenopausal patients with ER-positive or ER-unknown metastatic breast cancer clearly showed letrozole to be more effective than tamoxifen. Letrozole was superior to tamoxifen in time to treatment progression, reducing the risk of progression by 30% (hazard ratio 0.70; 95% CI, 0.60-0.82, p = 0.0001). Median time to treatment progression was prolonged by 57%, 41 weeks for letrozole and 26 weeks for tamoxifen. Letrozole also was significantly superior for the secondary endpoints: time to treatment failure, objective response rate, rate of clinical benefit (complete responses + partial responses + stabilization, no-change lasting at least 24 weeks), with a similar median duration of objective response, and similar duration of clinical benefit.

The results of the supportive multivariate analysis with treatment comparison adjusted on key baseline co-variates (receptor status, prior adjuvant anti-estrogen therapy and dominant site of disease), showed superiority of letrozole over tamoxifen for all strata. In particular, the odds ratio for achieving objective response and disease progression were 1.83 (95% CI, 1.12-2.97, p = 0.02) and 0.69 (95% CI, 0.55-0.87, p =0.001), respechvely in favor of letrozole.

An updated analysis at a median follow-up of 32 months confirmed the previous results: time to treatment progression was significantly longer with letrozole than with tamoxifen (p < 0.0001; median time to treatment progression 9.4 months for letrozole, 6.0 months for tamoxifen), as was time to treatment failure (p < 0.0001; median time to treatment failure, 9.0 months for letrozole, 5.7 months for tamoxifen). The rate of objective tumor response (complete + partial response) was 32% for letrozole, 21% for tamoxifen (p = 0.0002) and the rate of overall clinical benefit was 50% for letrozole, 38% for tamoxifen (p = 0.0004). Duration of response and duration of clinical benefit both showed tendencies to be longer for letrozole than for tamoxifen (p = 0.05 and 0.08, respectively).

Most importantly, the final analysis of overall survival showed a significant survival advantage for letrozole over the first 2 years following randomization in the overall population (64% vs. 58% of patients alive at 2 years, p < 0.02), including patients who at first progression crossed over from tamoxifen to letrozole or vice versa. In the subset of patients who did not cross over and received subsequent therapy at physicians' discretion after first progression, the median overall survival was 33 months (95% CI 26-39) vs. 19 months (95% CI 19-23) in favor of letrozole, with 45% of patients surviving at 3 years vs. 32% with tamoxifen. Results are available also for trials regarding anastrozole and exemestane (Table 1; Buzdar, 2001).

A randomized, double-blind cross-over study compared tolerability, quality of life and patient preference between letrozole and anastrozole. More than

Table 1. Results of the randomized trials including the new inhibitors of the aromatase and tamoxifen (Tam) in terms of response rate (RR), clinical benefit (CB), time to treatment progression (TTP) and time to treatment failure (TTF)

	Anastrozole/Tam	Anastrozole/Tam	Letrozole/Tam	Exemestane/Tam
Patients	170/182	340/328	453/454	61/59
RR (%)	21/17	33/33	30/20*	41/14
CB (%)	59/46	56/56	49/38	56/42
TTP (months)	11/6*	8/8	9/6*	9/5
TTF (months)	8/5	6/6	9/6*	-

* $p < 0.05$

twice as many women (68% vs. 32%) preferred to take letrozole rather than anastrozole as a result of a significantly higher quality of life (5.1 difference, $p = 0.02$) and fewer side effects (particularly lethargy 8% vs. 19%, headache 5% vs. 14%, joint pain 3% vs. 11%, abdominal discomfort 3% vs. 11%, nausea 10% vs. 22%, loss of appetite 2% vs. 8%; Thomas, 2002).

An exploratory uncontrolled study was conducted to evaluate letrozole as maintenance therapy in patients responding to or with disease stabilization after standard chemotherapy. Preliminary results in 46 patients are encouraging: 4/38 patients (10.5%) with less than complete response to chemotherapy have improved their response status (from stable disease to partial response or from partial to complete response) and CA 15-3 levels significantly decreased in 17 patients who had abnormal markers at the end of chemotherapy ($p = 0.01$; *t*-test baseline vs. nadir): 65% of patients were still free of progression after 18 months follow-up, with a median time to progression of 15 months. Performance status improved in 54% of cases and tolerability was excellent. These data suggest that letrozole as maintenance therapy can possibly maximize response to chemotherapy with no added toxicity (Merlano, 2002).

On these bases letrozole, among the new inhibitors of aromatase, seems to be particularly active in inducing response and clinical benefit.

Treatment of Metastatic Breast Cancer

For treatment of metastatic breast cancer, the general attitude is to utilize hormonal and chemotherapy in sequence, according to the patient's likelihood to respond to each specific therapy. Preservation of patients' quality of life as long as possible is of importance, particularly for patients in which a survival advantage is unlikely (Robertson et al., 1997; Thurlimann et al., 1999).

The current clinical practice for front-line treatment of metastatic breast cancer of patients positive for well-established predictive factors for response to endocrine therapy (ER-positive, bone or soft tissue disease, long disease interval from first diagnosis to relapse) includes a trial of hormonotherapy. Based on response to first-line therapy, a second-line hormonotherapy or a first-line chemotherapy is then administered at the time of tumor progression.

Several lines of salvage treatment, including drugs not completely cross-resistant with front-line treatment, are commonly employed in sequence with a palliative intent.

In cases of visceral involvement, chemotherapy is in many instances preferred as initial therapy, even in ER-positive patients, despite a lack of certainty about its efficacy relative to hormonal therapy. Literature data indicate that anthracycline-based chemotherapy regimens achieve higher response rate and improve time to treatment progression and overall survival as compared to non-anthracycline-containing regimens. Taxanes have also proved to be highly active agents in metastatic breast cancer.

Only a few trials have been published comparing endocrine therapy and chemotherapy as initial treatment strategies for metastatic breast cancer, and no firm conclusions can be drawn. Based on data from old trials indicating no advantage on overall survival of combined chemoendocrine therapy over chemotherapy, the association of chemotherapy and hormonal therapy is not usually adopted in clinical practice.

The above data, however, have been generated using tamoxifen and old chemotherapy regimens. Newer hormonal agents and chemotherapy regimens are now available that have proved superior to agents tested in the past:

- Letrozole proved to be more effective than tamoxifen in ER-positive patients with visceral metastases in terms of response rate and time to treatment progression, and in providing survival advantage.
- Letrozole proved to be well tolerated and improved quality of life and/or performance status, both as a single agent and when administered in combination wiyh chemotherapy or after chemotherapy as maintenance therapy. The toxicity of chemotherapy should not substantially increased by letrozole, and adverse effects observed with chemoendocrine treatment in the old studies with tamoxifen and progestins (weight gain and thromboembolic events) are not expected using letrozole.

Data from a randomized study evaluating the effectiveness and tolerability of a combination of docetaxel and mitoxantrone with or without letrozole indicate that letrozole is well tolerated, with no negative impact on response rate (69% vs. 59%, respectively, in patients receiving chemoendocrine or chemotherapy only) when administered in association with taxane-based chemotherapy in postmenopausal patients with metastatic breast cancer.

Treatment of Locally Advanced Breast Cancer

In contrast with the traditional approach in which the treatment of breast cancer was based on a local therapy followed by a systemic adjuvant therapy, in recent years the so-called neoadjuvant approach has been developed. In the neoadjuvant approach, chemotherapy or hormonotherapy are administered before surgery in order to anticipate action against the tumor (also in occult micrometastases) and to reduce the bulk of the tumor, allowing a more limited surgical intervention. This strategy has been extensively studied more with chemotherapy; nevertheless, an important study has been car-

Table 2. Response rate according to clinical evaluation, ultrasound, mammography and application of breast conserving surgery in a trial comparing neoadjuvant tamoxifen or letrozole

	Clinical response (%)	Ultrasound response (%)	Mammography response (%)	Breast-conserving surgery (%)
Letrozole	60	39	38	48
Tamoxifen	41	29	20	36

ried out with neoadjuvant hormonotherapy, specifically with letrozole. In this study (Eiermann et al., 2001; Ellis et al., 2001), 337 postmenopausal patients were randomly assigned to letrozole or tamoxifen. All patients had ER-positive tumors not amenable to conservative breast surgery. The response rate was superior in the letrozole group (55% vs. 36%) and 45% of patients treated by letrozole were able to receive a breast-conserving surgical procedure (against 35% in the tamoxifen arm). The results (Table 2) should be considered very favourable, even though chemotherapy does better in the neoadjuvant setting, and therefore the neoadjuvant letrozole may be considered in selected cases.

Conclusions

Letrozole and the new aromatase inhibitors represent a new important tool in the treatment of breast cancer. Many studies are in progress on the adjuvant application of these drugs, and a first trial of anastrozole vs. tamoxifen or a combination of both has been published [The ATAC (Arimidex, Tamoxifen Alone or in Combination) Trialists' Group, 2002], with favourable results for anastrozole in terms of reduction of the risk of breast cancer recurrence. Furthermore, the new aromatase inhibitors may overcome the problems related to tamoxifen administration (mainly the risk of endometrial carcinoma and the occurrence of thromboembolic events: Day et al., 1999; Demissie et al., 2001; Fallowfield et al., 2001; Ganz et al., 2001; Mortimer et al., 1999). Further studies are warranted concerning a large series of issues:

- Anticipation of hormonal treatment in case of rising blood tumor markers in the absence of evident metastases.
- Maintenance hormonotherapy after the induction of chemotherapy.
- Combination of chemotherapy and hormonotherapy as front-line treatment of metastatic disease or locally advanced tumor.
- Combination of LHRH analog and aromatase inhibitors in premenopausal women.
- Best employment of aromatase inhibitors in the adjuvant setting (sequences with tamoxifen, short or long duration, selection of responsive cases).
- Long-term side effects, mainly on lipid and bone metabolism (Elisaf et al., 2001).

References

The ATAC (Arimidex, Tamoxifen Alone or in Combination) Trialists' Group (2002). Anastrozole alone or in combination with tamoxifen vs. tamoxifen alone for adjuvant treatment of postmenopausal women with early breast cancer: first results of the ATAC randomised trial. Lancet, 359, 2131-2139.

Buzdar A.U. (2001). A summary of second-line randomised studies of aromatase inhibitors. J Steroid Biochem Mol Biol, 79, 10-114.

Day R., Ganz P.A. and Constantino J.P. (1999). Health-related quality of life and tamoxifen in breast cancer prevention. A report from the National Surgical Adjuvant Breast and Bowel Project P-1 study. J Clin Oncol, 17, 2659-2669.

Demissie S., Silliman R.A. and Lash T.L. (2001). Adjuvant tamoxifen: predictors of use, side effects, and discontinuation in older women. J Clin Oncol, 19, 322-328.

Dombernowsky P. (1998) Letrozole, a new oral aromatase inhibitor for advanced breast cancer. Double-blind randomized trial showing a dose effect and improved efficacy and tolerability compared with megestrol acetate. J Clin Oncol, 16, 453-461.

Early Breast Cancer Trialists Collaborative Group (1992). Systemic treatment of early breast cancer by hormonal, cytotoxic or immune therapy. 133 randomised trials involving 31,000 recurrencies and 24,000 deaths among 75,000 women. Lancet, 339, 1-15.

Eiermann W., Paepke S. and Appfelstaedt J. (2001). Preoperative treatment of postmenopausal breast cancer patients with letrozole: a randomized double-blind multicenter study. Ann Oncol, 12, 1527-1532.

Elisaf M.S., Bairaktari E.T. and Niolaides C. (2001). Effect of letrozole on the lipid profile in postmenopausal women with breast cancer. Eur J Cancer, 37, 1510-1513.

Ellis M.J., Coop A. and Singh B. (2001). Letrozole is more effective neoadjuvant endocrine therapy than tamoxifen for ErbB-1- and/or ErbB-2-positive, estrogen receptor-positive primary: evidence from a phase III randomized trial. J Clin Oncol, 19, 3808-3816.

Fallowfield L., Fleissig A. and Edwards R. (2001).Tamoxifen for the prevention of breast cancer: psychosocial impact on women participating in two randomized controlled trials. J Clin Oncol, 19, 1885-1892.

Ganz P.A., Day R. and Ware J.E. Jr (2001). Tamoxifen and depression: more evidence from the National Surgical Adjuvant Breast and Bowel Project prevention (P-1) randomized study. J Natl Cancer Inst, 93, 1615-1623.

Gershanovich M. (1998). Letrozole, a new oral aromatase inhibitor: randomised trial comparing 2.5 mg daily, 0.5 mg daily and aminoglutethimide in postmenopausal women with advanced breast cancer. Ann Oncol, 9, 639-645.

Goss P.E. and Strasser K. (2001). Aromatase inhibitors in the treatment and prevention of breast cancer. J Clin Oncol, 19, 881-894.

Gruber C.J., Tschugguel W., Schneeberger C. and Huber J.C. (2002). Production and actions of estrogens. N Rugl J Med, 346, 340-352.

Hamilton A. and Piccart M. (1999). The third-generation non-steroidal aromatase inhibitors: a review of their clinical benefits in the second-line hormonal treatment of advanced breast cancer. Ann Oncol, 10, 377-384.

Lipton A. Ali S.M. and Keitzel K. (2002). Elevated serum HER-2/neu level predicts decreased response to hormone therapy in metastatic breast cancer. J Clin Oncol, 20, 1467-1472.

Merlano M.C. (2002). Maintenace therapy with letrozole after first-line chemotherapy in advanced breast cancer: the MANTLE trial. 38th ASCO, Orlando (FL), May 18-21, Abstract 1996, 46b.

Mortimer J.E., Boucher L. and Knapp D.L. (1999). Effect of tamoxifen on sexual functioning in patients with breast cancer. J Clin Oncol, 17, 1488-1492.

Mouridsen H., Gershanovic M. and Sun Y. (2001). Superior efficacy of letrozole vs. tamoxifen as first-line therapy of postmenopausal women with advanced breast cancer: results of a phase III study of the International Letrozole Breast Cancer Group. J Clin Oncol, 19, 2596-2606.

Robertson J.F.R., Willsher P.C., Cheung K.L. and Blamey R.W. (1997). The clinical relevance of static disease (no change) category for 6 months on endocrine therapy in patients with breast cancer. Eur J Cancer, 33, 1774-1779.

Rose C. (2002). Letrozole (Femara) vs. anastrozole (Arimidex): second-line treatment in postmenopausal women with advanced breast cancer. 38th ASCO, Orlando (FL), May 18-21, Abstract 131, 34a.

Thomas R. (2002). Empowering patients to make informed treatment decisions based on tolerability, quality of life patient preference. A comparison of letrozole and anastrozole in a multicentre randomised, single-blind cross over study. EBCC, Barcelona, Spain, March 2002, 200, Abstract 171.

Thurlimann J.B., Hsu Schmitz S.F. and Castiglione-Gersch M. (1999). Defining clinical benefit in postmenopausal patients with breast cancer under second-line endocrine treatment: does quality of life matter? J Clin Oncol, 17, 1672-1679.

Yamauchi H., Stearns V. and Hayes D.F. (2001) : When is a tumor marker ready for prime time? A case study of c-erbB-2 as a predictive factor in breast cancer. J Clin Oncol, 19, 2234-2356.

Subject Index

MIX
Papier aus verantwortungsvollen Quellen
Paper from responsible sources
FSC® C105338

If you have any concerns about our products,
you can contact us on
ProductSafety@springernature.com

In case Publisher is established outside the EU,
the EU authorized representative is:
Springer Nature Customer Service Center GmbH
Europaplatz 3, 69115 Heidelberg, Germany

Printed by Libri Plureos GmbH
in Hamburg, Germany